T0321945

THE
DARK SIDE
OF
HEALTHCARE

Issues, Cases, and Lessons for the Future

Highly Recommended Titles

Pioneers of Medicine Without a Nobel Prize
edited by Gilbert Thompson
ISBN: 978-1-78326-383-7
ISBN: 978-1-78326-384-4 (pbk)

How Medicines are Born: The Imperfect Science of Drugs
by Lisa Vozza and Maurizio D'Incalci
translated by Andreas Gescher
ISBN: 978-1-78634-297-3
ISBN: 978-1-78634-298-0 (pbk)

Nobel Prizes that Changed Medicine
edited by Gilbert Thompson
ISBN: 978-1-84816-825-1
ISBN: 978-1-84816-826-8 (pbk)

Longevity in the 2.0 World: Would Centenarians Become Commonplace?
by Jean-Pierre Fillard
ISBN: 978-981-120-116-5
ISBN: 978-981-120-203-2 (pbk)

Medicine My Vocation, Fishing My Recreation: Memoirs of a Physician and Flyfisherman
by Gilbert Thompson
ISBN: 978-1-78634-811-1

THE
DARK SIDE
OF
HEALTHCARE

Issues, Cases, and Lessons for the Future

Brian Edwards
University of Sheffield, UK

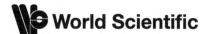

World Scientific

NEW JERSEY · LONDON · SINGAPORE · BEIJING · SHANGHAI · HONG KONG · TAIPEI · CHENNAI · TOKYO

Published by

World Scientific Publishing Co. Pte. Ltd.
5 Toh Tuck Link, Singapore 596224
USA office: 27 Warren Street, Suite 401-402, Hackensack, NJ 07601
UK office: 57 Shelton Street, Covent Garden, London WC2H 9HE

Library of Congress Cataloging-in-Publication Data
Names: Edwards, Brian, 1942 February 19- author.
Title: The dark side of healthcare : issues, cases, and lessons for the future / Brian Edwards.
Description: New Jersey : World Scientific, [2021] | Includes bibliographical references and index.
Identifiers: LCCN 2020051837 | ISBN 9789811231377 (hardcover) |
    ISBN 9789811231384 (ebook for institutions) | ISBN 9789811231391 (ebook for individuals)
Subjects: MESH: Delivery of Health Care--standards | Delivery of Health Care--organization &
    administration | Patient Harm--prevention & control | Professional Misconduct |
    Safety Management | Organizational Case Studies
Classification: LCC RA427.3 | NLM WA 530.1 | DDC 362.10289--dc23
LC record available at https://lccn.loc.gov/2020051837

British Library Cataloguing-in-Publication Data
A catalogue record for this book is available from the British Library.

For any available supplementary material, please visit
https://www.worldscientific.com/worldscibooks/10.1142/12136#t=suppl

Desk Editor: Jiang Yulin

Typeset by Stallion Press
Email: enquiries@stallionpress.com

Printed in Singapore

Foreword

As the global COVID-19 pandemic takes its toll, people in countries around the world have expressed their thanks and support to health and care workers who have been at the epicentre of the crisis. Our collective admiration for the doctors, nurses and carers who have helped others in the most difficult of circumstances whilst putting themselves in harm's way has been uplifting. We should not be surprised. In the UK, people standing on their doorsteps 'clapping for the NHS and care workers' may be an unusually visible response to the acuteness of the coronavirus crisis, but it exhibits a deep affection for the NHS and more generally our understandable vulnerability in the face of an infection which has and continues to cause so much illness and death. We want, and need, to believe that our healthcare systems can help and protect us, and in response, we want to express our thanks and support to those to whom we will turn when the need arises. This is not blind faith. Healthcare services do a great deal of good, and all of us have personal stories that bear witness to their positive benefits.

How then should we interpret the events narrated by Brian Edwards in this book? All of them are troubling. Many are shocking and deeply disturbing and untold numbers of people have suffered greatly as a consequence of them. Fortunately, these events occurred over many years and in many different places around the world. However, this contextual perspective should create no room for complacency.

A common feature found in many of the cases is that they occurred in circumstances, where hitherto, those closest to the events did not heed or understand the warning signs or found some plausible alternative explanation for their observations. Alarm bells sounded but were not heard and all of these troubling events happened in advanced countries that may have believed, 'this couldn't happen here'. Perhaps the main lesson of *The Dark Side of Healthcare* is, 'yes it can!' A second lesson is that there are usually multiple interacting causative factors that hinder detection until it is too late to prevent harm being done.

There are no simple, single answers to the prevention of dreadful events occurring in healthcare settings. Scientific advances and changes in professional practice simultaneously bring benefits and unforeseen risks to us all. In spite of honest commitments to learn lessons, to modify policies and practice and to implement new safeguards, other adverse events are likely to emerge when new evidence comes to light or hindsight enables conclusions to be drawn that were not visible at the time. Fortunately, over the past decade and more, changes have been made to healthcare governance that have been designed to reduce the possibility of harm occurring to patients: professional regulation has been reformed; clinical governance is now an integral part of health and care management; explicit standards and inspection processes have been extended and improved; patient concerns are increasingly acknowledged and recognised as warning signs and there has been a welcome and positive embrace of patient safety as a priority in service delivery. But risks remain. Diligence in the practice of evidence-based care and vigilance in identifying and investigating the unusual may provide some protection. However, the greatest safeguards are to listen — both to the voices of patients and to those of the people who care for us, the vast majority of whom do so because they have a vocation to help others. We must support them and provide them with the necessary tools to be our custodians of safety and quality in our healthcare services in order to mitigate the bad outcomes that this book brings to light.

Kevin Woods
Former Director-General for Health and
Chief Executive of the National Health Service (NHS),
Scotland, and Director-General of Health and
Chief Executive of the Ministry of Health, New Zealand

Contents

Foreword   v

Chapter One   Failing Hospitals and Healthcare Systems   1
Chapter Two   Angels of Death   27
Chapter Three   Unsafe Clinical Practice and Its Impact
                on Patient Safety   45
Chapter Four   Struck Off   99
Chapter Five   Medical Negligence   133
Chapter Six   Mental Health   157
Chapter Seven   Fraud and Corruption   183
Chapter Eight   The Sexual Exploitation of Children:
                The Health Response   207
Chapter Nine   Managerial Scandals and Problems   219
Chapter Ten   Social Care   269
Chapter Eleven From Darkness into the Light   287
Endnotes   307

Index   355

Chapter One

Failing Hospitals and Healthcare Systems

Hospitals are very complex organisations that can, on occasion, suffer catastrophic failures. This chapter will examine some of the key examples of such occurrences. The collapse of entire healthcare systems, outside of war zones, is extremely rare, but in 2020 some healthcare systems were reported to be close to the edge of economic collapse. In addition, the severe stress placed on hospitals and healthcare systems as a result of the COVID-19 pandemic has revealed additional fault lines in the resilience of many countries to such health emergencies. This chapter examines case studies from different healthcare systems and failing hospitals in the UK, Australia, USA, Japan, Sweden, Ireland and Venezuela in a search for some common underlying causes of this malaise. The chapter concludes with an early review of how hospitals and healthcare systems have responded to the current pandemic.

The Mid Staffordshire NHS Trust, 2005–2013

Stafford General Hospital, opened in 1983, was an acute hospital with approximately 350 inpatient beds serving the people of the West Midlands of England. It has now been renamed County Hospital. The hospital was a public sector organisation typical of many NHS hospitals with around 350 beds — unremarkable in many respects but with leaders that had ambitions to make it greater. However, by 2004, it had lost all its performance stars and was struggling to recover. The Mid Staffordshire NHS Trust (which ran Stafford General along with another smaller hospital) wanted to secure NHS Foundation Status and the financial and other freedoms that came with this. Once this had been secured, they aimed to enlarge their clinical footprint and compete with the other hospitals around them in the NHS internal market. In order to balance the books, an essential component of a Foundation bid, they reduced nursing staff numbers in a misguided and badly managed ward reconfiguration exercise. They tried to move away from traditional wards to separate floors for medicine and surgery without sufficient medical and nursing support.[1] What they did not acknowledge were external reports that patients were already receiving very poor care and the hospital was generating many more avoidable patient deaths than might have been expected for a hospital with Stafford's case mix and size. Patients had been voicing their individual concerns for some years, but their representative body, the Forum for Patient and Public Involvement, dismissed them as troublemakers and instead defended the hospital. They were, said one critic, 'more like a League of Hospital Friends than a voice of patients'.[2]

The early warning signs of a full-blown crisis came in January 2006 when the local newspaper carried reports of an inspection of the Accident and Emergency Department under the headline 'Town Hospital in squalid state'. The hospital managers rejected the criticism. Further negative stories followed until eventually, Julie Bailey, a local businesswoman deeply upset at the treatment of her mother created the pressure group CURE the NHS to press for a major inquiry. As her campaign gained momentum, other people came forward with their stories. Bailey commented: 'We have launched this campaign and we have found each other. Through very sad circumstances we now intend to ensure something is done. We are ordinary people who have witnessed the abuse/neglect of vulnerable people. We have put our trust in others who have let us down. We have all seen our loved ones suffer and we all know unless we do something together more will suffer'.

An 86-year-old patient was referred by her family doctor to the hospital with symptoms of recurring vomiting. Accompanied by her daughter, she was sent to the emergency assessment unit where although she received care, the patient, who was hard of hearing, struggled with the number of junior doctors who were constantly in and out of the unit. The daughter had to explain her mother's symptoms to a number of different clinical staff. After three days the patient was taken to Ward 10 — a mistake, as she was expected on Ward 11. She was left unattended for some time until later that evening she eventually arrived on Ward 11; a ward described by her daughter as being in complete chaos. This chaos intensified at night with few staff and patients wandering around and bedside buzzers constantly being activated. Weekends were worse with even less nursing staff and no doctors. The patient was taken to another ward for a gastroscopy without her oxygen supply. The porter said he was in a hurry and she would have to go without it. There was then a delay in bringing the patient back to Ward 11 whilst nursing staff argued about whose responsibility it was to organise the move. On her return she was not reconnected to her oxygen supply and subsequently collapsed. A doctor was eventually found to examine her. After a cursory examination he asked her daughter to sign a 'Do-not-resuscitate order' (DNR) as her prognosis was so poor. The family vowed to stay with her around the clock. Some weeks later, after the diagnosis had changed to heart problems, she was ready to be discharged when a healthcare assistant, attempting to lift her on her own, dropped her and she banged her head. A day or two later the family were told that their mother needed a blood transfusion. The clinical records later showed that the transfusion had been bodged. The daughter then asked for a doctor to re-examine her mother. The nurse in charge said she would decide if and when doctor should be called. The patient died the following day.[3]

Meanwhile, the patient group CURE the NHS was talking to local politicians and eventually got traction with the government. The hospital, however, still regarded them as the enemy.

An independent inquiry by the Health Commission[4] was undertaken that confirmed how deep the problems were and highlighted the high number of avoidable deaths at the hospital. The standard mortality ratio for patients admitted as an emergency to the hospital was between 127 and 145, when the expected rate would have been 100.[5] There was only a 5% chance that these rates were the result of a statistical aberration or chance. The Trust argued that this was down to inaccurate coding. They told local politicians that there was nothing to worry about.

The Trust secured its Foundation status in February 2008, despite the early warning signs of serious problems — an issue that would arise during the later inquiry.

The doctors at Stafford were not an easy group to manage. They did not have a close relationship with the Board of the Trust, its managers or with each other. They each thought that they should have the freedom to do what they thought was right for their patients. Surgery had been a problem for some years. Concerns had been expressed on a number of occasions by a surgeon about the performance of one of his colleagues. Some theatre staff had refused to work with the surgeon concerned. A review by the Royal College of Surgeons (RCS) confirmed the dysfunctional relationships between the surgeons. Following a serious incident in March 2009, the RCS were called back in.

> *The problem centred on the treatment of a patient with bowel cancer. A multidisciplinary team had discussed the case and agreed that the patient should have chemotherapy or palliative radiation treatment and a colostomy. Instead the surgeon had performed an abdominal perineal resection and the patient died two hours after the procedure.*

This time they pulled no punches: 'This is either a weak clinician giving in to unrealistic patient expectation or one who has a lack of clinical insight. It shows a complete disregard for nationally accepted best practice of multidisciplinary working and a complete disrespect of other professionals' advice. This was 1970's medicine being practiced in 2009'.[6] The surgical division was seen as still being dysfunctional: 'its members are polarised and this caused problems for nursing and other staff and crucially put patient safety at risk'.[7] The case note review found significant concerns with the cases of four of the five surgeons. The mortality from gallbladder removal was 10–15 times the expected rate. The local surgeons argued about the findings and delayed its report by some months. Poor results from laparoscopic cholecystectomy (keyhole surgery used to remove the gallbladder) continued. Eventually one of the surgeons concerned was suspended from clinical practice. The reason this took so long to happen, according to a former medical director, was that the evidence of poor performance was weak. 'Bring me the evidence and I will act', she said. One could certainly argue that if the safety of patients had been her overriding concern, challenges to the surgeons concerned might have come sooner.

Meanwhile, nursing in some parts of the hospital was poor and, in a few cases, later judged to be unprofessional.

> *We got to the hospital at about 10.00 am and I could not believe my eyes. The door was wide open with people walking past. Mum was in bed with the cot sides up and she did not have a stitch of clothing on. I mean she would have been horrified. She was completely naked and if I said covered in faeces it was everywhere. It was in her hair, eyes, nails and cot sides so she had obviously been trying to lift herself up and move about as the bed was covered. It was literally everywhere and dried. It would have been there a long time. It was not new.*[8]

The Trust explained away or ignored comments about poor clinical governance, disagreements amongst the surgeons and poor clinical outcomes following surgery, an understaffed Emergency Department and a badly managed reorganisation of the wards.

This first Inquiry came and went, and the Trust still secured their Foundation status. Some remedial actions were taken but the deep-rooted problems of a bad culture and low morale remained. How could government ministers have given their approval when the warning signs were already flashing? This question was asked in the formal Inquiry that was to follow.

However, for the Chair and Chief Executive of the Trust, their success at retaining Foundation status was short-lived as both were forced to resign in the wake of the Health Commission Inquiry and pressure from CURE and the NHS trust regulator.[9]

CURE the NHS had not gone away and kept pressing for further action. They held candlelit vigils outside the hospital and mounted a wall of shame in a local cafe featuring the hospital managers and senior clinical staff. In 2009, this public pressure led to an Independent Public Inquiry chaired by Robert Francis QC. Officials at the Department of Health had advised Ministers against such an inquiry, arguing that the problems had already been exposed and a newly constituted Trust needed time to make improvements.

In the first of his two inquiries, Francis examined the patient stories and found most of them to be accurate. He exposed once again the persistent problems with surgery — it remained a very dysfunctional clinical division — and the poor performance of one of the younger surgeons had still not been fully addressed. The hospital was, of course, not all bad and some patient relatives reported good care on some wards and by some clinical teams. However, the forceful management style used at the hospital was perceived as being toxic and bullying by many of the staff. Morale was poor and employee turnover high. Francis examined in detail the allegations about high avoidable death rates and found that the claims had a solid foundation. The national press put the number of such deaths as high as 1000.

Francis' principal conclusion was that the problems resulted from a poor organisational culture that did not foster excellent care both at the Trust and within the wider NHS. A common witness comment to the Inquiry was: 'How could all this happen and we not see it'. Organisational blindness is a common phenomenon in complex organisations. Incoming management teams tried to repair the relationship with CURE without success. The distrust ran too deep.

Francis' second inquiry reviewed the role of those outside the Trust including the Department of Health and the responsible government Ministers. Ministers and senior civil servants had to give evidence under oath as they struggled to explain why they had not seen the problems earlier and forced corrective action.

The result was that, far from forming a basis for improvement, the report ignited a national political storm and badly damaged the reputations of many of those caught up in the events at Stafford. The unanswered question was 'how typical was Stafford Hospital?' Could there be many more hospitals with the same uncovered deficiencies? Inquiries followed into any hospital with a high avoidable death rate. Politicians pronounced that to them quality mattered more than a slavish adherence to the financial bottom line and managers became more likely to be sacked for quality breaches than overspends. The financial barriers to recruitment were removed resulting in rapid increases in nursing numbers all over England with the inevitable consequence of increased costs on hospital balance sheets. The seeds of a future financial crisis had been sown in the response to Stafford, and by 2017–2018, the NHS was heading for a financial deficit of £5.9 billion.[10]

As for changing the inherent culture that had led to the situation in Stafford, it was to prove extremely challenging for the large number of organisations that made up the NHS. Politicians can rarely influence culture in healthcare systems. Government attempts to impose common values made little impact. It requires more than new inspectors and statutory duties. It demands exceptional professional and managerial leadership.

The government pumped huge sums of money into Stafford Hospital but its full range of services came under serious challenge as it merged with its bigger neighbour in Stoke-on-Trent and moved to a much-diminished satellite status handling, in the main, non-emergency care. This merger forced the new Trust (University Hospitals of North Midlands NHS Trust, created in November 2014) into special measures[11] as it struggled to absorb its now infamous neighbour. There was a very mixed public reaction as some in Stafford blamed the patient group CURE the NHS for what was happening to their local services and the fact that they now needed to travel further for specialist care and treatment.

Queensland Public Hospitals, Australia, 2004–2006

At around the same time as events were unfolding in Stafford, a Committee of Inquiry was reporting in Queensland, Australia.[12]

In fact, this report was the outcome of the second inquiry into the Queensland Public Hospitals — the first had been shut down by the Queensland Supreme Court because of what was referred to as 'apprehended bias' by the Inquiry Commissioner and his team.

Bundaberg Base Hospital

Complaints had surfaced about the judgement and competence of Dr. Jayant Patel and the failure of the administrators at Bundaberg Base Hospital — the main community hospital in Northeast Queensland, 239 miles north of Brisbane, employing around 4000 staff — and officers at Queensland Health to address these concerns. Bundaberg Base Hospital had once been an efficient, safe hospital providing reasonable care but had markedly deteriorated to becoming both inefficient and unsafe. It was into this environment that Dr. Patel was recruited as a senior medical officer in general surgery. If the administrators had properly checked, they would have discovered that his practice had been previously been restricted in a former post in Oregon, US and that he had also surrendered his licence to practise in New York following disciplinary proceedings against him. He performed a large number of operations at Bundaberg between April 2003 and early 2005 and his high throughput helped the hospital achieve its elective surgery targets. He had, however, delayed the transfer of patients to other tertiary hospitals where his patients should have been treated. The subsequent Inquiry reported that Dr. Patel had made himself so valuable to the hospital that administrators were plainly reluctant to offend him let alone investigate him. External medical examiners would later conclude that his professional conduct was very deficient. His assessment of presenting patients was inadequate, his surgical techniques were defective and his post-operative management was poor as was his follow-up. There were at least 13 deaths in which an unacceptable level of care on the part of Dr. Patel contributed to the adverse outcome. Dr. Patel's results were, according to one expert witness, not 10 times worse than one would have expected — but 100 times worse. There had been no attempt at peer review by his colleagues. In a striking parallel with the Stafford Inquiry, the results for laparoscopic cholecystectomy were

28 times worse than the national average. Dr. Patel was later convicted of manslaughter at the Queensland Supreme Court.[13] Once again, the early warning signs from a nurse whistle blower and patients' relatives had been ignored.

Hervey Bay Hospital, Fraser Coast

At Hervey Bay Hospital in Queensland, another large hospital accepting tertiary referrals from other smaller hospitals, two Fijian surgeons were performing orthopaedic operations well beyond their competence resulting in extremely unfortunate outcomes. There had been complaints about their performance, but these had been rejected or ignored. The hospital needed to keep the orthopaedic service open. Eventually the services were closed down once it repeatedly failed to recruit sufficient trained surgeons.[14] The service had always been under-resourced and unsafe.

Townsville Hospital

Townsville Hospital is one of the largest in Queensland. The Queensland Inquiry concluded that the District managers' refusal to replace rusty surgical instruments was unreasonable. The Inquiry did, however, commend the hospital for introducing compulsory clinical oversight by experienced doctors for all overseas trained doctors. In effect, this established a probationary period.

The hospital had also employed a Russian psychiatrist with bogus qualifications. He had claimed he had qualified at the Voronezh State Hospital in Russia but when the hospital was asked to confirm this they reported that they offered no training in his speciality. Concern for the hospital's reputation impeded further action or patient recalls. The doctor was quietly sidelined.

Charters Tower Hospital, Brisbane, Queensland

Another doctor at the Charters Towers Hospital in Queensland was also appointed without any peer review of his competencies. He was a South African trained doctor who claimed to be experienced in obstetrics and anaesthesia. He was found to be negligent in applying an anaesthetic to a patient as a result of which she died. He quickly returned to South Africa and was never prosecuted.

Rockhampton Hospital, Brisbane, Queensland

Rockhampton Hospital was found to have a serious problem with its emergency department. Instead of deploying its most experienced staff to the department it was instead used as a dumping ground for underperforming doctors and was consistently understaffed. Patient safety was being compromised.

Prince Charles Hospital, Brisbane, Queensland

The problems at Prince Charles Hospital centred on an under-resourced cardiac service. Queensland Health had decided to transfer the service to the Princess Alexandra Hospital contrary to the advice of the cardiologists at Prince Charles. Funding was transferred to Princess Alexandra but was plainly inadequate and waiting lists grew ever longer. The cardiologists who complained were told that they could all be replaced by foreign doctors and should refrain from further criticism.

The overall conclusions of the Queensland Inquiry were strikingly close to those at Stafford. The hospitals were all operating with inadequate and poorly administered budgets and medical recruitment did not properly include proper reviews of clinical competence. There was a failure to monitor the performance of doctors or to properly investigate complaints and there was a pervasive culture of concealment. The public and professional pressure to keep services open at all costs overrode all patient safety concerns.

Maidstone and Tunbridge Wells NHS Trust, UK, 2004–2006

Poor infection control features in a number of failing hospital inquiries. Stafford Hospital, for example, had 420 cases in 2006. In 2007, the Healthcare Commission in England produced a highly critical report on the management of *Clostridium difficile*[15] (also known as *C. difficile* or *C. diff*) outbreaks at the Maidstone and Tunbridge Wells NHS Trust.[16] Between April 2004 and September 2006, there had been over 1000 cases in the three hospitals the Trust managed. A Health Commission Inquiry later reported that the infection had killed at least 90 patients and was a factor in the deaths of a further 241. However, they qualified this conclusion by adding that some of the infected patients would have died even if they had received excellent care. The fundamental problem was infection control.

The Trust had experienced a troubled history after it was created as the result of a merger in 2000. The Chair, Chief Executive and other senior staff had all left the Trust in 2003 after serious criticism about the management of waiting lists. It was also struggling to balance its books. The main hospital was only cleaned in the morning and not at all at night despite the fact that it was extremely busy, with bed occupancy levels consistently over 90%. Initially, at least, the hospital had no isolation facilities so infected patients were nursed in open wards. Bed spacing was tight and a shortage of nurses contributed to the spread of infection because they were too rushed to undertake hand hygiene, empty and clean commodes, clean mattresses and equipment properly and wear aprons and gloves appropriately and consistently.

The Trust also relied heavily on agency staff. A managerial focus on achieving targets in the Accident and Emergency department created chaos in the rest of the hospital as patients were moved around at short notice.[17]

The subsequent inquiry blamed poor professional and managerial leadership. The lack of organisational stability, with numerous structural changes and a high turnover of senior managers meant that managers could not settle into their roles and focus on the key issues. The Infection Control team had no strategic direction and there was an unresolved difference of opinion between microbiologists that led to inconsistent action. The Board appeared to be insulated from the realities and problems that were being experienced on the general wards. The Chief Executive quickly left the Trust with a large financial settlement (that was unsuccessfully challenged by the government). The Chief Medical Officer for England wrote to all doctors telling them to ensure that, in future, hospital infections were routinely included on death certificates so that the problem could be effectively measured going forward.

Infection Control Internationally

Poor infection control became a smoking gun for deeper problems of low professional standards, including something as basic as hand washing. Indeed, infection control is a challenge for all hospitals and there are wide variations in performance. The Secretary of State for Health in England reported that the best NHS hospitals had an infection rate of 1 in 500 patients while the worst experienced a rate of 1 in 25. Australia has a target of 2 cases per 10,000 patient days, though in 2018–2019 they were well below this target but with local variations.[18] In the EU, 9 million patients a year catch infections in hospitals and care homes, most of which were avoidable.[19]

Stephen Parodi, Chief of Infectious Diseases for 21 hospitals in Kaiser Permanente's Northern California system said of his organisation: 'The attributable mortality one year out from having the original infection is 16.7% and that's pretty high. Almost one sixth of the people are not alive in a year. And remember, it's not the thing the patient originally came in with'.

A media inquiry in May 2008 reported that 131 patients at the Vale of Leven Hospital in Scotland had been diagnosed with C. difficile between January 2007 and June 2008. A public Inquiry chaired by Lord MacLean followed. The hospital had been the subject of prolonged speculation about its closure that had had a damaging effect on recruitment and staff morale. The physical environment had been compromised including a lack of hand-wash basins and unsatisfactory repairs. There had also been a managerial reorganisation that had materially weakened local management. MacLean concluded that this had led to a hospital culture that had lost sight of its purpose 'to be a caring and compassionate environment dedicated to the highest levels of care'. The infection control team should have declared an outbreak (i.e. two or more linked cases) but they did not do so, and seven out of 28 death certificates failed to mention C. difficile as a cause. Clinical record keeping was poor as was the shortage of isolation rooms.

This is yet another example of a problem that should have been identified and dealt with far earlier than it was. The inquiry concluded with surprise at 'how many managers at different levels within an organisation like the Greater Glasgow and Clyde Health Board failed in one of the most fundamental aspects of management, namely to ask questions'.

Common Problems in Failing Hospitals

All of these hospitals had problems in common. All were very busy and struggling to live within budgets that put a special strain on quality standards. All had, in desperation to keep services running, recruited poor doctors who practised with little supervision. Pre-employment checks were minimal and ineffective. Nurse staffing levels were always at the margins of safety and this led to poor professional practice. All had administrators who repressed or ignored criticism in an attempt to protect the hospitals reputation or failed to ask the right questions when alarm bells began to ring. Complaints by patients and patient groups were ignored, as were those of whistleblowers amongst the staff. Boards were out of touch with the realities of what was actually happening on the wards and in operating theatres. Complaints by patients and patient groups were ignored. The pervading defensive culture did nothing to encourage best practice.

The problems are widespread. Even the most famous hospitals can run into trouble.

Karolinska University Hospital, Sweden

Karolinska University Hospital in Stockholm, Sweden, and its partner University has a long and distinguished reputation for specialised medicine and research, but in the last decade it has run into serious problems in the wake of a complicated merger with a rival hospital, major cost overruns at its new hospital, IT systems that have proven to be defective, a serious research scandal and a huge financial deficit that threatens jobs. All of these events coincided with a radical change in the way in which the hospital was organised and managed.

Gone are traditional hospital departments; healthcare at Karolinska is now organised in patient flows. For example, patients with heart and vascular conditions are treated in an integrated manner, with specialists from functions such as emergency medicine, imaging and cardiology working together — often in the same building or corridor. This new management approach was termed 'Value-Based Healthcare'. It aimed to align physician and hospital profit and loss with cost, quality, and outcome measures based on outcome studies. There would be a high degree of standardised diagnosis and treatment. According to Boston Consulting Group, who were contracted to manage this change process, this would make Karolinska a model for the rest of the world. However, not everybody was convinced: 'Stockholm has got the world's most expensive hospital but not the world's best hospital', said Magdalena Andersson, the Swedish Finance Minister, as it emerged that the building costs had increased from US$1.8 billion to US$7.5 billion.[20]

The research scandal centred on the recruitment in 2010 of Paolo Macchiarini, a star surgeon and ground-breaking stem cell researcher. He claimed to be regenerating human windpipes by seeding plastic scaffolds with stem cells from the patient's own bone marrow — one of the holy grails of medicine as the body will not reject its own cells. Colleagues concerned about Macchiarini's work and results launched their own investigation that showed that the synthetic tracheas had not worked, the data had been falsified and critical information had been supressed. As a result, patients were dying a lingering and agonising death. Initially, the opinions of the whistleblowers were ignored or rejected, and plans progressed to build a stem cell centre in Hong Kong. In fact, the hospital reported the whistleblowers to the Swedish police for violating Swedish law and patient privacy.[21] In April 2015, the Karolinska Ethics Committee acquitted Macchiarini of all charges of scientific misconduct. In January 2016, a Swedish television programme called 'The Experiments' documented the death of a Russian woman who had received one of Macchiarini's implants. The same month, a devastating article appeared in *Vanity Fair* about his personal life.[22] In February 2016, the President of Karolinska Institute stepped down and a number of top officials followed him. Macchiarini was sacked the following month. The controversy continued into 2018 when seven researchers who had worked with Macchiarini were found guilty of scientific misconduct in research.[23] The University took steps to remedy matters but Karolinska's reputation for medical research had been seriously tarnished.

The management system has been more difficult to operate than promised. According to Rostlund and Gustafsson,[24] the new systems are slow and proven routines are lost. Medical staff began leaving, and bureaucracy has increased. The hospital has a sterile, soulless atmosphere of suppressed fear and anger, but people will not speak up; they fear reprisals and bullying. There are no waiting rooms for patients or offices for consultants (who must book a room if they need one). The manager recruited to lead the changes resigned unexpectedly in September 2018.

By the end of 2019, the budget deficit at Karolinska had climbed to US$167 million. The hospital announced that they would need to slash 550 administrative posts, 250 doctors and 350 nursing assistants. Unless new funding can be provided, further major job cuts are inevitable despite the fact that demand is increasing from an ageing population.

Hospitals like Karolinska can recover from disasters like these but to do so will take years of trouble-free operation. If they do not resolve the deep-seated financial problems, they will limp along from crisis to crisis and fail to recruit the international clinical stars they had planned. A slow decline into mediocrity will follow.

So, what is the future for Value-based Healthcare? As we will see in Chapter Nine, it has not gone away.

Healthcare System Collapses

Political unrest and economic crises always affect healthcare systems, sometimes with catastrophic results. The strongest evidence of a full-scale healthcare system collapse in recent years has been seen in Venezuela[25] as a result of political tensions and a rapidly worsening economic climate. Vaccine-preventable diseases such as measles and diphtheria spread rapidly as did infectious diseases such as malaria and tuberculosis. Medicines were in short supply and became extremely expensive, while at the same time, high rates of inflation eroded personal savings and investments. The Pharmaceutical Federation of Venezuela claimed that the country had an 85% shortage of medicines. Infant mortality rose by 30% in the country in 2016. Many doctors and nurses fled the country. Public hospitals were hit particularly badly and some lost their electrical supply.

Things are so bad that, according to Dr. Paul Spiegel, from Johns Hopkins School of Public Health, patients who go to hospital need to bring not only their own food but also medical supplies like syringes and scalpels as well as their own soap and water. The Venezuelan government no longer publish health data. Other healthcare systems are also reported to be on the verge of collapse in the 2020s. Some commentators allege that the NHS in the UK and healthcare services in most of the rest of Europe are now in serious crisis and on the edge of collapse. This is an exaggeration but highlights deep-rooted problems. Every country has to respond to the challenge of making new and expensive treatments available to its citizens, dealing with economic downturns and managing demographic realities. The healthcare choices that governments have to make can be extraordinarily difficult and some countries are better at managing these tensions than others.

However, citizens in countries such as the Russian Federation find that their healthcare systems really are close to collapse because of historical low levels of investment, a rapidly ageing population and a moribund healthcare system that has resisted reform. The Russian system had improved radically throughout the 2000s but then deteriorated as the Russian economy experienced a sharp downturn. Russia has nearly double the OECD average number of hospital beds but only invests 6.5% of its GDP in health. Its low level of investment is also not deployed in what many observers would regard as an effective manner. The alarm bells are ringing but is anybody listening?

Hospital closures are also not uncommon in the US, with rural hospitals particularly at risk. One study estimated that 20% of rural hospitals were struggling to stay open and that 172 have closed between 2010 and the time of writing.[26] Funding is at the heart of the problem, with many rural communities dependent on state-sponsored health programmes. Many families are simply uninsured. But finance is not the only problem. Rural hospitals are often too big and insufficiently focused on community or ambulatory care. They are rarely at the forefront of modern medical science and have difficulty recruiting and retaining good staff.

Larger hospitals have also closed, including the Hahnemann University Hospital in Philadelphia. This hospital, located in the centre of the city, had 496 beds and a major trauma centre serving a poor inner-city community. The hospital had huge debts, and when it closed in 2019 it was losing US$5 million a month. The hospital ecosystem in Philadelphia was consolidating and reducing beds with inevitable consequences. Most large cities in the developed world are going through the same cathartic experience. This process represents a dangerous time for patients if the changes are not managed well.

Changes to the method of funding healthcare services quickly impact on care. In 2006, Massachusetts decided to provide health insurance to all its citizens. The so-called Romney plan was to stop subsidising hospital care and redirect the money to ensure that all citizens had at least minimal health insurance. It succeeded in the sense that 98% of citizens secured some level of health insurance coverage. However, the programme steadily expanded from minimum cover for catastrophic events to a more generous health insurance coverage that stimulated demand with inevitable consequences for the now underfunded hospital system. This, in a country that invests twice the average percentage of its GDP, as compared with other developed countries, on health.[27] Unintended consequences are typical in healthcare funding decisions.

How to fund modern healthcare systems with a rapidly expanding science base and growing public demand is an international problem. If politicians get it wrong, they put their citizens at a serious risk of harm.

Physician Morale

Primary care, the planned bedrock of modern healthcare systems, at least according to the World Health Organization, is also showing signs of strain in some countries, including the UK. It is now proving difficult to retain physicians even when they are well paid.

Japan's healthcare system was reported to be on the verge of collapse in 2008 because Japanese physicians are utterly demoralised.[28] The reasons were complex but included underinvestment, overwork, a hostile media, an increasing number of lawsuits against doctors and violence by patients. *Karojisatso* (suicide due to overwork) was increasing amongst healthcare professionals. Physicians felt undervalued. Demoralised physicians are much more likely to leave the profession and their dissatisfaction, if prolonged, results in health problems for the physicians themselves. Investment levels in the Japanese healthcare system had fallen to the lowest in the G7 countries as the country battled its way through a long period of austerity.[29] Japan had been reluctant to increase the number of physicians to avoid 'physician-induced demand' on the system. Shortages were particularly apparent in rural areas.

In 1999, a nurse at Tokyo Hiroo Hospital mistakenly injected the disinfectant chlorhexidine into a 58-year-old female patient instead of the correct drug. The patient died of acute heart failure. In the same year at Yokohama City Hospital, a 74-year-old male with cardiac valve disease was confused with an 84-year-old male with lung cancer due to a mix up in the surgical centre. The former underwent lung resection while the latter underwent mitral valve plasty. These two cases made shocking headlines and were followed by media allegations that such cases were common. The reputation of Japanese physicians was badly tarnished, and they were acutely affected by it.[30]

Low physician morale has been reported in other countries, including the US. According to a group of doctors from Dallas, physician autonomy is under siege and morale is declining: 'Insurers, government and hospitals dictate how doctors can treat patients. If we continue to devalue the experience and skills of our physicians, they will become the most expensive data entry clerks in the nation'.[31]

Physicians with signs of depression make more medical errors and those who report errors have more depressive symptoms later on.

The association appears to be bidirectional, with reported errors affecting mental health and vice versa.[32]

Danger at the Boundaries

It is very common for healthcare system failures to have catastrophic ramifications on individual patients and their families. This often occurs as a result of the various component parts of a healthcare system failing to integrate their services around an individual patient. A recent Irish case[33] centred on a hospital that discharged a patient that needed oxygen support to a care home that could not provide it. The patient quickly died. The most common problems appear to manifest themselves in the boundaries between primary and secondary care and their links with social services.

The Victoria Climbie case[34] in the UK illustrates these dangers.

Victoria Climbie was an eight-year-old girl, born in the Ivory Coast, who was tortured and murdered by her guardians in London, allegedly after a preacher from the Universal Church of the Kingdom of God convinced her aunt that the child was possessed by the devil. The pathologist who examined her body noted 128 separate injuries and scars and described it as the worst case of child abuse she had ever seen. The guardians were found guilty of murder and child cruelty and sent to prison for life. The judged described the social workers involved in the Climbie case as 'blindingly incompetent'.

The subsequent Inquiry discovered numerous instances where Victoria could have been saved, noted that many of the organisations involved in her care were badly run, and considered the racial issues involved in the case, as many of the participants were black. Victoria had been presented to hospital staff on a number of occasions with multiple injuries, including severe scalding. Social services were involved at various times as were the police, when allegations were made (and later denied) about sexual assault. Everybody assumed that someone else was looking after Victoria's interests. Alan Milburn, who was the Minister of Health at the time said, 'this was not a failing on the part of one service, it was a failing on the part of every service'. Dr. Liam Fox, the Shadow Health spokesman said that this was 'a shocking tale of individual professional failure and systemic incompetence'.

The Climbie case was one of many inquiries into child abuse that has been held in the UK over the years. Child sexual abuse will be considered at greater length in Chapter Eight of this book.

Hospitals exist in complex local health economies. If primary or community care moves into crisis, it quickly impacts on secondary care and vice versa.

> *Basildon and Thurrock Hospital in the East of England had been a worry for statutory regulators and inspectors for some years. It was under constant attack by local media, many staff felt ashamed when asked where they worked and patients arrived at the hospital with low expectations. A new Chief Executive began to address these problems by first getting the hospital to recognise and acknowledge its problems. She then placed safety and quality at the heart of the organisation's culture. Some problems were not of the hospital's making as the health economy in which it was located was inherently weak. Hospitals in the system were keen to talk about collaboration but did little to advance potential projects when they realised that one or more of them might lose clinical services or income. Under pressure to get quick results the new Chief Executive emphasised that this was not possible and that turning around an institution as complex as a hospital took time and could not be achieved by command and control.[35]*

Avoidable Deaths

Most definitions of a healthcare system collapse include a measure of avoidable deaths. These are deaths that were avoidable in the presence of timely and effective healthcare or public health intervention. In the UK, in 2017, 23% of deaths were considered avoidable.[36] This issue was at the centre of the Francis Inquiries into Stafford Hospital. A follow-up review by the Medical Director of NHS England found that 11 of the 14 hospitals with the highest avoidable death rates required urgent reform. High still birth rates were also being ignored. Hospital Boards were struggling to analyse clinical data, operating theatres were below standard and patient warnings were not being heeded. Avoidable death rates are a highly contentious measure of hospital competence but nevertheless a powerful indicator of potential problems.

Patient Safety

Reports from around the world indicate that medical error is a major problem. In the US, it is the third leading cause of death after heart disease and cancer. Often, the problem lies with the system rather than individual practitioners. Reporting of adverse events rather than deaths is very patchy and almost certainly under-reported. A Johns Hopkins study[37] led by Dr. Martin Makary blamed the system more than individual practitioners: 'Medical care workers are dedicated, caring people, but they are human. And human beings make mistakes'.[38]

> *Emily Jerry was two years old when she lost her life after a pharmacy technician filled her intravenous bag with more than 20 times the recommended dose of sodium chloride. On the day Emily was given her fatal dose, the hospital pharmacy was short staffed; the pharmacy computer was not working properly and there was a backlog of physician orders. This tragedy led to Emily's Law that specified the required educational background and training for pharmacy technicians.[39]*

Countries have responded in different ways to the challenge of ensuring patient safety. Mandatory clinical protocols have been adopted by many nations, as have targets and definitions of 'never' events: clinical errors that should never occur.[40] Clinical audits have become routine in the best healthcare systems, as have patient death reviews. 'No blame' reporting has been adopted with apparent success in some countries.[41] This concept is associated with what are termed High Reliability Organisations where small errors can have catastrophic results. The National Transport Board in the US, which supervises all domestic air traffic, is now underpinned by the belief that errors are inherent in human activity rather than causally linked to poor performance. Other countries, such as the UK, and Australian states such as Victoria, have created a legal duty on healthcare providers: a 'Duty of Candour', to be open and honest with patients when things go wrong.

Patient empowerment in its various forms also appears to be a great aid to safety. As Dr. David Classon, a Consultant at the University of Utah, puts it: 'The system of care is fragmented. Any tools that enable patients to manage their own healthcare needs will be a game changer'.

Commercial companies are emerging that design ways to increase patient safety and improve clinical reliability. New computer-based quality systems should help as they introduce multiple checking at every stage in the treatment process.

Accreditation systems of various types, which measure and report quality and fitness to operate have undoubtedly helped improve services but have not solved all of the problems. As we will see in a later chapter, such systems cannot identify serial killers or incompetent practitioners who move between healthcare providers. Some, like the Care Quality Commission in England, have moved in the direction of self-improvement rather than just inspecting and reporting.[42] Inspection can be good at identifying problems and risk but is often focussed on blame rather than finding solutions. In the US, hospitals that lose their accreditation are thrown into an immediate financial crisis. The usual response is to bring in external management consultants and change the leaders.

Computer systems have been developed, often using artificial intelligence, which increase patient safety and improve clinical reliability. In time it will become mandatory to install them.

The reporting of adverse events and near misses is very patchy and is almost certainly under-reported. One Canadian study estimated that as many as 23,000 Canadian adults die annually because of preventable adverse events. In Canada, there is no routine public documentation of one common cause of healthcare harm: malfunctioning medical devices that are linked to dozens of deaths and hundreds of serious injuries each year.[43] Many experts contrast this with the airline industry, where near-miss reporting is routine. Such a transparent approach is not deeply rooted in most healthcare systems. These issues are explored in greater detail in later chapters.

The 2020 COVID-19 Pandemic

The 2020 pandemic may prove to be a huge stimulus for positive change. Some regional systems in developed countries such as Italy found its hospitals overwhelmed by the numbers of patients with the disease in urgent need of intensive care beds. New York was also seriously challenged. Other countries, like the UK, have (at least at the time of writing) survived the crisis but only after the most radical action to reshape their services and expand intensive care capacity. Large new temporary hospitals emerged around the world in conference centres and sports stadia in a matter of weeks, and industries quickly switched to the production of urgently needed ventilators and personal protection equipment. Hygiene protocols had to be rapidly reworked. Funding streams also had to be changed or simply left in place to be sorted out later. Cancer surgery in England was switched to coronavirus-free hospitals rented from the private sector. In many areas of healthcare, what had been previously unthinkable suddenly became eminently possible.

Radical changes were also made to primary care in the UK and other European countries as consultations by phone, email and videoconferencing systems like Skype, Zoom and Teams largely took over from crowded surgeries and face-to-face contact. The same effects were also evident in the US and Canada.

The managerial response to the pandemic is considered further in Chapter Nine.

Lessons for the Future

The widening gap between what modern medicine can achieve for patients and the levels of investment we are prepared to make into healthcare systems is a policy question confronting all governments. Even countries with the highest levels of investment, such as the US, are struggling to match patient and physician expectations. For all practical purposes, the demand for healthcare is infinite. The advance of medical science will not slow but it is unlikely to result in a reduction of costs. The proliferation of austerity policies, as a result of the financial crisis of 2008, has resulted in falling levels of investment and increased risks for patients and, should this continue, it will need to be handled carefully and skilfully. The difficult priority decisions that often manifest themselves in such circumstances need to be effectively addressed. For example, hospital reorganisations or the threat of cuts or closures has, as we have seen, an extremely detrimental effect on staff and managers. Similarly, the almost inevitable trend to consolidate hospital services onto fewer sites increases risks. This trend is driven largely by economics but in some circumstances it is to enable closer cooperation between specialists. Local communities and their politicians, however, often prioritise having local care above promises of better clinical outcomes following such consolidations.

Whenever change is initiated there are warning signs when the strain begins to threaten patient safety. These warnings are often ignored in the heat of local politics. Organisational blindness is commonplace in complex organisations and uncomfortable signals are filtered out leaving critics as the uninformed enemy. A strong national lead is necessary in this area to encourage and enforce local initiatives.

Recruiting competent clinical staff is a high-risk area particularly for services in rural areas. This risk increases sharply when the applicant is from another country. Hospitals, in particular, need robust and open systems of clinical audit that identify poor performance early. Leaders must be effectively empowered to act once problems emerge. Supportive corrective action rather than playing the blame game appears to be a far better way forward. The best and safest hospitals have a policy of learning from accidents and mistakes rather than covering them up. Concealment of problems is common in hospital systems that are under pressure and this includes hiding the truth about their financial status.

System failure is relatively common at the interface between hospitals and primary care. To be effective, patient safety must become an overriding priority for Hospital Boards and deeply embedded in an organisation's culture. A public crisis usually provokes demands for immediate action, but fundamental change takes time.

Of course, we are now experiencing the biggest public health crisis that we have seen in our lifetime. The 2020 pandemic may provide an opportunity for the radical reshaping of healthcare systems. If nothing else, it demonstrates the urgent need for the disparate parts of healthcare systems to work together far more effectively. Operational independence is no longer as important as some had claimed. Caring for healthcare staff has always been important but the number of doctor and nursing staff deaths whilst working on the 2020 pandemic has shocked politicians and managers alike. Safe working policies and ideas will need a radical review. This is explored in more detail in Chapter Nine of this book.

Chapter Two
Angels of Death

There are sadly numerous examples of healthcare professionals using their clinical skills and knowledge to deliberately end the lives of their patients. The motives range from the mercy killing of patients with terminal illnesses to the act of murder for theft or personal sexual gratification. Such deaths have proven difficult to prevent and the killers difficult to identify mainly because it is almost unthinkable that healthcare professionals would either murder or deliberately end the life of their patients. Such actions are completely contrary to professional ethics that stress the sanctity of life. Of course, murder by doctors is very rare indeed but there are numerous examples from the nursing profession (although again, statistically, the numbers are extremely small). The unthinkable does, however, sometimes happen, and is often devastating as the killers may be responsible for multiple deaths. These cases deserve review in order to learn how to prevent such occurrences in the future and maintain the essential trust that patients must have in all healthcare professionals.

The cases of many offenders have raised difficult ethical and legal issues and finally result in convictions only after lengthy police investigations and difficult prosecutions. In what circumstances can a doctor or nurse, through easing the pain of a dying patient, be accused of murder? Usually there is a trail. If the warning signals from irregular events had been picked up earlier, many deaths might also have been avoided. Let us look at some of the key historical examples from around the world.

Dr. John Bodkin Adams

One of the oldest documented cases is that of Dr. John Bodkin Adams, who practised medicine in Eastbourne on the South coast of England. He had many famous patients on his list, including the 10th Duke of Devonshire who died suddenly in his presence. Between 1946 and 1956, more than 160 of his patients died in what could be deemed suspicious circumstances. Of these 132 left him money or other items in their wills.[1] He was tried but acquitted of one murder in 1957 on the grounds that the expert witnesses had not conclusively proven the case. The trial established the doctrine of 'double-effect' whereby a doctor, providing treatment with the aim of relieving pain, may lawfully, as an unintentional result, shorten life. In a later trial, Bodkin Adams was found guilty of prescription fraud, lying on cremation forms, obstructing a police search and failing to keep a register of dangerous drugs. He was fined and struck off the medical register but reinstated four years later. For several years afterwards, rumours circulated about the conduct of the politicians, lawyers and policemen involved. Some had been quite close to Bodkin Adams. Expert opinion remains divided about him. Many are convinced he was an unconvicted mass murderer. Others have speculated that he was a serial killer and probably schizophrenic. The judge in the second case, Sir Patrick Devlin, later suggested that Bodkin Adams was a mercenary mercy killer prepared to sell death. Many of his patients, convinced of his innocence, remained with him until he died in 1983.

Dr. Harold Shipman

The doctor with the most recorded and proven murders practised in the UK. Over 24 years in practice as a general practitioner (GP) — from 1974 to 1998 — Harold Shipman murdered at least 200 patients. His victims were mostly elderly women, though nowhere near death. They were killed either in their homes or in his surgery with a large dose of diamorphine.[2]

He signed all of the death certificates himself so there was no need to involve a coroner. Fellow GPs, to whom he gave plausible accounts of the deaths, countersigned cremation certificates without making their own inquiries. He falsified patient records to explain sudden deaths.

He was loved by many of his patients but proved to be a difficult colleague with dominating views about medicine. The pharmacists and nurses who worked closely with him were groomed until the thought of questioning his actions and decisions did not even cross their minds.

The first murders probably occurred in Todmorden, in Yorkshire, and it was here that the first warning signs about his character began to appear. He was caught forging Demerol prescriptions for his own use. He was addicted to the drug, a powerful opioid painkiller, essentially a cleaned up version of heroin. After two years of treatment at a drug rehabilitation clinic, he was allowed to practise again and moved to a partnership in Hyde, near Manchester, where the murders continued. He eventually ended up with his one-person private practice. As he continued to avoid detection, he moved on to stealing from his patients. He was finally noticed when one of the practice staff, encouraged by the local undertaker, passed on concerns about the number of cremation certificates signed by Shipman to the local coroner. A police investigation followed but they were unable to find sufficient evidence to bring charges. Shipman went on to murder three more patients before he was apprehended after falsifying the will of one of his patients in his favour. The patient had died in his presence and the death certificate recorded old age as the cause of death. The deceased woman's daughter, a lawyer, challenged the will and when the body was exhumed it was found to contain traces of diamorphine. Shipman was re-arrested and a new investigating team uncovered a pattern of unexplained deaths amongst his patients. Shipman was charged with 15 murders, found guilty of all of them and sentenced to life imprisonment. He committed suicide in Wakefield prison four years later.

There is general agreement that Shipman was a psychopath and a narcissist, He had a 'God Complex' and became addicted to killing. Dame Janet Smith, who chaired the subsequent inquiry,[3] explained that: 'Shipman rode a cart and horses through our systems of regulating the use of controlled drugs by GPs and our systems of death certification. He made a detour around the coroner's system of death investigation and undermined confidence in the medical profession'. There were many recommendations for system change.[4] Had a system for effectively monitoring deaths been in place he might have been detected earlier. At his practice there were 67 excess deaths of women age over 65 years in 1996 and this had increased to 119 by 1998. A system of professional validation, now in place in the UK, might also have identified him earlier.

Dr. Maxim Petrov

Theft was the dominant motive driving Dr. Maxim Petrov to target patients at a local healthcare centre in St. Petersburg, Russia, between 1999 and 2000. His early offences were robberies but in 1999 he was interrupted during a robbery at the house of a patient he had anaesthetised. He stabbed the patient's daughter with a screwdriver and then strangled the unconscious patient. His later modus operandi was to inject his victims with a variety of drugs at their home that quickly led to unconsciousness and death. Petrov would then steal whatever valuables were available and set fire to the homes to destroy any evidence. He was suspected of committing 19 murders but tried for just 17. He was found guilty and sentenced to life imprisonment. In this very strange case we have a thief who used his clinical skills to facilitate his robberies.

Edson Izidoro Guimarães

Corruption may have been the underlying cause of multiple deaths at the Salgado Filho Hospital in Brazil. Edson Izidoro Guimarães worked as a nursing assistant and was seen by a co-worker filling a syringe with potassium chloride and injecting a comatose patient who immediately died. The police were informed and uncovered a higher-than-average death rate in his ward. On his arrest, he confessed to five murders. 'I don't regret what I did', he said, adding 'I did it to those in irreversible comas and whose families were suffering'. He was sentenced to 76 years in prison. One possible motive for the murders was thought to be the fact that he was paid US$60 each time he informed local funeral homes of a patient's death so that they could contact the relatives of the deceased. According to Josias Quintal, Rio Secretary for Public Security: 'He may have begun doing it to make money and just lost control'. He is thought to have killed up to 131 patients.

Donald Harvey

Donald Harvey began working as an orderly and sometimes autopsy assistant at Marymount Hospital in Kentucky in 1970.[5] He later confessed to killing at least a dozen patients in his first year at the hospital out of empathy for his victims. He used many methods to kill his victims, including poisoning with arsenic, cyanide, insulin or morphine, as well as turning off ventilators. His killing spree continued until 1987 when he was arrested in connection with the unexpected death of a patient who had been on life support following an accident on a motorcycle. A post-mortem examination had uncovered large amounts of cyanide in his system. Harvey had become a person of interest when police had discovered that he had been stealing body parts for occult rituals. When challenged, Harvey confessed that he had 'euthanised' the patient. On the evening of his arrest, nurses told a TV reporter that they had reported a spike in the death rate over the past few months to hospital administrators but had been told to keep quiet. In the search for a plea bargain, to avoid the death penalty, Harvey told his lawyer of another 70 cases. He explained that he had started killing to ease the pain of his victims but, as time progressed, he had begun to enjoy it more and more and became a self-described 'angel of death'. He died in prison in 2017.

Dr. Michael Swango

Dr. Michael Swango was identified as a potential problem on numerous occasions in his career but continued to poison his patients and colleagues until his final conviction for murder in 2000.

Swango had qualified in medicine in Illinois, but only after taking an extra year because he had been found to be cheating in his exams. After qualifying, he took up a residency in neurosurgery at the Wexner Medical Centre, Ohio State University.

Nurses reported that healthy patients in his care died in mysterious circumstances. Their concerns were ignored even after one nurse caught him injecting some 'medicine' into a patient who then suddenly became ill. His residency was quickly ended after his internship. This should have been a major warning sign, but those in charge did not want a lengthy external inquiry and instead simply removed him from the hospital. They may not have had firm evidence of his misdeeds but they must have had a high level of suspicion.

He moved on to an ambulance service where staff noticed that whenever he made coffee or brought in food, several of them became violently ill. He was subsequently arrested, convicted of aggravated battery and sentenced to five years' imprisonment. Police investigated his previous history but decided not to proceed with more serious malpractice charges for want of physical evidence.

On his release from prison, he worked in a number of places, including a job as a laboratory technician, where again, fellow workers suffered from mysterious stomach problems. In 1991, he changed his name and forged legal documents to re-establish his medical credentials and minimise his prison record.[6] He went on to work as a doctor in South Dakota at the Sanford Medical Centre and appeared to be performing well until he made the mistake of applying to join the American Medical Association. Their checking was more rigorous than the hospital and they discovered his previous identity and conviction for poisoning, which led to him being fired.

He next surfaced at a psychiatric residency programme in New York where again, patients began to die for no explicable reason. The poisoning had continued. When challenged about his earlier poisoning conviction, Swango admitted that he had lied in his application and resigned. The Dean wrote to all medical schools in the US, blacklisting Swango from ever again getting a medical residency in the US.

In 1994, he fled to Zimbabwe and worked as a doctor at the Lutheran Hospital in Bulawayo. Again, his patients began to die in mysterious circumstances. His colleagues became suspicious and he was suspended. At this time, he was renting a room from a widowed woman who became violently sick after a meal. A local doctor suspected arsenic poisoning and sent samples of her hair to the regional forensic centre. The results confirmed toxic levels of arsenic and a police investigation commenced. Through Interpol, the US authorities became aware of his location and began their own investigation. Swango, however, continued to move. He crossed the border into Zambia and later Namibia where he worked as a locum doctor. In Zimbabwe he was charged in absentia with a number of poisonings. Swango was finally arrested in 1997 at Chicago O'Hare International Airport when he was in transit to Saudi Arabia.

There was still insufficient evidence to bring charges of murder but he was convicted of fraud and sentenced to three and a half years in jail. The sentencing judge ordered that Swango not be allowed to prepare or deliver food or have any involvement preparing or distributing drugs during his sentence. Whilst he was in jail, the investigations continued and bodies of his former patients exhumed. Poisonous chemicals were found and murder charges followed in both the US and Zimbabwe. In order to avoid the death penalty, he pleaded guilty to three charges of murder and was sentenced to life imprisonment. His modus operandi with co-workers was to poison their food and beverages, usually with arsenic. With patients, he usually administered an overdose of whatever drug the patient had been prescribed.

The FBI believed that he had been involved in as many as 60 deaths. He had attracted suspicion throughout his career but until his final conviction no investigation had been thorough enough to provide enough evidence to stop him. Hospitals that had suspicions about his activities, but no concrete proof, simply moved him on. Some were worried about the legal and financial consequences of not finding the evidence to confirm his crimes. Professional and institutional reputation took precedence over patient safety. During his trial, the contents of his notebooks were read out to the court in which he expressed his pleasure at the crimes he had committed. His defence lawyers offered no proof of mental health issues in mitigation for his actions.

Arnfinn Nesset

Poisoning was also the method used by Arnfinn Nesset, a Norwegian nurse. During the summer of 1981, a series of suspicious deaths were uncovered at the nursing home in Orkdal where Nesset was working as a manager. Local journalists received a tip off that Nesset had ordered a large quantity of curacit, a strong muscle-relaxing drug. When questioned by police, he confessed to the murder of 27 patients. 'I have killed so many I'm unable to remember them all', he told police. He later retracted his confession but was nevertheless convicted of murder and sentenced to 21 years in prison. Over a 20-year nursing career, he was thought to have murdered 138 patients but proof was difficult to secure as curacit becomes increasingly difficult to trace with the passage of time. He gave a number of motives for his actions: mercy killings, schizophrenia and morbid pleasure in the act itself. However, he was also found guilty of embezzlement and forgery. His lawyers claimed that he was mentally ill but four independent psychiatrists pronounced him sane and fit for trial. He was released from prison in 2004.

Jane Toppan

Sexual gratification has sometimes also been the motive that has driven medical serial killers. More than a hundred years ago, Jane Toppan, a nurse from Massachusetts confessed to 31 murders at her trial in 1901. She was a psychopath who poisoned her victims, many of whom she was close to. She would fondle her victims and attempt to see the inner working of their souls by staring at their eyes as they died. She claimed to derive a sexual thrill from being with patients who were near death, coming back to life and then dying in her arms.

Petr Zelenka

At Havlickud Brod Hospital in the Czech Republic, concerns had been raised about the suspiciously high number of deaths of patients from internal bleeding in the intensive care unit between May and

September 2006. Petr Zelenka had been the head of the unit throughout this period. As local investigations continued, the hospital decided that Zelenka should leave and negotiated a deal to terminate his contract. There was no proof at that stage that Zelenka was the cause of the deaths but the hospital must have had some suspicions. He subsequently managed to secure another job in East Bohemia. When finally interviewed by the police, he admitted injecting patients with heparin, an anticoagulant drug, excessive doses of which can cause excessive bleeding and become lethal.[7] He was charged with the murder of seven patients and the attempted murder of 10 others. In 2008, he was found guilty and sentenced to life imprisonment. He explained at his trial: 'The first impulse to kill came out of nowhere. As if a voice inside kept telling me, "give it to them"'.

Healthcare experts and patient's right groups blamed the system. Some argued that careful documentation of the amount and number of drugs each patient is given would have prevented this tragedy, as would a rule that drugs should only be administered to patients in the presence of two healthcare professionals. Others took a different view: 'These were the criminal acts of one person. You can't blame it on the system. I don't think there exists any safety measures anywhere in the world that can protect patients against a determined murderer'.[8] The Hospital Director was sacked for taking so long to remove Zelenka from the intensive care unit. The Minister of Health, Tomas Julinek, explained: 'Such people enjoy killing the helpless, those who need to rely on the help of others. They think and feel differently than the rest of us and get enjoyment from deciding over life and death. That is when they gain the most pleasure'.

The Lainz Angels of Death

For some serial killers, the motives are more mundane and include the targeting of patients who simply snored or soiled their beds. In the 1980s, four Austrian nursing assistants (aides) decided to make their tough job a little easier by eliminating some of their patients. They eventually confessed to murdering 49 elderly patients over a six-year period between 1983 and 1989. The slightest annoyance would trigger the wrath of the aides. Patients who complained, snored, soiled their beds, refused medication or buzzed the nurses' station too often would be placed on a kill list. 'This one gets a ticket to God', one was reported to have said to her colleagues. Their method of murder was to either administer an overdose of drugs or employ the 'water cure' where the patients nose was pinched closed, the tongue held down and water poured into the lungs. As their trial progressed it became clear that whilst mercy might have been the motivation for the first killings, this was clearly not the case for the majority of their crimes. They were eventually caught when a local doctor overheard them giggling about their latest victim in a bar and reported them to the police. All four were imprisoned, but by 2008 all had been released for good behaviour despite public protests. Senior staff at the hospital where they worked were disciplined for not detecting what had been happening or acting to investigate when the excessive death rate should have been obvious.

Christine Malevre

The case of Christine Malevre from France opened up the argument about the distinction between mercy killing and euthanasia even though the former was, and still is, illegal in France. She had confessed to helping about 30 terminally ill patients to die at the Francois Quesnay hospital in Paris between 1997 and 1998. This was all done, she claimed, with the patient's or family's consent. Her actions had been uncovered following an investigation into the abnormal number of deaths in the department in which she worked. Murder charges followed and she was found guilty and sentenced to 10 years in prison.[9] The prosecution had argued that she had a morbid fascination with death. Euthanasia activists, on the other hand, argued that the trial helped highlight the problem of clandestine mercy killing that happened regularly in French hospitals. She eventually served four years in prison. In 2016 the law in France changed; while euthanasia still remained illegal doctors could, in certain circumstances, put terminally ill patients into continuous deep sedation until death.

Stephan Letter

A German nurse, Stephan Letter, confessed to killing patients but insisted that he had acted out of sympathy and a desire to end the suffering of the sick. The prosecution challenged this assertion as many of those who died were in a stable condition and ready to be discharged. During his employment at a hospital in Bavaria from January 2003 to July 2004, a pattern of more than 80 deaths occurred on his shifts. He became a suspect after large quantities of drugs, including the muscle relaxant, Lysthenon,[10] had gone missing from the hospital. Unsealed medication vials were found in Letter's apartment. He was sentenced to life imprisonment.

Charles Cullen

An American nurse, Charles Cullen, confessed to killing up to 40 patients during his 16-year career at healthcare facilities in New Jersey and Pennsylvania between 1986 and 2003. He had had a troubled childhood and a subsequent spell in the US Navy resulted in a number of admissions to the Navy Psychiatric Service after attempts at suicide. Shortly after his discharge he commenced his training to be a nurse. On qualifying he took up a post at the Burns Unit at St. Barnabas Hospital.

His first murder, in 1988, followed his administration of a lethal dose of intravenous medication to a patient. Several other murders followed. He left the hospital when the authorities began investigating who had the contaminated IV bags, which had led to dozens of patient deaths. Cullen moved to a new post in Phillipsburg where he murdered three elderly patients by giving them overdoses of the heart medication, digoxin. The breakdown of his marriage led to more suicide attempts and more changes of jobs. Meanwhile, the murders continued, usually through overdoses of digoxin.

In 1998 he moved to a hospital in Pennsylvania but was fired after being accused of giving drugs to patients at unscheduled times. He had also been observed entering a patient's room with syringes in his hand in very suspicious circumstances. His next move was to a cardiac unit at St. Luke's hospital in Bethlehem, where it was later confirmed that he had murdered at least five patients.

Suspicions had been aroused when a co-worker found vials of medication in a disposal bin. These were drugs that would not be used for recreational use so the theft was unusual. Cullen was the suspect. He was offered a deal by the medical faculty; resign and be given a neutral reference or be fired. He resigned and was escorted out of the building in June 2002.

In September of the same year he began working in another critical care unit in Somerville, New Jersey, where more deaths followed. This time, however, the alarm bells were loud and clear. The hospitals' computer system showed that Cullen was accessing the records of patients that he was not involved in nursing. Co-workers began to find him in the rooms of patients where he had not been assigned. His drug requests were strange. In July 2003, state officials warned the hospital that at least four suspicious overdoses indicated that there was a possibility that an employee was killing patients. The hospital delayed contacting authorities until October, by which time Cullen had murdered another five patients.

The hospital finally acted because of the death of a patient with low blood sugar who Cullen had been nursing. This was to be Cullen's last victim. The hospital fired him for lying in his job application but a fellow nurse voiced her suspicions about his activities to the police. The police kept Cullen under surveillance for some weeks. They sent the nurse to talk to Cullen wearing a wiretap and with this as subsequent evidence they were able to bring charges of murder. Cullen promised to cooperate with police authorities if they did not seek the death penalty and admitted killing 40 patients. His defence was that he had given patients overdoses so that he could end their suffering. The jury did not believe him and he was sentenced to life imprisonment. Many of the relatives of the patients he murdered sued the hospitals concerned.

There were multiple signals and warnings about Cullen but the healthcare system did not pick them up as he moved from hospital to hospital. New laws followed in 37 states that gave employers legal protection against prosecution when they provided a truthful reference for an employee — Cullen had made deals to receive what were essentially false references that enabled him to keep on offending.

Cullen was also a major reason for the passing of the Federal Patient Safety Act in 2005 that required hospitals to report serious preventable adverse events and keep complaints and disciplinary records relating to patient care for at least seven years.

Beverly Allitt

The idea of a nurse deliberately taking the lives of children under her care is almost unthinkable but it has happened. The most widely reported case is that of Beverly Allitt, a state-enrolled nurse who was convicted of murdering four children and attempting to murder three others on a children's ward at Grantham and Kesteven Hospital in Lincolnshire in the UK. During the months of February to April 1991, there was a series of unexpected events at the children's ward at the hospital. Three children died suddenly on the ward, and a baby died at home not long after discharge. Nine other babies and children collapsed unexpectedly, some more than once. All but one of them had to be transferred urgently to the specialist children's unit in Nottingham. In many of the cases, it seemed to the doctors at both Grantham and in Nottingham that what had happened was unusual, but could be explained on the basis of each child's medical history. As time went by, more children collapsed unexpectedly. Medical and nursing staff in Grantham, at first bewildered by these events, grew deeply alarmed. Post-mortem results on the decreased children yielded no clues. However, a blood test result indicated that one child had been wrongly injected with insulin. Once the possibility that this could have happened accidentally had been ruled out, suspicion grew that somebody was deliberately harming the children. After some pressure from the doctor in charge of the children's centre at Nottingham where many of the seriously ill children had been referred, the police were called in to investigate. Some of the local professionals continued to reassure police that everything that had happened could have been due to an unhappy sequence of natural but tragic events. So, the first challenge the police faced was to prove that a criminal offence had taken place.

As events were gradually pieced together, a picture emerged of one person, Beverly Allitt, as the likely culprit. The police discovered that Allitt was the only nurse on duty for all of the unexpected deaths and other incidents where attempted murder was suspected. However, finding the proof of murder was not easy and took time as Allitt claimed her innocence. In addition, it did not seem to make any sense. One of the parents whose child had been attacked by Allitt had been so impressed with the care that the nurse had given that they had invited her to become the child's godmother.

Eventually, it was proven that Allitt had injected a large dose of insulin to at least two victims and a large air bubble was found in the body of another. She was charged with murder, found guilty and sentenced to life imprisonment.[11]

An independent inquiry later reported, 'We were struck throughout our inquiry by the way in which fragments of medical evidence which, if assembled, would have pointed to Allitt as the malevolent cause of the unexpected collapses of children, lay neglected or ignored all together'. The Inquiry added: 'civilised society has little defence against the aimless malice of a deranged mind'.

In its search for similar international cases, the Allitt Inquiry team found two examples. In a Canadian case, a nurse was arrested following a dramatic increase in the mortality rate in a cardiology ward at a children's hospital. The deaths were consistent with digoxin poisoning. A nurse was arrested but charges dismissed when it was discovered that digoxin had been administered to another child when she was not on duty. The second case occurred at the paediatric intensive care unit of the San Antonio University hospital in Texas where there had been an unusual increase in the number of deaths and cardiac arrests. Most of the instances occurred during the evening shift and in the presence of one nurse. She was charged and convicted of one charge of attempted murder.

In an interesting epilogue, the Allitt Inquiry stated: 'when some great disaster befalls the human race the instinctive reaction of most people is to seek its cause and try to prevent a reoccurrence. But behind this civilised response there lies a darker motivation old as time — the urge to lay blame. The ancient notion of a scapegoat, to bear the guilt for disastrous happenings and thus relieve feelings of rage and frustration, is still with us'.[12]

Victorino Chua

Another recent case illustrates the difficulties of first identifying criminal acts and then finding sufficient proof to bring charges. Victorino Chua, a nurse at Stepping Hill Hospital, Stockport, England, embarked on a killing spree of mostly elderly patients in Summer 2011.[13] He secretly loaded drips with insulin in order to put his patients into hypoglycaemic shock. He had also tampered with saline bags before they were used on patients. He selected his victims at random. As the number of attacks increased, medical staff became concerned until a nurse discovered a number of saline bags that were leaking and had clearly been tampered with. Once insulin was found in the contaminated bags the police were informed. They then discovered that the bags had been punctured with a hypodermic needle. An 18-month police investigation followed[14] at the end of which they arrested the wrong person who was later released.[15] Chua halted his killing spree during this period. The hospital was effectively in lockdown, with armed guards on duty and a rule that medication could only be given by two healthcare professionals working together. Despite this, Chua became active again in January 2012 by altering patient prescription charts. Fortunately, other nurses noticed the crude alterations and reported him. He was arrested. By this stage the police were investigating 22 cases of patients who had been poisoned as well as seven deaths. Chau was found guilty of two counts of murder and multiple counts of grievous bodily harm. He was sentenced to 25 life sentences with a minimum of 35 years in jail. The police stated that he was a narcissistic psychopath. Whilst in prison he continued to claim his innocence but lost his appeal against his sentence in 2016.

Dr. Louay Omar Mohammed al-Tael

One setting, war, presents a very different environment in which healthcare professionals have to be judged. Hospitals, in particular, have become targets for hostile action by rogue doctors. Triaging wounded patients can be a tough and at time brutal process. One case illustrates the problem. In 2006, Dr. Louay Omar Mohammed al-Tael, an Iraqi doctor, moved among the puddles of blood and crowds of family members in al-Jumhuriya Hospital's hectic emergency unit quietly dispatching police officers, soldiers and officials who had been wounded, some only slightly, by insurgent attacks. His favoured killing method was the injection of a fatal cocktail of drugs. He was himself a member of a Sunni insurgent group and part of a wider network of doctors and nurses supporting Sunni militants in Iraq. At the end of his filmed confession he is asked whether he betrayed his profession. 'We thought we could do something to liberate the country', he said. 'Later our network went astray, but we had to keep working, and we had to keep committing these crimes.' In his own warped community, he was a hero. To the police chief of Kirkuk he was something else: 'I can understand a doctor may have personal sympathies with the insurgency but to use his professional position to become an instrument of death turns sense and humanity on its head'.

Lessons for the Future

The key message from these cases is that the unthinkable does sometimes happen. Healthcare professionals do on very rare occasions kill or harm their patients. A close recording and regular review of adverse events in all healthcare settings is a key defence against such actions. In addition, the monitoring of unexpectedly high death rates is essential. Very high rates of unexpected deaths can be identified at either national or state levels and then investigated locally within a culture of discovery rather than blame. The signals of an inherent problem with excessive numbers of avoidable deaths were visible at a national level in the Mid Staffordshire case (discussed at length in Chapter One) but local managers and doctors invested their energies in trying to challenge the data rather than search for another explanation.

But national surveillance is not enough. For the most part, high-level information systems will not pick up suspicious deaths in multiple locations. They are also hospital-focused and ignore primary care. The best identifiers are found at a more local level. As can be seen in the cases discussed in this chapter, the alarm bells are usually rung by whistleblowers and the relatives of patients. These people need to be listened to. An anonymous reporting system that some might consider distasteful and disruptive needs to be considered. A recent development in England has been the requirement to appoint a medical examiner at each hospital to review all deaths. This should materially strengthen the defences for patients, particularly if the examiners can find a way of sharing data with each other.

Tracking professional careers has also been suggested as a means of stopping medical serial killers in their tracks but this idea seems impracticable. To be of any use, the tracking information would have to include more than what can be found on a traditional curriculum vitae. It might include licence violations and imposed conditions of practice but could never incorporate suspicions of misconduct when those were not proven.

We consider regular revalidation by licensing bodies in Chapter Four of this book but this is not a process designed to identify serial killers. There is no reliable psychological profile that could be used to identify in advance healthcare professionals who might harm their patients.

What is increasingly being recognised as a major problem is the unacceptable but nevertheless common practice by some employers to allow problem professionals to move on, often quietly, to another post in another place. Concern for the reputation of the affected institution or company too often takes precedence over patient safety as does the fear of legal proceedings for the defamation of a suspected offender. The law should protect those who act in the interests of patient safety. This problem is compounded when recruiting authorities fail to properly validate references from former employers or check licensing credentials. The Allitt Inquiry was of the view that nobody should be allowed to enter a School of Nursing when there was evidence of a major personality disorder and that all nurses should be formally screened with a health check before taking up a post on qualification. This could be applied to all healthcare professionals, despite the evident challenge of identifying individuals with personality problems who might pose a danger to patients in the future.

'Bring me proof and I will act' is a common defence of inaction by managers and medical and nursing directors. This is understandable when suspicions are being raised about the conduct or performance of senior members of staff. If the suspicions turn out to be unfounded, relationships may have been irreparably damaged. The culture of an organisation needs to be open enough to allow suspicion to be a sufficient cause to initiate sensitive but thorough investigations in the interests of patient safety. An innocent member of staff should have nothing to fear and participate fully in an investigation on the understanding that this is being undertaken in the higher interests of patient safety. They should be involved in the process rather than suspended.

Identifying a serial killer in a healthcare setting is extraordinarily difficult. It remains an extremely rare occurrence and healthcare authorities almost always first search for other explanations when unexplained events occur. They need always to remember that when no other explanation is available there are clear precedents for the worst-case scenario to be true.

Police authorities are usually only involved when, in the absence of any other explanation, criminal activity has to be a possibility. The first challenge for the police is to establish that a crime has actually been committed. All that is usually handed to the police are suspicious deaths or injuries to patients. Such cases often involve long and complex inquiries that would be better handled by experienced teams operating at the highest levels of police organisations such as the FBI or the National Crime Agency in the UK.

Chapter Three

Unsafe Clinical Practice and Its Impact on Patient Safety

Unsafe clinical care is one of the top 10 leading causes of death in the world. It accounts for more lives lost than lung cancer, diabetes or road accidents. According to one report,[1] in low- and middle-income countries, unsafe care claims the lives of 2.6 million people each year. Many of the practices that create such dangers for patients are avoidable.

The largest population studies of such events come from the US and Australia. The Harvard Medical Practice Study is the reference for estimating the extent of medical injuries occurring in hospitals. A review of the medical charts of 30,121 patients admitted to 51 acute hospitals in New York State in 1984 reported that preventable adverse events occurred in 3.7% of hospital admissions.[2] A later international review covering 27 countries over six continents, published in 2018, recorded a median adverse event rate in hospitals of 10%, half of which were avoidable, and a death rate of 1.1% for medical errors.[3] The authors of this study described their own results as shocking.

The three most common types of adverse events are operative/surgical related, medication or drug/fluid related and healthcare associated infections.

In 2008, the economic cost of such failings in the US was thought to be US$1 trillion which, if extrapolated, would result in a global figure in the multi-trillions of dollars — a sizeable slice of global GDP investment in health.[4] Experts in healthcare systems have known about this for years but it is only in recent times that the evidence about the scale of the problem has emerged and entered the public domain. Medicine is not an exact science and relies significantly on physician experience and instinct. Psychologists who have studied 'how doctors think' have concluded that 10%–15% of initial diagnoses are wrong.[5] This appears to have been confirmed by 'mystery patient' studies when real or simulated patients with classical presentations of common diseases such as rheumatoid arthritis or COPD[6] are sent into real practice settings.[7] Patients, of course, expect all diagnoses to be 100% correct.

Since 2019, the World Health Organization (WHO) has had a World Patient Safety Day, and there is now an active international research programme on patient safety. The variations between countries rank in regard to patient safety is very wide. One measure, mortality due to adverse medical treatment, ranks Finland, the Netherlands, New Zealand, Norway and Singapore as the best global performers, with the US and Canada at the bottom end of the developed country rankings. Most developed countries now have national organisations focussed on patient safety with data collection systems monitoring adverse events. Many hospitals also now have safety committees.

The sheer size of the problem and the fact that many of the adverse events that occur are avoidable makes it disastrous for public confidence in healthcare professions and the systems in which they work. If hospitals were factories, they would have long since been closed down on health and safety grounds!

> *Whenever a doctor cannot do good, he must be kept from doing harm.*
>
> One of many versions of the Hippocratic Oath

Although practitioners do make mistakes that harm patients, many adverse events happen as a consequence of either system failure or when organisational pressures place staff in unreasonably stressful situations.

So, we need to maintain a proper sense of proportion and look for ways of improving systems rather than just concentrating on scapegoating individuals that make bad decisions. The focus should be on those areas that create the greatest danger for patients and staff. As Paul Barach, an American doctor, explained to a conference in London:

> *Health care should learn from the team work of other high reliability organisations (special forces, aviation and space flight). The lessons will be hard; egos are sacrificed for the good of the team, safety before hierarchy, and radical changes to the educational curricula for the health professions. Continuous in-service training and education is a must.*[8]

One underused safety resource is the patients themselves who can be encouraged to check their own progress through a clinical pathway and alert their carers when things are missed or go wrong. Pathways can be complicated but for standard procedures, such as a hip replacement, or diseases like diabetes, it ought to be possible to provide patients with a pathway that they can both understand and check. Finland has appointed an ombudsman to help patients to understand and navigate a safe clinical pathway.

Creating new bureaucratic structures might help spur and inform action but, according to another American physician, Joel Nobel, caution should be exercised in an uncritical acceptance of data about patient safety:

> *During the 1960's spurious research, falsified data, charlatans, gullible biomedical engineers and imaginative media types ushered in America's first widespread patient safety campaign, flawed reporting systems and poorly considered medical device regulations. Hundreds of millions of dollars were spent by US hospitals defending patients and themselves from a risk that had been immensely exaggerated. To this day, there are disproportionate efforts expended by biomedical and electrical engineers on improving the electrical safety of medical devices. Yet the real risks are mechanical problems; plumbing, gas line mix-ups and a failure to connect ventilators properly to patients are examples. Patients have died because oxygen and nitrous oxide lines have been interchanged during construction or renovation. A further 50% of adverse events have been caused by operator error which needs to be remedied by training and human factor design-areas that get inadequate attention or investment.*[9]

Sometimes widely accepted clinical practice can later be found to be of harm to patients. The challenge is how quickly individual practitioners and healthcare systems respond to early warning signs.

Drug Safety

Thalidomide was originally marketed as a mild sleeping pill, safe even for pregnant women. It had an inhibiting effect on morning sickness. It was produced in Germany by Chemie Grunenthal, and by the late 1950s, 14 pharmaceutical companies marketed thalidomide as a prescription-free, over-the-counter drug in 46 countries using at least 37 different trade names. In the UK, it was marketed by The Distillers Company. In the US, the Food and Drug Administration (FDA) took another view and refused a licence because of doubts about its safety. William McBride, an Australian obstetrician, first raised a serious alarm in 1961. He reported that some patients had suffered nerve damage in their limbs (many of which were shortened) through taking the drug. Thalidomide was removed from European markets in November 1961.[10] Later estimates suggested that as many as 10,000 babies had been born with birth defects as a result of their mothers using the drug.[11] Critics argued that the pharmaceutical companies should have seen red flags far earlier. The companies later apologised for both producing the drug and remaining silent about the birth defects. Most countries ensured that victims and their families received substantial financial compensation from funds provided by both the companies involved and governments, although 50 years later, some victims were still fighting for adequate damages.[12] The scandal also resulted in tougher rules for the testing and licensing of new drugs in many countries.

In 2019, an Australian Senate Committee was sympathetic to calls by the Thalidomide victims for more compensation, but the final decision lay with government. Thalidomide was later found to be effective in the treatment of Hansen's disease (leprosy) and is now in use in many developing countries. Researchers and licensing authorities will be watching closely.

> *Two pills were all it took. Lisa McManus was left physically disfigured and emotionally scarred by one of the world's worst pharmaceutical disasters. When Lisa was born in Queensland, Australia, the midwife assisting in her delivery fled the room in tears. Her mother, Beryl, was taken to a ward and left alone. Lisa's tiny body had severely malformed arms, only three fingers and no thumbs. Lisa's mother had taken only two tablets to relieve anxiety during her pregnancy. She took the pills seven months after the Australian government had been alerted of the risk of Thalidomide to pregnant women by the company that had marketed it. The then Minister of Health had decided not to issue a public warning 'as it would serve no useful purpose'.*[13]

They will also be watching the outcome of the charges made in 2020 against Sanofi, a major French pharmaceutical company, for its failure to warn thousands of pregnant women about the risks associated with its epilepsy drug, Depakine, which is thought to produce birth malfunctions and slow neurological development when taken during pregnancy.[14] Sanofi claims that it has always complied with its duty to inform and be transparent.

Breast Implants

Silicone breast implants, produced by Poly Implant Prostheses (PIP), were first introduced in France in 1991 and used extensively over the next 20 years. In 2001, PIP started to use unapproved industrial grade silicone in their implants. It gradually emerged that these implants were rupturing at double the industry average. When compromised, the silicone gel was known to cause inflammation and possible scarring, and this also raised questions about the possibility of other long-term effects. PIP went into liquidation in 2010 after the French Medical Safety Agency ordered it to recall its implants. The French government recommended that 30,000 women with PIP implants had them removed as a precaution. The European Commission issued new medical device regulations and the directors of PIP were prosecuted.[15] Jean-Claude Mas, the founder of the company, was sentenced to four years in prison but died in 2019 without having served his sentence.

In another breast implant case, women complained that they had not been sufficiently informed about the risks associated with textured implants produced by the Irish-headquartered pharmaceutical company, Allergan. These had been withdrawn from the US market in 2018 at the request of the FDA, and a worldwide recall followed in July 2019. The recalls were issued after a link was established between the textured implant and anaplastic large cell lymphoma (ALCL), a rare blood cancer. Whilst the risk was judged to be low (one in 24,000 women with an implant), the FDA reported that at the time of the recall, 481 cases of ALCL had, at the time of their diagnosis, an Allergan implant, and that there had so far been 12 attributable deaths.[16] The company offered to replace the implants and contribute to the costs of surgery and cancer treatment.[17] Legal actions continue.

The PIP scandal was partly responsible for a crackdown on cosmetic surgery in England and a review of non-surgical cosmetic treatments that remain almost entirely unregulated, both in the UK and in many other countries.[18] This booming industry was worth US$94 billion in the US alone in 2019.

Blood Contamination

Blood transfusion has produced a number of serious contamination problems over the years. In 1991, a journalist published an article claiming that the French Blood Transfusion Service had knowingly distributed blood products contaminated with HIV to haemophiliacs in 1984 and 1985. Commercial interests were at the heart of this scandal.[19] An application to sell equipment for blood testing by Abbott Laboratories, a US multinational was, it was alleged, delayed as the government waited for a rival French product manufactured by Diagnostics Pasteur to become available.[20] The French Transfusion Service had also been allowed to use up old stocks of blood products for haemophiliacs even though it was known they might have been contaminated. Patient groups alleged that up to 500 patients died.

Prime Minister Laurent Fabius and two of his ministers were accused of manslaughter in 1999. Though he and the Minister for

Social Affairs were acquitted, the Minister of Health was found guilty but received no sentence. Four officials were later charged, including employees from the National Blood Bank and the Blood Transfusion Research Bureau. Two were sentenced to periods in jail.

Patients in other countries, including Australia, Ireland and Canada, have experienced similar problems with blood supply. In Ireland, a Tribunal of Inquiry rejected criticism of Ministers for their handling of a Hepatitis C scandal between 1994 and 1996 but criticised the National Haemophiliac Centre for being slow to respond to the risk of HIV infection.[21] A Royal Commission in Canada that reported in 1997 concluded that blood and plasma from unpaid donors were safer than blood and plasma from donors that had been paid. The Commission based this conclusion in part on the Canadian experience of purchasing what turned out to be tainted blood from an American company that collected blood from prisoners in Arkansas. The WHO took the same view, premised on the belief that well-informed altruistic donors would not donate if there was a possibility that their donation would do harm rather than good.

In 2018, the Infected Blood Inquiry[22] began its work in the UK. It was established to investigate how thousands of people with a bleeding disorder called haemophilia came to be infected with HIV and/or Hepatitis C through a clotting medicine, commonly known as Factor 8, some of which was imported from the US. Leaders in the NHS were well aware of this purchase but were assured by experts that it was safe. The Inquiry will investigate whether this purchase was a reasonable course of action and address allegations of a cover up by individuals and government departments. As was the case in France, senior Ministers and officials are likely to be called to give evidence.

Problems with tainted blood re-emerged in Ireland in 2020 when the Crumlin Hospital in Dublin recalled 70 former patients who were given blood products between 1991 and 1994 that were not adequately screened for Hepatitis C. At the time, Crumlin was taking blood donations for use in its blood platelet treatment for child cancer patients. However, it emerged in 2020 that the test it was using to screen blood for Hepatitis C was inferior to the one being used by the Blood Transfusion Service.[23] This might potentially have led to Hepatitis C-infected blood received from donors not being detected and therefore passed on to children as part of their treatment. A consultant paediatric oncologist told the press that the hospital's failure at the time to introduce a more sophisticated blood-screening test was due to funding shortages.[24]

Hospital-acquired Infections

One of the greatest dangers to patients is an infection acquired whilst in a hospital or care facility. We have already seen some examples in Chapter One of this book. International comparisons have to be made with care as national definitions vary. A commonly reported range (including Switzerland, France, Belgium, Italy and the UK) is that between 5%–7% of hospital admissions result in an infection. In the US, The Centre for Disease Control and Prevention (CDC) estimates that roughly 1.7 million hospital-associated infections, from all types of microorganisms, including bacteria and fungi, together cause or contribute to up to 99,000 deaths a year. WHO estimated that 7% of hospitalised patients in developed countries would acquire a healthcare-associated infection and this number was even higher in underdeveloped countries. WHO recently stated that there are 37,000 deaths attributable to hospital-acquired infections (HAIs) a year in Europe.[25]

The most common infection is MRSA,[26] which is serious but treatable with antibiotics. Gram-negative infections are proving much more difficult to treat as many are resistant to all modern antibiotics. The spread of infection can be prevented with basic hygiene such as handwashing between patient contacts, although in some clinical settings protective clothing is also needed. Some countries have tried both incentives and penalties to encourage hospitals to improve their infection control discipline.

The State of Maryland developed a programme of penalties and incentives in an attempt to improve infection rates. Poor-performing hospitals lost up to 3% of their inpatient revenues and good performers could earn up to 3% in rewards. In the first two years of the programme, infection rates reduced by 15% with an estimated cost saving of US$110 million.[27]

Other countries, including the UK, have published advice on prevention and reducing HAI rates and the performance of infection control teams are now a central feature of external quality reviews. There has been progress, but for measures to be successful actions need to be sustained and embedded into day-to-day practice.

In 2014, an entire family caught MRSA after admission to a hospital in north England for the delivery of a baby. The family presented with symptoms shortly after discharge and were prescribed antibiotic therapy by their General Practitioner (GP). The adults had achy joints, skin lesions and boils and mild depression secondary to MRSA. The outbreak was linked to a member of staff who was colonised with MRSA and who was also suffering with dermatitis.[28] A claim for compensation from the hospital was settled for £10,250 plus costs.

A minor-league pitcher in his younger days, Richard Armbruster kept playing baseball recreationally into his 70s until his right hip started to bother him. He was admitted to a hospital in St. Louis for a routine hip replacement but died from a blood stream infection that sent him into shock and resisted treatment from antibiotics.[29]

The statistics on hospital-acquired influenza are not well quantified, but New Zealand reported 132 cases in 2019 — probably introduced by visitors — with at least five mortalities.[30] Hospitals will have to rethink their policies with regard to visitors as they are now doing with the coronavirus. Should they only be allowed in exceptional circumstances?

In all countries, the economic consequences of HAIs are considerable in terms of increased lengths of stay and far outweigh the costs of more stringent cross-infection control. There will be much to learn from the response to the COVID-19 pandemic.

Unnecessary Treatments and Tests

In recent years, several countries have attempted to reduce the number of treatments judged to be ineffective or, as the Medical Director of NHS England put it, 'futile'. Two leading US physicians claimed in 2009 that if unnecessary care was defined as services that show no demonstrable benefit for patients, then 30% of US care was unnecessary.[31] Almost all clinical procedures carry some degree of risk — usually this is very small but nevertheless there are risks that can be avoided. Subjecting patients to treatment that cannot possibly help them is rooted in outmoded clinical habits, supply-driven behaviour and an ignorance of current science.

In 2020, NHS England had 13 procedures on its list that would only be offered to patients when certain conditions were met. These included breast reduction, removal of benign skin lesions, grommets for glue ear, tonsillectomies, varicose vein treatments and haemorrhoid surgery. Other procedures that would only be performed at the express request of patients included snoring surgery, knee arthroscopy for osteoarthritis and injections for non-specific back pain.[32]

Australian governments have also been active in seeking to reduce the number of unnecessary tests and treatments. These have ranged from reducing the use of antibiotics for patients with upper respiratory infections to imaging for non-specific lower back pain.

A new organisation, 'Choosing Wisely', launched in 2012 by a consortium of medical associations helps its subscribers (mainly physicians and healthcare authorities) first identify and then reduce unnecessary interventions. Two examples are:

> *Leaders at the San Francisco Health Network wanted to address overuse of diagnostic imaging such as CT scans, MRIs and ultrasounds for outpatients as per the recommendations of various medical societies. They began displaying the relative cost and radiation exposure for selected imaging at the point of physician electronic ordering to help raise physician awareness about risks and costs. It worked.[33] The interesting feature of this study is that the data about radiation was more influential with physicians than the data about cost.*

Another Choosing Wisely advisory lays out the top five actions recommended by the UK Royal Colleges of Anaesthetics and Surgery:

(1) Day surgery should be considered the default for many elective surgical procedures;
(2) With appropriate preoperative assessment and preparation, patients do not need to be admitted to hospital the day before surgery;
(3) Healthy patients having planned minor or intermediate surgery do not need routine preoperative tests;
(4) Patients at high risk of death after their surgery (greater than 1% of predicted rate) should have a shared decision-making consultation;
(5) Patients should be helped to stop smoking, reduce alcohol consumption, improve fitness and modify weight before surgery.[34]

Economics play some part — maybe a major part — in drives to reduce these treatments, but patient safety is also a factor. These measures have, however, had the unintended consequence of intruding deeply into the clinical freedoms of physicians and there is some resentment of that. The Australian initiatives led to a major investigation into how healthcare professionals' fears of being sued can lead to them prescribing low-value care. It also exposed the problems that can result from fee-for-service funding methods that can stimulate unnecessary tests and treatments.

It has been claimed that Canadian citizens undergo more than 1 million potentially unnecessary medical tests or treatments every year. This represents 30% of all the tests, treatments and procedures performed.[35] The Canadian Institute for Health Information focussed on eight types of tests and procedures that were commonly ordered by healthcare professionals and found to be unnecessary and of no value to patients. These included imaging tests for lower back pain, mammograms, blood transfusions and drug treatment for insomnia. Most physicians blame patient demand and a fear of litigation for such unnecessary testing.

Arguments about reducing unnecessary or futile treatments have been the most intense in the US where market forces play a major role in stimulating patient demand. This has also led to demands to make over-treatment an ethical violation. However, insurers using physicians to review the work of other doctors have not been very successful. An initiative by the American Board of Internal Medicine to publicise tests and treatments that are often overused may have a greater long-term impact. Patient safety committees, charged with reviewing the quality of care, can view over-utilisation as adverse events.

Diagnostic Errors

Modern medicine is heavily influenced by diagnostic test results from laboratories and imaging centres. Audits suggest that 2%–4% of laboratory test results are misleadingly wrong, and roughly the same error rates are found in radiology and imaging. In the US, where 13 billion tests are performed each year in 250,000 certified testing laboratories, the error rate is thought to be as high as 1 in 20 adults.[36] Thanks to enhanced quality control systems in laboratories, most errors originate in the pre-analytical and post-analytical phases, namely, physician ordering, sample collection and interpreting the results. Reliably communicating abnormal test results is a universal problem, even in systems with advanced electronic medical records.[37] Diagnostic uncertainty is rarely disclosed to patients, but laboratory tests are not always right, and they are not always useful. As we will see in Chapter Five, diagnostic errors represent 34% of all cases of medical malpractice.

Screening Errors

Medical screening has been in operation for over 100 years. One of the early programmes was designed to pick up psychiatric disorders in potential recruits to the US Army. Later programmes screened for cancer and tuberculosis. As population screening has been extended, so has the number of reported errors. Some errors have been due to a clinical misinterpretation of the screening tool whilst others are administrative errors in the reporting and call-up processes.

Problems were reported at the East Devon Breast Cancer screening unit in the UK in 1997 when a clinician reported that a significant number of patients had been misdiagnosed. A government minister sent the Chief Medical Officer (CMO) to investigate. An independent review of 2000 cases followed that found that of 229 cases sent for further assessment, 61 patients had received a delayed diagnosis and 11 women had subsequently died. In many of the cases doctors had diagnosed lumps in the breast as benign tumours or cysts and had failed to recognise the features of malignant cancer. An expert witness at a later General Medical Council hearing said that this was: 'A unique catalogue of screening assessment failure the like of which I have never come across before or since'. Dr. John Brennan, the Director of the Unit, explained that the screening process had its limitations and doctors were fallible. He had missed eight cancers, all of which were very small and at an early stage of development. He and a colleague were found guilty of serious professional misconduct but did not have their licences to practice revoked provided that they no longer worked in the screening field.[38] The CMO concluded that the screening unit had been an island within the hospital and so had escaped the scrutiny of colleagues in other disciplines.

Cervical cancer screening is a method of detecting pre-cancerous changes in a woman's cervix or the neck of the womb. It is a common cancer amongst women under the age of 35 years. In England, the national screening programme started in 1988 is thought to have prevented up to 3900 cases a year and heralded a dramatic fall in death rates. Australia has an ambitious plan to eradicate the disease altogether. In real-world situations, the majority of screening examinations are normal. Under these conditions, a second expert reviewer would only detect a critical abnormality within the range of 2%–5%.[39]

A number of screening programmes have had problems.

Kent and Canterbury Screening Programme.

Ninety-one thousand women were recalled for more tests after errors were spotted in 1996. At least eight women were thought to have died as a result. An Inquiry found that the service had poor and confused management, was understaffed and training was inadequate. There had also been a breakdown in working relationships between the clinicians. The Trust Chair and Chief Executive resigned.[40]

Republic of Ireland

In June 2018, a terminally ill woman with five children settled a case against the Irish Health Executive and a US laboratory contractor for €7.5 million. She had received an all clear from a smear test that proved to be wrong. She was, it transpired, not alone and it later emerged that 18 other women had been given incorrect tests and died. The Irish government also agreed a comprehensive package to support the 209 women who had been diagnosed with cervical cancer but had audit results that differed from their original smear tests. The Chief Executive of the Irish Health Executive resigned a few weeks earlier than he had planned as a result of the controversy.[41]

False negatives are evident in all screening programmes according to a report prepared for NHS England, and this remains true even if the quality of the service provided is high. The Royal College of Pathologists put the acceptable error rate at 1.6%. A false-negative result is judged to be more serious than a false positive that can be picked up by further tests prior to treatment. The evidence about the consequences of false-negative results is limited but it is clear that there is a potential danger in delaying the detection of breast and cervical cancer.[42] It is perhaps not surprising that dual testing is now becoming more commonplace. As we will see in Chapter Five, 'a second test may be more valuable than a second opinion'. Artificial intelligence may, it is hoped, improve the rate of test accuracy. E-trigger algorithms, for example, look to be a promising way forward.

The Ethics of Clinical Trials

In New Zealand, an inquiry[43] established by the Minister of Health in 1987 investigated whether there had been a failure to adequately treat patients with cervical carcinoma. It had been alleged that Dr. Herbert Green had been withholding medical treatment from some patients without their consent, as part of a clinical trial. According to Green, 'The only way to settle finally the problem of what happens to *in situ* cancer is to follow indefinitely patients with a diagnosis but untreated lesions'. He and his colleagues were roundly condemned for their actions and the case hastened the introduction of cervical cancer screening in New Zealand. Thirty years later, the patients received a comprehensive and unqualified apology from the Auckland District Health Board,[44] admitting past mistakes and making a firm affirmation that it would never happen again.[45]

Long before the cervical cancer scandal (between 1949 and 1983), New Zealand had experienced another problem that had barely caused a ripple. A technique to help premature babies survive inadvertently caused an epidemic of blindness. At the National Women's Hospital in Auckland, extra oxygen was given to babies in incubators because it was thought they were at risk of brain damage due to the lack of oxygen they had received in the womb. However, there was little control over the amount of oxygen given to the babies in the hospital, resulting in infants going blind from a disorder called retrolental fibroplasia where fibrous tissue forms behind the lens of the eye. Not every incubated baby received extra oxygen, and in a nearby hospital no babies had the condition. The practice had been widely used throughout the Western world but was abandoned as a 'well-intentioned but misdirected therapeutic intervention'.[46]

Antibiotics

The overuse of antibiotics is likely to become a major international scandal. Antibiotics are used extensively throughout the world to treat or prevent many types of bacterial infection but do not work for viral infections. First discovered in 1928 by Alexander Fleming, their overuse has led to some bacteria developing a resistance to them that WHO has classified as a major health threat. Experts predict that by the mid-21st century, 10 million people will die of antibiotic-resistant infections. Dame Sally Davies, former Chief Medical Officer for England, puts it rather more starkly: 'If we do not act now, anyone of us could go into hospital in 20 years for minor surgery and die because of an ordinary infection that cannot be treated with antibiotics'.[47]

Governments have reacted to the problem, but progress has been slow and there are few new antibiotics currently in the pharmaceutical industries' discovery pipelines. Australia has some of the highest rates of resistance in the world, and resistance to vancomycin, one of the reserve antibiotics used in the most complex cases, was approaching 50% in 2016.

The CDC in the US reports that at least 28 million people are infected with antibiotic-resistant bacteria each year, leading to 35,000 deaths. Patients at particular risk are those being treated for cancer, advanced kidney disease and organ transplantation. The picture in the European Union (EU) varies by country, but the number of predicted deaths that could not be treated with anti-microbial drugs now stands at 33,000.[48] Since 2013, Denmark, Latvia, the Netherlands and Romania have reduced their antibiotic consumption by almost 9% whilst large increases in usage have been recorded in Italy and Spain. The principal line of defence against resistance is to prevent the use of antibiotics in inappropriate cases. In many countries, these drugs remain on unrestricted sale to the public. If no decisive action is taken, antibiotics may need to become controlled drugs.

The EU estimates that the extra healthcare costs and productivity losses caused by resistance to antibiotics amounts to at least €1.5 billion a year while the Organisation for Economic Cooperation and Development (OECD) predicts cumulative losses by 2050 of US$2.9 trillion.

Opioids

Another developing problem is the so-called opioid crisis. In the late 1990s, pharmaceutical companies reassured the medical community that patients would not become addicted to opioid pain relievers and, as a result, their use expanded rapidly. It later became clear that these medicines were, in fact, highly addictive. In the US, more than 2 million people use opioids and overdoses now account for 47,000 deaths a year. Michigan was the first state to sue major distributors of opioid drugs under a liability law that is typically used to target drug dealers.[49] Pharmaceutical companies are currently paying out large sums of money to settle claims for damages. Opioid use in Europe is on the rise but nowhere near the levels reported in the US.[50] Australia has also sued some companies for the improper advertising of opioid drugs.

New Drugs

All new drugs and devices carry some degree of risk for patients. The ethical dilemma is to decide what the appropriate risk threshold is. Regulators are constantly raising the risk barrier, sometimes against the wishes of desperate patients who are prepared to take the unquantifiable risks involved.

New drugs and medical devices undergo extensive clinical trials before they are licensed for use. However, the pharmaceutical industry and governments constantly apply pressure to speed up the approval process. This has happened and will continue to happen with regard to the COVID-19 pandemic in 2020, where trade-offs had to be made between effective safety screening and increased treatment options. Safety thresholds were lowered in an attempt to mitigate the number of short-term deaths. The negative effects of this trade-off will not emerge for some years.

In an attempt to simplify medical trials, process companies often recruit patients who will only be taking that particular drug. In real life, many patients, particularly the elderly, will be taking multiple drugs. Researchers at the Yale School of Medicine reported that nearly a third of drugs approved for usage from 2001 through to 2010 had major safety issues years after the medications had been made available to patients. Drugs ushered through the US FDA's accelerated approval process were amongst those that resulted in higher rates of safety interventions.[51] The FDA approves new drugs faster than its counterparts in Europe, partly in response to governmental pressure. The FDA also often uses surrogate end points, such as tumour size, rather than survival rates.

Benoxaprofen (Opren)

One drug that slipped through the safety net of clinical trials was Benoxaprofen, marketed in the UK by a subsidiary of Eli Lilly[52] as

Opren, a new wonder drug to treat arthritis. It was a non-steroidal anti-inflammatory drug (NSAID). Other products in this class of drug include aspirin and ibuprofen. Opren had one distinctive advantage over its rivals: it remained in the patient's system longer than other drugs and was heavily promoted as a breakthrough in the treatment of arthritis. Some media reports even described it as a cure for the disease (which it was not). Unfortunately, it had some severe (but relatively rare) side effects that only emerged once the drug had become widely available. Eli Lilly had lowered the recommended dose after consultation with the regulator. The problems began to be reported in the medical press and via the Committee on the Safety of Medicine's yellow card warning system. Lord Jack Ashley described the issues in a UK parliamentary speech, asking for compensation for the victims as follows:

> *The agony, disfigurements and deaths are akin to a battlefield. They have been cynically and systematically played down by the company, yet some of them are horrific. They include rashes that blister and bleed, ulceration and haemorrhages of the stomach, bladder incontinence, liver jaundice, kidney damage, acute eye sensitivity, detached finger nails and skin photosensitivity. The company is distorting the truth. The clinical trials conducted before marketing were hopelessly inadequate, according to some experts. They were too small, conducted for too short a period, the participants were given too small a dose and there were too few older people.*[53]

Eli Lilly challenged these allegations. The drug had, after all, been licensed in both the UK and the US in 1980. In August 1982, after reports of 61 deaths and 3500 adverse events, the UK English Health Minister withdrew the drug's licence on the advice of the regulator and Eli Lilly withdrew it from the market. It never returned.

Over 1000 patients sued for damages in the UK, and Eli Lilly came to an out-of-court settlement reported to be worth £2.2 million. There was a much larger settlement in the US.

There has been much debate in the academic community about the rights and wrongs in this case.[54] Were Eli Lilly right to give Opren the benefit of the doubt after its trials, and were the regulators justified in keeping it available to patients until August 1982? Did Eli Lilly withdraw the drug too early or too late? Officials from the company, Dista (Lilly's UK subsidiary), the UK's Committee on the Safety of Medicines (CSM) and the FDA put forward several arguments for keeping Benoxaprofen on the market. They challenged the strength of the evidence from the case reports. In each case, the patients had other ailments other than rheumatoid arthritis and were taking medicines other than Opren. The case reports were unexpected because one of the key side effects — cholesteric jaundice — had not occurred in the trials. They suspected that causation might have been misattributed. Even if Opren was responsible, the number of cases reported was still quite small as a proportion of the 500,000 patients taking the drug in the UK — even comparable to the adverse event rates of other well-accepted NSAIDS such as aspirin. If such side effects were comparable in scale, then some liver damage might become accepted as the price of treatment. An Eli Lilly director argued that despite the side effects, withdrawing the drug was a worse option: 'You have to consider the case of that elderly person who has been literally crippled by the disease and finally found something that worked for her'.[55] Finally, had the side effects been blown out of all proportion by public and media hysteria? The experts disagreed. Kenneth Clarke, the minister who took the decision to suspend the licence for Opren felt that the episode was a tragedy but not a scandal.

Mediator

In December 2009, French drug regulators withdrew the licence given to the pharmaceutical company Servier to market a drug named Mediator (benfloure) because the anti-diabetic, on the market for more than 30 years, had fatal side effects. It may have been responsible for up to 1800 deaths and 4200 hospital admissions. A whistleblower had been involved in exposing the problem. A decade later, the company is to face criminal charges, as it is accused of covering up the side effects. The trial will also focus on the role of France's regulator, who allowed Mediator to remain on the market from 1996 until 2009 despite the fact that it was suspected of causing heart and pulmonary failure.

Servier will deny the charges when the trial takes place in 2020/2021 and no doubt point out that that it has already paid out €132 million in compensation and offered total compensation worth €164 million to 3732 patients.[56] An associated problem has been that the national body responsible for compensating French patients harmed by Mediator has been swamped by claims and, in the view of some observers, has been using a compensation rate that is too low. Patients have complained that the decisions it has taken are unfair and unethical.[57]

Pharmacovigilance in the EU operates through cooperation between the EU Member States, the European Medicines Agency (EMA) and the European Commission. The system is seen as being quite strong, and their database of suspected adverse drug events is an open system. Serious problems for patients should therefore emerge with reasonable speed. However, the underlying problem remains. It is possible to establish that a new drug can work but it takes very long trials to demonstrate its safety for all patients. In addition, safety nets are not of much value when people purchase medicinal products online from unlicensed providers.

Medication Errors

Medication errors are common in all healthcare systems. In England it has been reported that there are an estimated 237 million medication errors per year with 66 million of these potentially clinically significant. Some 712 errors were recently estimated to have resulted in death each year.[58] Similar rates have been recorded in other countries, although comparison is difficult as there is no internationally agreed definition of a medication error. A study by Davis and Cohen published in 1981[59] found an error rate in American hospitals of around 12%. A later study, in 2020, put the number of US deaths at between 7000 and 9000 a year.[60] The Massachusetts State Board of Registration in Pharmacy estimated that 2.4 million prescriptions were improperly filled each year in Massachusetts and 88% of these errors involved giving patients the wrong drug or the wrong strength.[61] A WHO review in 2016[62] reported wide variations in the rate of medication error reporting, including one study that suggested that the error rate in primary care in the UK (with a population of 68 million) was around 12%. The error rate in care homes in England is thought to be even higher than that. An Australian study reported that errors occur in 9% of medication administrations in hospital[63] and 2%–3% of all hospital admissions were medication related.

Irrespective of the exact number of errors, it is certain that it is far too high, affects very many patients and can and should be reduced. The economic costs of these errors are enormous. In England, definitely avoidable adverse drug reactions are estimated collectively to cost the NHS £98.5 million per year.[64] In the US, the estimated cost in 2020 was US$40 billion.

In 2017, WHO launched its third global patient safety challenge: 'medication without harm'. It highlighted that mistakes happen at every point in the medication delivery chain starting with the naming, labelling and packaging of drugs. If a drug is marketed in multiple strengths e.g. 5 mg, 10 mg, and 25 mg doses, the labels of each container should be easy to differentiate. Prescribing the right drugs for a patient is the next stage where things can go wrong, and WHO stated that decision support systems with integrated safety alerts can be helpful in this area. Making sure that the patient actually receives the correct dose of the prescribed drug is evidently essential. However, incorrect ordering accounts for almost 50% of all medication errors. In addition, the dispensation of drugs by a pharmacist, although subject to tight professional rules, still generates errors. Bar code scanning has been helpful in reducing errors in this part of the process, but in many cases medication errors are caused by distraction in busy wards, clinics and departments.

Non-prescription drugs sold directly to the public can produce side effects for some patients that increase the importance of clear patient information leaflets. Patients are well-advised to clearly understand what their medication is and to undertake their own checks. In fact, NICE (UK) reports that between a third and a half of all medicines prescribed are not taken as recommended.[65] Regular drug reviews by physicians, nurses and pharmacists are increasingly common although in some countries, such as Australia, only the patients' medical practitioner can initiate a domiciliary medication review. In England, commercial pharmacies can undertake reviews (and claim a fee) although the number they are allowed to conduct is limited.[66] This is both good practice and good business for pharmacies that can normally be relied on to provide a skilled and safe service.

Medication errors are also common in other healthcare professions that, in recent years, have been allowed to prescribe medicines. A study of prescribing nurses in Iran reported that a majority of reported errors and near misses, the most common being related to dosage.[67] However, a Cochrane Systematic Review found that, with appropriate training and support, nurses and pharmacists performed just as well as physicians.[68]

Medication errors represent a major system failure that can be radically reduced. Open and honest reporting in a no-blame culture would, in the view of many experts in the field, help immensely in lessening their prevalence.

Vaccines

WHO plays a major international role in identifying the spread of new diseases and risks. Their role in the management of pandemics is covered in Chapter Nine of this book. WHO has reported that the two public healthcare interventions that have had the greatest impact on improving the world's health are improved access to clean water and the development of effective vaccines.[69] Vaccines are extensively used to immunise people — and particularly children — against diseases and secure the benefits of herd immunity. As Bill Gates has said: 'vaccines are magic'. The WHO target is for 95% of a population to have coverage. If high rates are not sustained, protection levels against a disease fall.

> *In 1998, a study appeared in the Lancet claiming that the MMR (measles, mumps and rubella) vaccine had caused autism in 12 children. It was later condemned as a fraudulent piece of research. Andrew Wakefield, a gastroenterologist at a London hospital and his fellow authors had picked and chosen data that suited their case and falsified some of the facts. Their investigation of the children had also been undertaken without the appropriate ethical clearances. Despite the small sample size, the uncontrolled design and the speculative nature of the conclusions, the paper received widespread publicity and MMR vaccination rates began to drop as parents became increasingly concerned about the risk of autism after vaccination. The next episode in the saga was a retraction of the interpretation of the original data by 10 of the 12 authors of the paper. The Lancet completely retracted the paper in 2010. Wakefield was later struck off the medical register for serious professional misconduct.[70,71]*

After the Wakefield affair, the MMR vaccination rate in England remained below the WHO recommended level until 2017. Few countries have compulsory immunisation policies although the issue appears to be under constant review. Almost all US states require children to be immunised before entering school but there are many exemptions and enforcement is mixed. The challenge is to build and then sustain public trust in vaccination programmes.

China has recently had problems with the production of vaccines. In October 2018, Changchun Changsheng Life Sciences was fined US$1.3 billion. An inspection by the Chinese National Medical Products Administration discovered during an on-site probe that the company had mixed different batches of active vaccine ingredients, including time-expired ones, failed to conduct proper efficacy tests, fabricated production dates and destroyed original records to cover their tracks. This case lead to inspections of all other vaccine production companies in China and a review of the regulating bodies involved.[72]

Medical Equipment

Modern medicine uses a wide range of very sophisticated equipment that can sometimes go wrong. Recent problems reported by the FDA in the US have included inadequate sterilisation for orthopaedic surgery tools, ventilators with defective components, assembly errors in infant respirators, guide wires that have the potential for the coating to flake off in use, a tracheal tube that kinked, faulty pacemakers, batteries failing on life support machines and patients dying after a faulty dialysis machine pumped too much liquid into their bodies. In 2013, badly maintained wheelchairs caused injuries. In 2018, 260,000 packs of diabetes test strips were recalled because of a risk they might give false high or low readings.

The Medicines and Healthcare products Regulatory Agency in England estimated that 300 patients die and 5000 people suffer harm each year as a result of equipment failures and that number was rising.[73] In the US, the FDA has collected 5.4 million adverse event reports over a 10-year period.

Fifty-five patients at Hawke's Bay Hospital in New Zealand had to be recalled for HIV and Hepatitis tests after surgical equipment used in their operations may have been inadequately sterilised. A batch of equipment had been thoroughly cleaned, heated to a high temperature and dried, but failed to go through the final sterilisation process overnight. In this case, managers did react quickly when a nurse noticed that the colour coding on a surgical tools pack was wrong.[74]

The Institute of Mechanical Engineers in London recommends that every large hospital has its own Chief Biomedical Engineer to ensure that quality standards are high.

Medical Devices

All medical devices need approval before they can be marketed, but still, they have a mixed safety record. In England at least 400 people die or are seriously injured in adverse events involving medical devices each year.[75] Some problems relate to design and others to manufacturing standards.[76]

> *Theranos was a medical device company that produced a product called 'Edison', a blood test device that claimed to be able to test for hundreds of things by taking only a small amount of blood. The technology it used was never peer reviewed and when tested by the Cleveland Clinic was found to produce erroneous results about 1.6 times more than other tests. The FDA licence for the device was revoked, and the company was closed. The owner was fined.*[77]

> *GE Healthcare recalled a number of infant resuscitators in 2014 after discovering a serious error in the assembly process. The FDA said 'these recalled products may interfere with oxygen delivery resulting in inaccurate oxygen regulation in neonates and may lead to low blood oxygen (hypoxia) or high blood oxygen (hyperoxia)'.*[78]

Joint replacements

Joint replacements are now commonplace in most developed countries, but the procedure carries risks which patients rarely appreciate.

In fact, according to Deborah Cohen, investigations editor of the *BMJ*,[79] hundreds of thousands of patients around the world may have been exposed to toxic substances after being implanted with poorly regulated and potentially dangerous hip devices. This problem relates to metal-on-metal implants (MoMs). The head of the implant and the lining of the cup that it fits into are made of a cobalt–chromium alloy rather than ceramic or polypropylene. MoMs first arrived on the orthopaedic scene in 1997 when they were marketed as the most advanced hip replacements and targeted at young active patients who needed a hip to last a lifetime. However, average failure rates at seven years were much higher than implants made from other materials. They were also thought to release metal ions that can seep into local tissue causing reactions that destroy muscle and bone and leave patients with long-term disability. They can also leech into the blood stream, spreading to the lymph nodes, spleen, liver and kidneys before being excreted with urine. There were also warnings raised about their carcinogenic potential although the link to cancer has not been proven.

The first serious alarms were raised in 2006 but resulted in no significant action by the regulatory bodies. Further studies followed showing generated metal debris between the stem taper and head. In 2011, the British Orthopaedic Association advised that large-diameter MoM total hip replacements should be 'carefully considered and possibly avoided'. In the same year, the National Hip Register in the UK also reported its concern about higher-than-expected revision rates. There were fewer reported problems with the metal components of hip resurfacing. In the US, the FDA demanded long-term surveillance. Johnson & Johnson pulled their DuPuy MoM model from the market in 2010.

A UK medical device alert in 2017 warned that 'whilst the majority of patients with MoM hip replacements have well-functioning hips some patients will develop progressive soft tissue problems due to wear debris'. Regular check-ups were recommended. Similar advice had been given in Canada and Australia. By 2020, the MoM hips had been radically redesigned but were rarely used.

This is an example of industry and regulators responding to clinical data as it became available. But some critics have complained that regulators should have acted far more quickly. Nick Freemantle, Professor of Clinical Epidemiology and Biostatistics at University College London, went much further: 'If it were the pharmaceutical industry developing a new chemical entity, it would be abandoned early on if it metabolised in the wrong bits of the liver. We would not be in this position where we do not know and there is so much uncertainty. The stability of a compound should have been ascertained before it was widely used in people. As yet we do not know the consequences of this'.[80]

Registers of orthopaedic implants are now commonplace. The National Joint Registry for England, Wales, Northern Ireland and the Isle of Man reported in 2017[81] that the revision rate for hip replacements at 14 years had reduced to 2%. Patients are now being offered risk calculators as part of a shared decision-making process.

Vaginal mesh

Another device implant problem has arisen with vaginal mesh, used as a treatment for urinary incontinence or organ prolapse. As women began to complain of problems, the FDA began to express its concerns and demanded new studies because it was 'concerned about potential safety risks'. In 2019, one of the largest US manufacturers, C.R. Bard, withdrew its Avaulta mesh from US markets and ended the production of mesh implants altogether. They had been fighting lawsuits for years and claimed that the decision to withdraw from the market was a commercial rather than a safety issue. At or around the same time, 90% of mesh manufacturers discontinued their products in the US or changed the products' indication for use.[82] Australia and New Zealand banned mesh devices in 2017. In England, the use of vaginal mesh implants was paused until investigations by NICE had been concluded. The Royal College of Obstetricians and Gynaecologists recommended that only specialist surgeons should undertake vaginal mesh operations.

The *Lancet* commented that whilst for some women vaginal mesh surgery would still be the best option, the risk of complications must be documented and communicated clearly to patients. The evidence (about potential harm) should have been energetically accumulated before vaginal mesh surgery became so irresponsibly fashionable.[83]

SPG Law, a unique law firm whose mission is to achieve justice for complainants around the world, put it rather more starkly: 'Mesh manufacturers failed to properly research, design and test their products and then sold these unreasonably dangerous devices without adequately warning women and the medical community about the risk of vaginal mesh failure'.

Linda Gross and the US$11 million verdict

Johnson & Johnson lost the first bellwether trial involving its transvaginal mesh implants. In February 2013, a New Jersey jury returned a US$11 million verdict against Ethicon for injuries caused by its Gynecare Prolift. Linda Gross claimed that she required 18 revision surgeries after receiving the mesh implant. She said she could not sit comfortably and had to take pain medication after her device caused complications. The jury agreed that Johnson & Johnson had failed to warn of the risks associated with the device and that it made fraudulent representations about the product. Gross was awarded US$3.35 million in compensation and US$7.76 million in punitive damages.[84] Johnson & Johnson appealed this decision but lost in 2016.

So, what happened?

'Nobody involved in the mesh revolution emerges covered in glory — not the companies who aggressively hustled the products into widespread use, not the regulators who aided and abetted them on the flimsiest of evidence, and not the medical profession, which failed to ensure surgeons were properly trained or that patients were carefully selected and properly informed of the risks and perhaps most importantly, failed to set up comprehensive registries for the new procedures that might have identified unforeseen complications far sooner'.[85] One startling number is that over a 10-year period, nearly 500,000 patients across the world had explants.[86]

Despite all these problems, there are still very few national medical device registers, although pressure to create them is growing.

Radiotherapy

Radiotherapy is now a standard clinical option for treating cancer and other diseases, but if the machines are not properly calibrated, they can cause harm to patients. A hospital in Philadelphia gave the wrong radiation dose to more than 90 patients with prostate cancer and then kept quiet about it.[87] In 2005, a Florida hospital disclosed that 77 patients with brain cancer had received 50% more radiation than prescribed because one of the most powerful and supposedly precise linear accelerators had been incorrectly programmed for a year. Dr. J. Feldmeier, a radiation oncologist from Toledo in the US estimates that 1 in 20 patients suffer unintended injuries from radiation treatment. Most are normal complications from radiation rather than mistakes, but in many cases, the dividing line between the two is uncertain.[88]

> *As Scott Jerome-Parks lay dying he clung to this wish; that his fatal radiation overdose, which left him deaf, struggling to see, unable to swallow, burned, with his teeth falling out, nauseated, in severe pain and finally unable to breath be talked about so that others might not live his nightmare. A New York City hospital, treating him for tongue cancer failed to detect a computer error that directed a linear accelerator to blast his brain cell and neck with an errant beam off radiation. Not once but on three consecutive days, He died aged 43.[89]*

In Canada, a machine named Therac-25 experienced at least six accidents in the 1980s, and patients were given massive radiation overdoses. Inadequate software was largely to blame.[90]

> *In Stoke-on-Trent in England, over a 10-year period, more than 1000 patients received a dosage less than that prescribed (perhaps up to 35% less). This could have led to dozens of deaths and innumerable patient recalls. The problem caused by a mistake by a physicist causing an underdosage. An unnecessary correction factor was programmed into the radiotherapy computer in 1982 on her instructions. What the physicist did not realise was that the manufacturer had already written the correction factor into the software when the machine was delivered. The mistake was only spotted in 1991.[91]*

> *In Zaragoza, Spain, 27 patients were overexposed for 10 days in 1990 whilst being treated for tumours. Three months later 18 of the patients had died. The fault was identified as being due to poor maintenance, calibration problems and procedural violations.[92]*

A WHO report showed that between the years 1976 and 2007, 3125 patients were affected by radiotherapy incidents that led to adverse events. About 1% of the patients affected died of radiation overdose toxicity.[93] Misinformation or errors in data transfer constitute the largest percentage of incidents in modern radiotherapy services. New adaptive therapy which uses artificial intelligence to deliver personalised cancer care will be important in addressing these long standing issues. A patient undergoing treatment can expect patient setup, imaging, treatment planning, and dose delivery to occur within a 15-minute treatment session. This will, however, add new complexity to treatment programmes.

Nobody knows for sure how well the ancient linear accelerators still in use in developing countries are performing. We do know that 20% of the machines in the US were not listed in the database for the largest study with either the Radiological Physics Centre or the Radiation Dosimetry Services and therefore may not have an external source of dosimetry monitoring.[94] These machines need regular maintenance and should be replaced every 10 years or so. In 2016, more than 50% of the machines in use in England were found to be outdated, which led to a major reinvestment programme.[95] The question is how did this happen in a modern healthcare system and why did nobody blow the whistle? We may never discover whether any patients suffered serious harm as a result.

'Hospitals have become too trusting of new technologies and their integral computer systems', said Dr. H. Amols, Chief of Clinical Physics at Memorial Sloan Kettering in New York.[96]

Hospitals are now under pressure to employ biomedical engineers to maintain and conduct safety checks of the increasingly sophisticated equipment now in use. The same might be true of primary care, where an incorrect result from a blood pressure machine could be a danger to patients. In most countries, hospitals do receive hazard warnings when problems have been identified but reaction times vary enormously. This is clearly another item that should be added to patient safety checklists.

Maternity

The vast majority of pregnancies in developed countries are successful. The risk of clinical error is low. Maternal mortality has declined sharply in the past five decades. Italy and Poland have the lowest rates in Europe with only 2 fatalities per 100,000 births in 2017. Using the same measure, the UK had 7, Australia 6, France 8, Canada 12 and the US 19. Stillbirths and infant and neonatal mortality have also fallen sharply but there remains significant variation between countries. Japan, Sweden and Finland have the lowest global rates, while developing countries generally have relatively high occurrences of mortality. These disparities can be extremely stark. For example, a woman in Nigeria is more than 200 times more likely to die in pregnancy or childbirth than a woman in Sweden.[97] The UK compares poorly with the rest of Europe. In the three years from 2015 to 2017, 209 women died during or up to six weeks after giving birth. The principal cause of death was heart disease. Black women were five times more likely to die as a result of complications in their pregnancy than white women.[98] In 2016, 3000 infants died before their first birthday and there were over 2000 neonatal deaths and 3430 stillbirths.[99] There is a long-term plan in England to reduce the number of stillborn and neonatal deaths by 50% but it will need determined action and a major investment if this target is to be achieved.[100] The President of the Royal College of Obstetricians and Gynaecology points out that whilst the risks are small, 'one in every hundred births is problematic'. This is consistent with the results of a national outcome review programme which reported in 2019 that 1% of UK births led to a stillborn or newborn death.[101]

The US also now has a comparatively high maternal death rate of 17.4 per 100,000 births,[102] a sharp increase from 2000 that makes the US an outlier amongst developed countries — moving in the opposite direction to international trends. In 2018, 658 women died of maternal causes in the US. The maternal death rate for black women was more than double that of white women.

> *Jasmine E. Gant, an honour student and promising athlete entered St. Mary's Medical Center in Wisconsin in 2006, in labour. A nurse mistakenly gave her a dose of epidural medication in an intravenous line instead of the intended penicillin that had been prescribed to treat a strep infection in labour. The epidural medication caused cardiac arrest and Jasmine died within a few hours. Her baby son survived.*[103]

The CDC only started collecting data on maternal deaths in 1986 — a huge contrast with the UK who have had a Confidential Inquiry into Maternal and Child Health in operation since 1952.[104] There is also some doubt about the quality of the US data which is derived from State returns.

The explanation for the high rates prevalent in some countries is complex but two recent inquiries in England have pointed to insufficient staffing levels and poor interpersonal relationships amongst professional staff as two of the key causes.

Furness Hospital, Cumbria, England

An inquiry[105] into the maternity services at Furness Hospital in Morecombe in the northwest of England found that clinical competence was substandard, with deficient skills and knowledge; extremely poor working relationships between staff groups such as obstetricians, paediatricians and midwives; and efforts by overzealous midwives to pursue normal childbirth at any cost. Failures of risk assessment and care planning were identified that resulted in inappropriate and unsafe care. The response to adverse events was grossly deficient, with repeated failures to properly investigate and learn lessons. This lethal mix led to the unnecessary deaths of mothers and babies.

The first signs that there were problems at the maternity unit in Furness General Hospital appeared in 2004 when a baby died from the effects of a lack of oxygen due to a mismanaged labour. The investigation that followed was, in the view of the later Kirkup Inquiry, rudimentary, overprotective of the staff and failed to identify the underlying problems. Between 2006 and 2007 five more serious incidents occurred and provided more evidence of continuing problems, but little happened. The staff were in denial and the management team had other priorities. Five more cases emerged in 2008: a baby was damaged by the effects of a shortage of oxygen in labour; a mother died following untreated high blood pressure; a mother and baby died from an amniotic fluid embolism; and a baby died from an unrecognised infection. This time alarm bells did ring, and an inquiry was launched. When it reported, in 2010, it contained significant criticisms of the maternity unit including dysfunctional professional relationships, a poor working environment and a sub-standard approach to clinical governance. A small group of overzealous midwives, characterised as 'the musketeers', rejected much of the criticism. However, some of the parents continued their battle against the hospital and a 2008 Coroner's Inquest into the death of baby Joshua Titcombe returned a verdict critical of the hospital. He had died from sepsis, caught from his mother in her womb. A simple jab of antibiotics might have saved his life. In September 2011, Cumbria Police launched their own investigation into the deaths at Furness General Hospital but no prosecutions resulted.

The relatives of the affected mothers and babies were still not satisfied and their pressure and lobbying led to what was to become the final inquiry, led by Dr. Bill Kirkup. This time the inquiry got to the truth.

As a result of the Kirkup Inquiry, the most senior of the midwives secured a redundancy package, two others were dismissed, and a number of doctors and nurses were given written warnings about their future conduct by their regulatory bodies. The Nurses and Midwives regulatory body was heavily criticised for the delays in considering the conduct of the midwives involved and subsequently made major changes to its procedures.

Shrewsbury Hospital, England

An even greater maternity scandal was emerging in Shrewsbury, a market town close to the Welsh border, as an inquiry started to review 900 cases, some going back 40 years, after a series of tragedies including stillbirths, deaths of babies shortly after delivery, and the deaths of mothers and babies that had suffered brain damage after being starved of oxygen. It was, said one commentator, the largest maternity scandal in the history of the NHS.

An independent review led by Donna Ockenden, a senior midwife, was launched in 2017 after the local coroner and several bereaved families had raised concerns about the number of apparently avoidable baby deaths. The NHS Trust has been in special measures ever since amid reports of a toxic culture and professional tensions.

Many legal claims are anticipated once the final report is published. Criminal charges may follow. A number of maternity negligence cases are further described in Chapter Five of this book.

Regulation and policy

The tension between obstetricians and independent midwives in the maternity sector is well-documented, but in 2016, the Nursing and Midwifery Council (NMC) escalated the issue when it ruled that the professional indemnity of independent midwives, who are self-employed, was inadequate. This effectively restricted their practice to antenatal and postnatal care. They appealed to the High Court but lost. The NMC had not acted unfairly or illegally. The indemnity problem was finally resolved in 2018 and independent midwives returned to practice.

Healthcare policy about safe obstetric practice in England and other countries has shifted over years from the original position of arguing that a hospital was the safest place to deliver babies to a new viewpoint that recognised home deliveries as being perfectly safe for a normal birth. The final choice should therefore be left to the mother. In 2007, the Department of Health strongly endorsed midwife-led care and went as far as encouraging women to bypass their GP and self-refer themselves to midwives. Despite this, only 2% of UK births take place at home — marginally higher than most developed countries with the exception of Netherlands (although their home delivery numbers have now started to decline). A study of all serious English birthing incidents where children or mothers ended up injured found that the three most common reasons were: a delay following a call for assistance, a heavy workload and senior staff not available.[106]

There is still an unresolved argument amongst experts about the safety of home deliveries as compared to those that take place in a hospital setting. Establishing midwifery-led units next to major maternity units seems a sensible compromise for the future.

The Australian case below adds clinical competence to the list of problems experienced by patients in maternity wards.

There were significant failings in the obstetric care provided to three babies who died soon after being born at a rural hospital in Victoria in 2013. Each child was their parent's first. The deaths happened at the Bacchus Marsh and Melton Regional Hospital 50 kilometres northwest of the State capital of Melbourne but were only reported to the coroner in 2015 after a cluster of stillbirths and newborn deaths at the hospital were identified. An external investigator found seven deaths between 2013 and 2014 that could have been avoided. The Coroner described the handling of the three cases as 'sub-optimal' with the misinterpretation of the CTG, or foetal heart monitoring system, a feature common to each. All three babies required resuscitation after birth, but none had access to a paediatrician. A midwife who was linked to all three deaths was later struck off after admitting that she had failed to carry out appropriate clinical assessment and care and had inadequately interpreted the CTG scans. She also admitted failing to recognise and respond to an urgent situation.

A number of her colleagues also faced disciplinary action resulting in seven cautions, six practitioners having conditions placed on their licence to practise by the State licensing authority and five given interim restriction orders whilst further investigations continued.[107] In total the conduct of 40 professionals was investigated. The Director of Obstetrics first had conditions placed on his licence, retired a month later but was still struck off. The entire Djerriwarrh Hospital Board was sacked by the Health minister who said: 'this is one of the greatest clinical failures that we have ever seen in the Victorian health system'.[108]

This case led to a major review of patient safety in Victoria: 'Targeting zero: The review of hospital safety and quality assurance'. The new target was that no one should be harmed, with rigorous oversight and a new health information agency formed to analyse and share information across the system.[109]

The extent to which GPs remain involved in maternity care has been shifting around the world. In New Zealand, Australia and the US, they remain part of the picture, particularly in rural areas, but in the UK their role is now much more limited, and they almost never get involved in intrapartum care. Most of the local maternity units where GPs previously delivered babies have closed or been turned into midwife-led units.[110]

Caesarean sections

Concern has recently been growing about the increasing number of women who may be putting themselves at risk with unnecessary cae-sarean sections (C-sections) 'that have virtually nothing to do with evidence-based medicine'.[111]

Research published in the *Lancet*[112] showed that by 2015 the rate had almost doubled since 2000 to 21% of all births. It is only an appropriate clinical procedure in 10%–15% of deliveries. More than half of the deliveries in Brazil, Egypt and Turkey are now done via C-section.

C-sections are often marketed as an easy and convenient way to give birth and there are sometimes financial incentives for both the doctor and hospital to recommend them. Doctors are sometimes tempted to organise C-sections to ease the flow of patients through a maternity unit and medical professionals are thought to be less vul-nerable to legal action if they opt for an operation over a normal birth.

Improving maternity care

There is much evidence of plans to improve maternity care, but they will achieve little unless maternity services are better resourced and professional teamwork is re-established. If women are to be given a choice, it must be an informed choice and not one pressed on them by a doctor or midwife with a professional interest. All data about maternity care should be open to women and their families. Confidential inquiries need to get better at opening up their anonymised data banks. Triennial reports are also not good enough — shorter time frames to assess the state of care are needed. Good outcomes for a mother and her baby are also dependent on more than simply having skilled staff. Poverty, housing, environment and nutrition also play a significant role.

One unexpected consequence of the maternity scandals in England was the decision that from 2018 the Healthcare Safety Investigation Branch (HSIB) would investigate all reported maternity adverse events in England. The HSIB replaced local investigations although NHS Trusts are still responsible for exercising their duty of candour and for referring incidents to the national branch. This represents a major ramping up of the investigation of reported adverse events.

Centralisation of Specialist Services

There is good evidence that centralised specialist centres have better clinical outcomes than local hospitals, yet the move to create such centres has proven difficult in many developed countries. The case for focussing on volume and case variety in larger centres in order to preserve specialist expertise is now well-established, although some well-staffed smaller units can buck the trend. The evidence varies between specialties.[113] One study suggested that 453 children's deaths a year could be avoided in the UK if all paediatric patients requiring mechanical ventilation for more than 12–24 hours were transferred to specialist paediatric intensive care units.[114] A retrospective study of 20,000 non-surgical mechanically ventilated patients, reported by the same author, found that both ICU and in-patient mortality was significantly reduced in hospitals with a median of 600 inpatient beds compared to those with half that figure.

The arguments for centralisation are particularly strong in the field of cancer with a number of studies showing that hospitals with gynaecological oncologists on site can prolong the life of women with ovarian cancer.

Thousands of lives are potentially at stake as political arguments continue both between local politicians and within professional communities about planned change. Professional self-interest and political opportunism are both evident in some of these discussions.

Opponents of centralisation stress the importance of strong and viable local hospitals, particularly in rural areas. Many rural patients, they assert, would prefer to have their surgery with trusted physicians close to home, work, families and friends. They trust their local physicians to refer them onto a specialist centre if they judge a better outcome could be achieved. Responsible doctors do exactly that, but we have also seen examples in Chapter One of this book of overconfident physicians and surgeons who do not do this. Some local hospital managers also argue that their financial viability is dependent on providing as wide a range of care as possible to be able to recruit and retain doctors and nurses who need the stimulus of more complex treatment modalities. Studies from Australia suggest that patients are prepared to accept the increased risk of surgical mortality at their local hospital.[115]

A UK study in 2019 produced a rather different result. Whilst preferring local services and reduced travel time, people were willing to trade this off for high-quality emergency care in a centralised hospital.[116] The transport of critically ill patients to regional centres, whilst having a recognised risk, does not negate the other potential benefits.

New Zealand has taken the view that some of its hospitals will have to become more specialised in order to keep up with rapidly changing technologies, which allow for more sophisticated treatments. This creates a more limited but nevertheless important role for other hospitals and clinics to provide more routine care for their local communities. As a small country, New Zealand can only support a limited number of highly specialised tertiary hospitals because of the critical number of cases needed to provide sufficient volumes for sophisticated treatment and build up the necessary clinical experience and expertise. Large catchment areas are needed to attract staff in sufficient numbers and allow large teams to develop — an essential requirement for high-tech, and sometimes, high-risk procedures.[117]

Some case studies follow which illuminate the controversy and the evidence, both for and against.

Strokes are a leading cause of mortality and disability worldwide. Each year, an estimated 125,000 people in England have a stroke, of which 40,000 die. In 2010, acute stroke services in London were centralised. Before the changes, 30 hospitals provided acute stroke care. After the changes, specialist stroke care was provided in eight designated hyper acute stroke units around the clock. Patients were immediately assessed by specialist stroke doctors with access to immediate brain imaging and, when appropriate, thrombolysis. A total of 24 units were designated to provide stroke rehabilitation services and eight of these were attached to the hyper acute units. Five hospitals stopped providing care for stroke patients altogether. The results have been a reduction in both mortality (an estimated 400 lives saved in 3 years) and the length of hospital stays.[118]

In Denmark, the number of acute hospitals was reduced from 40 to 21 after a reform programme that started in 2007. The changes were driven by international evidence that hospitals with a small volume of surgical patients were not able to provide treatment of a high quality due to limited surgical experience. Treatment at a highly specialised level (e.g. surgery for lung cancer, heart surgery, transplants or the treatment of serious burns) is only performed at a small number of locations in the country. Urgent and emergency care is also only provided by a limited number of hospitals.[119]

In the United States 'hub and spoke' models have become popular as they offer the prospect of higher quality and lower costs. The Willis-Knighton health system, based in Louisiana, operates five hospital campuses with a total of 1290 beds and one retirement community. One hospital serves as the hub for four satellites. Medical staff work right across the system. Complex medical services, especially those that are technology and skills intensive, are centralised at the main campus or hub. The hub campus includes centres such as the Heart and Vascular Institute, the Spine Institute as well as Cancer, Transplantation and Eye Centres. The Willis-Knighton system provides services to communities living in three States. It operates on a not for profit model.[120]

In situations where geographical distance makes satellite to hub access impractical, an additional hub can be created to produce a multi-hub network.

Whilst these models have great potential to improve quality, consistency, efficiency and organisational agility, they have risks. These include congestion at the hubs, overextended satellites and staff dissatisfaction at the spokes, all of which are, with good leadership, manageable.

> *In Italy, the hub-and-spoke model of specialist service delivery is characterised by close links between regional referring hospitals and specialist centres and is exemplified by percutaneous coronary intervention networks. The introduction of such a network for cardiac surgery had a very positive effect on patient outcomes, with a 22% reduction in hospital mortality rates.*[121]

Hub-and-spoke models have also been deployed in India to provide modern healthcare services in rural settings.[122]

Paediatric cardiac surgery

Paediatric cardiac surgery has been a controversial issue in England for some years. The problems started in Bristol, where concerns about the apparently high mortality rate led to a major public inquiry.

The inquiry found that between 30 and 35 babies had died between 1990 and 1995 and, over that whole decade, up to 170 infants might have been saved if they had been operated on elsewhere. Sir Ian Kennedy, who led the Inquiry, found that there were staff shortages, a lack of leadership in the cardiac unit and that the unit was simply 'not up to scratch'. He also pointed to an old boys' culture amongst the doctors, a lax approach to safety, secrecy about doctors' performance and a lack of monitoring by management. John Roylance, the Chief Executive at the hospital (a radiologist by background) said he had no powers to intervene in the way that his surgeons were working. There was a mindset of 'professional hubris' that, as a teaching hospital, Bristol had to be at the leading edge and must always be right. Clinicians were actively collecting and discussing data but were quick to deny any adverse inferences that could be drawn from it. Roylance, however, had chosen to ignore warnings from a whistleblower (an anaesthetist). He was struck off of the medical register along with one of the cardiac surgeons.[123] What was needed, Kennedy argued, was a new culture of openness, a non-punitive system for reporting serious incidents and the end of clinical negligence litigation.

Many changes were to follow, including the publication of clinical results, but the key recommendation, that the number of specialist centres in England be reduced, was to take another 20 years to implement.

As this first review into paediatric cardiac surgery was underway, reports emerged that managers were trying to increase the number of children being treated at the John Radcliffe Hospital in Oxford in order to avoid the possibility of closure (at that time it was the smallest in the country).[124] The hospital had recruited an additional (but relatively junior) surgeon but four babies died after they had been operated on. The surgeon complained about the age of the equipment and poor working practices and asked to be relieved of his operating schedules. His concerns were ignored until a regulator got involved.

Across the country, arguments raged about the centralisation of paediatric cardiac services. At this point there were 13 units, 11 of which had only two surgeons. Almost everybody agreed that the number of centres had to be reduced but there was no agreement about which units should be merged or closed.[125] Was it clinical results or geography that should influence the decision? Ideally, units should be treating 400 children a year. Sir Bruce Keogh, the Medical Director of the NHS, himself a cardiac surgeon, expressed his frustration: 'It will be a stain on the soul of the profession if this is not resolved'.[126] A review in 2013 proposed to reduce the number of centres from 11 to 8 but was halted by ministers after a judicial review and protests by a number of hospitals and their patient support groups, who claimed that the analysis upon which the recommendations had been made was flawed. The matter was referred for further review and ended back with NHS England.

A former president of the Society for Cardiac Surgery put the problem in a nutshell: 'Can we really expect politicians to make difficult decisions which will lose them votes? Clinicians need to provide leadership in the drive to provide the best service for patients'.[127]

Three years later, three units were told to stop complex treatments unless they could meet the minimum safety standard of four surgeons working as a team treating a minimum of 125 patients a year. Medical staffing constraints were now driving change rather than clinical outcomes. However, this recommendation was consistent with international opinion.[128]

Survival rates are now openly available to the public but instead of directly comparing hospitals with each other, a hospital's survival rate is compared with what was predicted, taking into account how severe their cases were. The latest data available, for 2015–2018, shows that the 10 remaining units in England treated 10,694 children and recorded 165 deaths — a survival rate of over 98%.[129] All units were within or better than their predicted range.

Sweden, with a population of 9 million, reduced the number of centres undertaking paediatric surgery from 4 to 2 in 1993 after a long and difficult process and saw a sharp reduction in deaths[130] — from 9.5% to 1.9% — following open heart surgery.

Australia has also been through a difficult time trying to improve children's cardiac services, as the following case study shows.

The Children's Hospital Network in Sydney was created in 2011 through the merger of the city's two major children's hospitals: the Sydney Children's Hospital at Randwick and the Children's Hospital at Westmead. Some had hoped for an entirely new hospital but the decision was made to merge the management of the two hospitals, which are about 35 miles apart. Westmead is the larger and longer established of the two whilst Randwick is seen as the upstart vying for equal status. In summer 2019, the medical staff at Randwick complained that all paediatric cardiac surgery referrals were being sent to Westmead and, as a result, the accreditation of its intensive care unit had been downgraded as staff were not getting enough exposure to cardiac patients. The loss of paediatric cardiac surgery was also having a knock-on effect across all children's specialities and, they argued, could lead to the eventual downgrading of the whole hospital. The issue became so inflamed that one Randwick surgeon told the media that: 'the minister will have blood on his hands if a child dies'. A majority of senior doctors at Randwick threatened to resign over the issue. Westmead, they claimed was 'acting like a cartel to grow its empire'.

An independent review of the network in early 2019[131] *reported that the tensions between the two hospitals were the result of poor change management and resourcing when the merger took place. The Board was criticised for poor oversight as the rivalry continued under their management. In January 2020, after yet another review of cardiac services, ministers decided that surgery should continue at both sites and Randwick would get a new paediatric cardiology catheterisation laboratory. The cardiac surgeons at Westmead complained that the independent report was biased and the decision was political and not based on expert evidence. They repeated their argument that better clinical results would be achieved on one site despite the fact that their service was 'bursting at the seams'. They claimed that a two-site solution would result in three more deaths a year. One of their leading surgeons resigned and moved to a post in the US. However, the Health Authority said that their decision was final and would not be changed. The arguments continue. The most obvious solution is to introduce a more integrated way of working, perhaps with Westmead handling the most complex cases, but this will depend on the creation of greatly improved professional relationships.*[132]

Publish or be Damned

In recent years there has been an increasing international trend of publishing clinical outcome data in an anonymised form, including alarms and alerts when results fall outside expected boundaries. Cardiac surgery was an early topic for such an approach and over the years other specialties have followed suit. For example, the published data on joint replacements is very detailed. Most people judge this new trend to be a healthy state of affairs and of great assistance to those seeking ways to improve outcomes. However, others disagree, arguing that clinical audit is much stronger when conducted on a confidential basis.

In Leicester, England, the smear test history of 403 women who had developed cervical cancer between January 1993 and September 2000 was examined in a retrospective audit. The aims of the audit were to ascertain whether diagnosis could potentially been made sooner and to identify improvements that could be made to the screening service. About 80% of the women in the study had received a smear test prior to diagnosis and so their tests were re-examined. It transpired that 84 women had received a false negative and, in 38 other cases, the cytological abnormality had been undergraded. The consequences of these misinterpretations were extremely serious: 20 women had subsequently died, with diagnostic delay being an important factor in 14 of the deaths.

The managers of the service were informed about these results before any peer-reviewed papers were published. They informed the Department of Health. A minister then insisted that the data be released to the press and the women or their bereaved relatives be informed. The media demanded to know who was to blame and who had been disciplined. Some commentators thought that in this case the principle of confidentiality in clinical audit had been breached, exposed the NHS to litigation and adversely affected the confidence of the public in the value of screening programmes.[133]

Another case centred on the media reaction to early alerts of potential problems.

The Society for Cardiothoracic Surgery informed St. George's Hospital in London that analysis of its results in both 2017 and 2018 showed that early survival after cardiac surgery was lower than the expected level. The results were however still within the UK's accepted standard. The media had a field day and an independent report was commissioned. The inquiry report[134] *confirmed that the results were within acceptable limits but identified a toxic relationship amongst the consultants that was causing problems.*

A number of principles are in play in both of these cases. First, anonymised results with worrying conclusions should be reported to Managing Boards and published only after being checked and accompanied by an explanation and, if appropriate, an action plan to correct course. If patients can be identified, they, or their relatives, have a right to be informed under a Duty of Candour, if one exists.

Maintaining public confidence in screening programmes is a very real issue, as is admitting the fact that all programmes have a small in-built error rate. A false-negative smear result is, of course, a problem, but not necessarily evidence of negligence. The aim must be to reduce this error rate to an absolute minimum.

But should such alerts trigger a massive and critical media response? In the St. George's case, this was actually a second alarm and the toxic culture might not have emerged without the media scrutiny. There should be swift reactions by healthcare authorities to alerts with either a cogent explanation or the immediate implementation of corrective action.

Cancer Services

Cancer services have been through much the same sort of debate as cardiac treatment with regard to centralisation but perhaps with rather less passion. The clinical arguments are the same: larger, better-staffed units working in extended clinical networks generally get better results. For some types of cancer, the evidence for this is strong but for others, it is rather weak. A Cochrane study in 2012 found strong evidence to support the centralisation of services for ovarian cancer but less evidence for other gynaecological cancers.[135]

In 2020, Children's Cancer Services hit the headlines in England with an issue that was remarkably similar to the Sydney case study.

In January 2020, NHS England reviewed Children's Cancer Services in London and, in particular, the services provided by the Royal Marsden Hospital, a hospital with an international reputation for cancer care, on its two sites at Chelsea and Sutton some 40 minutes apart. The Sutton hospital did not have a paediatric intensive care unit. In one year, 22 children had been transferred to other hospitals for intensive care. Both sites had high-quality inspection scores and an international research profile. More than 330 sick children had been transferred from the Marsden to other intensive care units in London between 2000 and 2015. A series of incidents and deaths in 2009 and 2011 had triggered a number of inquiries and led to a recommendation in a report published in 2015 that London should create one specialist treatment centre. The current situation was deemed to be thoroughly unsatisfactory. However, the report was not made public, which led to allegations of a cover up. A former NHS Medical Director accused the hospital of burying concerns that had been raised.[136] *There were essentially three ways forward and two of these did not include the Royal Marsden at all. The professional advice was very clear: any major treatment centre should either have an intensive care unit on site or close by.*

To complicate matters, the Chief Executive of the Marsden had become the National Cancer Director. She properly declared an interest and recused herself from any decisions about the future of children's services.

One Board Director questioned whether a major, expensive and highly disruptive reconfiguration be justified to avoid a risk to 7–15 patients a year. Option appraisals were commissioned, which will no doubt lead to a further fractious public and professional debate during 2020.[137]

Wales has also had issues with the centralisation of specialist surgical services, which led the Royal College of Surgeons telling a minister: 'There is a clear need for the reconfiguration of services in Wales based on clinical need, particularly to address the sustainability of the current pattern of acute hospitals. This need is well recognised by the Welsh government. However, progress on service changes has been too slow, often hindered by a lack of local will and politicians campaigning against clinically necessary service changes. Political leaders need to spend as much time engaging with the clinical case for change as listening to public concerns'.[138]

The unspoken truth is that local politicians are often listening to local doctors who also want to protect local services.

These case studies tell us that securing patient safety is never easy and often means challenging powerful political, professional and commercial forces. In most cases, clear signals about problems are either ignored or missed. There are now many studies of safety risks and a growing number of reports about risk reduction. How to effectively build a safety culture is discussed in Chapter Nine of this book.

'Never' or Sentinel Events

There are some areas of healthcare that produce immediate learning opportunities and one of the most obvious of these is when 'Never' events occur. As the name implies, these adverse events should never happen if all the proper procedures and protocols are properly followed. For example, healthcare professionals should never transfuse a patient with the wrong blood, never operate on the wrong limb or have to return a patient to surgery to remove a missing instrument or swab. Yet these events do happen. There were at least 38 Never events in England in the financial year beginning April 2016. They included giving a pain-relieving injection to the wrong hip joint, the amputation of the wrong finger, an arthroscopy started on the wrong knee, a stent being placed on the wrong ureter and the wrong size hip being implanted. There were also a number of foreign bodies left in patients, including vaginal swabs, guide wires, plastic drain caps and a stainless-steel spring from a suction device. All of these cases were reported as Never events and subsequently investigated. The policy of fining organisations that reported such events was removed in England in 2019. Three of the cases are set out in more detail below.[139]

A patient attending for a follow-up after a cataract operation was asked to sit in a waiting area — shared by patients waiting for laser surgery — to undergo an OCT test to one eye.[140] The surgeon had a set of notes for a patient with the same first name who required surgery on the other eye and called for that patient (using the Christian name). The patient that required an OCT (not surgery) followed him. The surgeon explained the laser surgery and despite the patient telling him it was the wrong eye, it was performed. The later review reported that the surgeon did not properly check the patient's identity before the surgery, patient consent processes had not worked and the operating schedule was too tight allowing little time for the surgeon to carry out checks with the patient.

A patient was admitted for surgery on the left leg. The leg was marked with an arrow by the surgeon on the ward prior to the operation and the patient then seen by the anaesthetist. A trainee and the Operating Department Practitioner (OPD) completed the 'sign in'. The Consultant Anaesthetist then arrived and administered a general anaesthetic. The OPD and trainee left the room to collect other equipment and drugs. Working alone, the consultant then prepared the wrong leg for a nerve block and administered it. Luckily, the consultant realised his mistake and the patient was not harmed. The later review explained that the consultant had not checked which leg should be operated on prior to administering the block nor had he followed the failsafe 'stop before you block' convention, which had not been fully embedded into routine clinical practice.

A patient underwent an emergency laparotomy. During use, a stainless-steel suction device came apart. The surgeon reassembled the device and continued to use it, without the scrub practitioner being aware of this. The Central Sterile Department later informed the scrub practitioner that a spring was missing from the device. After a thorough search without success an X-ray was ordered. The spring was found in the abdominal cavity of the patient and later removed. The operating team might have spotted the problem had they all been fully engaged.

There are reports of similar incidents in other countries, sometimes called 'sentinel events', meaning that they signal the need for immediate investigation. The Joint Commission, a major accreditation organisation in the US, reported that the five most common sentinel events were: retention of foreign bodies, wrong site surgery, falls, on-site suicide and off-site suicide. A total of 436 sentinel events were reported to the Joint Commission in the first six months of 2019, though such reporting is not mandatory.[141]

When 16 Chief Executives of leading US hospitals were asked about their management of sentinel events, their responses were consistent. They included: a patient's relationship with their healthcare organisation is built on trust which demands honesty; always take patient complaints seriously; train staff for adverse event recovery; even when using protective equipment remember the power of a human face and a smile; patients should never die alone; Never events can include unexplained delays in treatment; and we need to think about patient experience as well as clinical process.[142]

More case studies about sentinel events that led to claims for damages can be found in Chapter Five.

The Safety of Women

The publication of the explosive Cumberlege report[143] in July 2020 exposed once again the shortcomings of the NHS and healthcare-related industries in respect to patient safety, particularly the safety of women. The Inquiry heard harrowing stories from almost 700 patients, many of them women who had been damaged and suffered for years without any acknowledgement of their problems or offer of compensation. It exposed in stark terms the dark side of healthcare for women in England. The Inquiry examined in detail three specific problem areas:

- Hormone pregnancy tests (HPTs), including Primodos, were introduced in the 1950s and withdrawn from the market in the late 1970s and are thought to be associated with birth defects and miscarriages. Distressing as the patient stories were and despite how obvious the damage was, the Inquiry could find no firm evidence to support a causal link between HPTs and physical malformation. One reason for this was the lack of data available for the period in question. A compensation scheme requiring evidence of harm, but not negligence, would have worked in this case.
- Sodium valproate is an effective anti-epileptic drug that causes physical malformations, autism and developmental delay in many children when taken by pregnant women. It is now a recognised disorder.[144] It was first licensed in 1972 but it was not until the 1980s that reports began to emerge of problems. Women were not warned about these risks. If known information had been shared they could have discussed a change of epilepsy medication with their physician before becoming pregnant. It was not until 1994 that the patient information leaflet for the drug advised that there was a slightly higher risk of having a child with an abnormality when using the medication. It took over 40 years for the healthcare system to put into place measures to ensure that women were fully informed of these risks prior to becoming pregnant.
- Pelvic mesh implants (as discussed earlier) are used in the surgical repair of pelvic organ prolapse and to manage stress

urinary incontinence. Their use has been linked to crippling and life-changing complications. The Inquiry recommended that patients should be made fully aware of the risks rather than a complete ban.

The Inquiry concluded that the English healthcare system was 'disjointed, siloed, unresponsive and defensive'. Recommendations included the creation of a Patient Safety Commissioner for England, a financial redress agency similar to that in France, changes to the yellow card alert system and a requirement for full declarations of interest about any financial relationships between clinicians and the pharmaceutical and medical device industries.

There are many vested interests that may attempt to block the implementation of some of these quite sensible recommendations.

Lessons for the Future

In this chapter we have seen that whilst almost all healthcare professionals are good people committed to their patients, mistakes, some of which are dangerous, do happen and cause harm to patients. Medicine is not an exact science, and as it becomes ever more sophisticated and complex, it also becomes more difficult to prevent breakdowns and mistakes. The key lesson is that vigilance must be used at all times, together with strict adherence to safety protocols. Never or sentinel events must always be investigated, and the results shared. Policies that get in the way of transparent reporting, such as fines, should be removed. Building a safety culture is vital and is explored further in Chapter Nine.

There is nothing wrong with attempts to eradicate futile and unnecessary treatment if the specific examples have the broad support of professionals. The San Francisco study demonstrates that physicians are more influenced by factors such as radiation levels than cost in reducing unnecessary tests.[145]

Tragedies such as the Thalidomide scandal highlight the need for prompt action when evidence emerges of harmful side effects. The issues with tainted blood demonstrate the need for open and ethical decision-making and to quickly provide help and support for patients who have been harmed. This process might be speeded up if it did not have to include or imply an admission of legal liability.

Well-intentioned but mistaken clinical practice requires speedy intervention as soon as problems are identified, and professional societies, as well as healthcare authorities, need to take full responsibility to respond and ensure such incidents do not reoccur.

There is an increasing need for biomedical engineers to become permanent members of hospital safety teams. Increasingly technical equipment with the potential to harm patients must be properly maintained and updated or replaced when they become outdated and not fit for the purpose. A single successful claim for damages from a patient that has been harmed by faulty equipment would likely far exceed the cost of any replacement. The growth of leasing particularly expensive equipment seems like a sensible way forward, as long as it also guarantees upgrades to the latest available model.

The centralisation of hospital-based speciality services to improve safety and overall outcomes remains problematic. Medical opinion alone is not winning the argument and even when clear evidence is available it can be overridden by local politicians (or physicians) who want to protect local services. Denmark is one of the few examples of countries that have succeeded in implementing comprehensive reforms, but this was achieved only as part of a wider reorganisation of government: 'larger regions meant that voter constituencies changed. This made it easier for regional politicians to balance the resistance in areas where hospitals were closing with additional support in areas where new hospital buildings were placed. Furthermore, regional politicians sweetened the bitterness of having to close down local hospitals by converting them into other types of health facilities'.[146] This is evidently not a solution that can work in every country, but we can distil some lessons from it. First, a national consensus needs to be built about the evidence for change supported by leading professional societies. Second, this evidence must be published in an easily understood format. Those arguing for the retention of local services must be listened to and allowed to engage in a conversation about alternatives. In particular, they will need reassurance (or in some cases, an honest opinion) about the impact the loss of one service will have on the rest of a particular hospital. Often, the central issue is as much about local employment and the local economy as it is with extended travel times for patients. Those promoting change with arguments that focus on how many lives will be saved must be very confident of their facts and take care not to exaggerate the consequences of decisions they do not support. Local professionals must also remain firmly connected to any major referral centre as they will be involved in the early stages of diagnosis and with continuing care after discharge. The process of change will be immeasurably easier if supported by local professional staff. If professionals cannot agree, it is of little use passing the problem on to politicians.

The exponential growth in technological advances should be embraced, but with the appropriate safeguards. The faith in computer systems needs to be balanced with caution and subject to regular checks. Artificial intelligence may improve the accuracy of diagnostic and screening programmes and should be trialled and potentially adopted, even if expensive, at the earliest opportunity. Real-time reporting of adverse events is now possible.

Those who want to shorten the time taken to authorise new drugs and devices need to be very sure that in so doing they are not unreasonably reducing safety standards. In the interests of patients, any suspicions about fault should always be enough to justify an investigation. Establishing and maintaining registers of implants and perhaps all medical devices seems a sensible thing to do in the interests of both patients and manufacturers.

Open, no-blame reporting systems are clearly important in moving many of these issues in the right direction, but, as we will see in Chapter Five, changes to medical negligence laws remain controversial.

Vigilance must be instilled as a core component of all good clinical and managerial practice. The creation of national or state investigation units to review reported adverse events sounds sensible but runs the risk of diminishing local responsibility for tackling problems and taking action. Indeed, it is difficult to see how a national system could operate on a no-blame basis. It may be better for such bodies to review local action (under a system of mandatory reporting) and only intervene when this is judged to be weak or inappropriate. The further the quality assurance systems are from the operational areas, the weaker they become.

Product licensing authorities have much to learn from these case studies. They should improve their responsiveness to reports of unexpected or unexplained problems and side effects. If legal concerns are preventing formal action, they should consider making whatever evidence they have available to clinicians without comment. This may have the effect of eliciting additional evidence. If patient safety is the principal driver, as it should be, then even the suspicion of a problem should be enough to prompt an investigation. Licensing authorities should listen more closely to patients and their stories and engage with them more actively.

Finally, it takes time to build a consensus on health-related issues. Healthcare systems need to be strong enough to withstand overreaching ambition from managers, healthcare professionals and hospitals that put their reputation ahead of patient safety.

Chapter Four
Struck Off

Healthcare professionals need a licence to practise in most developed countries. If they fail to live up to prescribed professional standards, this licence can be revoked or conditions (such as close supervision) may be enforced on their practice. Good practice, the standard against which all practitioners will be judged, is set out in some detail in most jurisdictions. Disciplinary processes are all designed to operate within strict legal guidelines, and in any action, the burden of proof lies with the regulator. The number of licensed health practitioners who are subjected to a sanction is very small indeed in all countries. Nevertheless, a few do fail to live up to the standard required and either harm patients or bring their profession into disrepute.

Practising without a licence is a criminal offence in all jurisdictions as is continuing to practise as a healthcare professional once struck off a register.

Professional Self-regulation

Some countries operate on the principle that the healthcare professions can be trusted to regulate themselves to protect the public from harm. Many of the key national regulatory bodies, such as the Australian and Canadian medical and nursing boards, are dominated by the medical and nursing professions, although other countries also have an extensive lay membership. The General Medical Council (GMC) in UK has equality between professional and lay members on its Council. The Medical Board of California has a medical majority of only one. New York has a much-admired single organisation for the regulation of over 50 professions, including healthcare professionals. However, this Medical Board, operating as the principal advisor on the licensing of doctors, has a membership of 24 registered practitioners and requires only a minimum of two public members.[1] The same principles apply to other professions.

Given that all of these bodies have a primary duty to protect the health and safety of the public, all of this is perhaps rather surprising. A recent trend has been for governments to put pressure on professional bodies that also act as trade unions to separate their role of representing the interests of their members with that of protecting the public. The Royal Pharmaceutical Society in the UK was obliged to give up its licensing role when the General Pharmaceutical Council was created in 2012 to handle those powers.

With the ever-accelerating pace of change in medical science, it is now becoming unusual to grant licence to practise for life, although this is still the practice in some US States, including New York. Most regulatory bodies are now insisting that evidence of continued professional development be intermittently provided.

The regulatory bodies also license and inspect the educational institutions that train healthcare professionals. This means that they have a heavy influence on the curriculum and control the entry-level educational requirements.

In 2011, the Governor of New York signed Chapter 410 of the laws of 2011 that established the entry-level degree required for a licence as a physical therapist at the master's level or higher in physical therapy or the equivalent. Applicants for licensure as a physical therapist must, since August 2012, meet the new standard of having a master's degree or higher.[2]

Good Professional Practice

The UK GMC defines good professional medical practice as always putting the patient first, keeping up to date, taking prompt action to protect patient safety, establishing good partnerships with patients and colleagues, speaking good English and being open, honest and acting with integrity.

The Australian version of good medical practice covers much of the same ground and refers to professional values as follows:

> *While individual doctors have their own personal beliefs and values there are certain professional values on which all doctors are expected to base their practice. Doctors have a duty to make the care of patients their first concern and to practice medicine safely and effectively. They must be ethical and trustworthy. Patients trust their doctors because they believe that, in addition to being competent, their doctor will not take advantage of them and will display qualities such as integrity, truthfulness, dependability and compassion. Patients also rely on their doctors to protect their confidentiality.*

The American Physician's Charter[3] lists 10 professional commitments that cover the same ground.

The General Dental Council (UK) published standards for the dental team rather than the individual practitioner where they distinguish between those duties that are compulsory and those that should be exercised with judgement by a professional. For example, a registered dentist *must* take appropriate action if they have concerns about the possible abuse of children or vulnerable adults and *should* only recommend products if they are best suited to meet a patient's needs.

The Spanish version of good medical practice[4] is interesting in that in addition to spelling out good standards it also gives examples of bad medical practice that should be avoided. These include: 'healthcare audits only serve to exert more control over doctors. I will avoid participating'; 'A second opinion is a smear on me and my team'; and 'Patient safety and quality of care are fashionable, but they are not my daily concern'.

The nursing professions have their own codes of good practice against which practitioners are judged. The nursing code of practice in the UK is structured around four themes: prioritise people, practise effectively, preserve safety and promote professionalism and trust. In the UK, the Nursing and Midwifery Council (NMC) registers both fully trained nurses and nursing associates.

The Hong Kong Nursing Council sets out nine domains that include infection control, informed patient consent and end-of-life care.[5] In Canada, four concepts underpin the discipline of nursing: the person or client, the environment, health and nursing practice. Of more practical use is the detailed Canadian code of ethics for nurses; a code that is echoed in different forms by other professional nursing organisations.

Canadian Nurses Code of Ethics for Registered Nurses[6]

Provide safe, compassionate, competent and ethical care
Promote health and well-being
Promote and respect informed decision-making
Preserve dignity
Maintain privacy and confidentiality
Promote justice
Be accountable.

These codes are not static, but evolve over time. Some aim to guide healthcare professionals through the ethics of medicine in a world of social media and deal with the increased use of new technologies, such as telemedicine, that cross state and national boundaries. Whenever any such code is reviewed, the specified standards of professional conduct are always raised and never lowered. Healthcare professionals are expected to maintain the highest moral standards along with adequate and well-practised technical skills.

China

In China, healthcare professionals (both native and foreign) are now licensed to practise after passing a specific licensing examination. The so-called 'barefoot doctors' — farmers, faith healers and students who received minimal basic training in medicine and provided care in rural villages — were phased out in 1981. These individuals had promoted basic hygiene, preventive healthcare and family planning as well as treating common illnesses, but were replaced by village doctors as China expanded the number of trained healthcare professionals and moved closer to the healthcare systems developed in other countries. Misconduct in China is largely dealt with at a local or workplace level.

Licensing Bodies and Their Spheres of Operation

The bodies that regulate and grant licences for individuals to practise in healthcare professions operate at different levels. Canada and Germany have bodies that operate at the state level. In the UK, the regulation body is national. In the US, although licensing is done at state-level, all doctors who possess a primary qualification in medicine are required to pass a three-step examination set by the national United States Medical Licensing Examination (USLME) before they can apply for state registration. Overseas graduates have to go through the same process.[7] Decentralised systems create problems in the US, as doctors who are forced to surrender a licence in one State can still go on to practise in another.

> *Dr. Larry Mitchell Isaacs agreed to surrender his medical licence for Louisiana in 2013 after facing disciplinary action for allegedly removing a healthy kidney during what was supposed to be a colon surgery. He moved to California, where he obtained a licence, and mistakenly removed a fallopian tube that he thought was the patient's appendix. Facing State sanctions, he surrendered his licence and moved to New York. There, regulators were moving to take action against him based on his problems in California, and he was eventually forced to surrender his third licence in 2017. He subsequently moved to Ohio and took a role at an urgent care clinic where he continued to practise.*[8]

In a response to this and other similar cases, some jurisdictions are moving their information systems above state and country level so that individuals can be tracked and their licences checked.

A European Professional Card is now available to three healthcare professions and supports free movement of professional staff within the EU.[9] An EU directive of 2005 required all member state registering bodies to inform all others when a licence is made conditional, suspended or revoked.[10] There is a similar clearinghouse in the US — the

National Practitioner Database (NPDB) was established by Congress in 1986. It is intended to prevent practitioners from moving from one State to another without disclosure or discovery of previous damaging performance. By law, hospitals and other healthcare institutions must report to the NPDB when doctors lose clinical privileges in connection with investigations of substandard care or misconduct. Insurers must also report any payments in a malpractice case, regardless of whether guilt was admitted.

Some States and organisations are better than others in accessing this data for pre-employment checks, but even when they do, some important events are not included. The reason for this is that it is easier for employers just to sack people or give them the chance to retire or resign. The way that States use the database also varies widely. Florida pays the NPDB to continuously monitor the licences of all its licensed physicians. California, on the other hand, has no fixed rules for accessing the database and it is not queried routinely. The database is also not open to the public.

Nurse RN applied to work at a small public hospital in the State of Nevada after moving from a mid-western State where she had qualified as a nurse but had been fired or resigned from a number of hospital and care home posts after a series of conflicted encounters with colleagues. The HR department in Nevada checked her status with the NPD and received a negative response; it had no derogatory information about nurse RN. Shortly after her appointment, drugs began to go missing from crash carts and patients began to die from Mivacron drug overdoses.[11] Nurse RN was identified as the likely culprit, indicted and charged with murder.[12]

Some countries, such as Saudi Arabia and Dubai, have bilateral agreements to allow the movement of healthcare professionals between their states.

Recruiting from Overseas

Recruiting badly qualified or incompetent healthcare professionals from other countries has generated many problems around the world, as was illustrated by the Australian cases in Chapter One. In fact, the majority of healthcare professionals struck off or sanctioned by the UK's GMC were trained at medical schools from outside of the UK.

> *Richard Karl, a British anaesthetist who reinvented himself as a minimally invasive spinal surgeon in the US after his UK conviction for gross negligent manslaughter and posing a danger to the public was later stripped off his licence by the State Board of Medicine in New Jersey.*

The Nurses and Midwives Council in the UK is processing over 6000 applications to practise each year from nurses who trained in other countries.[13] High levels of professional migration are putting licensing bodies under strain.[14]

Penalties

The majority of healthcare professionals who appear before disciplinary committees receive warnings or have conditions placed on their continued practice. These warnings usually have a time-expired date but, in the more serious cases, the professionals concerned have to demonstrate, before their licence is renewed, that they have taken steps to ensure that whatever unprofessional behaviour they have been sanctioned for has been addressed and will not be repeated or that that they have undertaken extra training.

Removal from a professional register is a penalty of last resort and only applied in the most serious cases. Even in these cases, the practitioner can apply for reinstatement after a period of years, although few of these applications are granted. In 2018 and 2019 of 27 applications for reinstatement made to the GMC in the UK, only six were granted.

Of the 409 cases reviewed by the UK's Medical Practitioners Tribunal Service in 2019, only 17% ended up with the practitioner being struck up.[15] Of those struck off, a total of two-thirds had qualified in medicine outside the UK.

There are many reasons for licensing bodies to take action against practitioners, ranging from incompetent practice to bringing the profession into disrepute. Criminal convictions almost always lead to a referral to a licensing body, as does the failure to disclose a previous conviction. Some examples follow.

Clinical Competence and Limits

It is an offence to practise beyond one's clinical limits in non-emergency situations. It breaks the Hippocratic Oath to practise beyond one's skills. This is a difficult legal area as the boundaries between medical specialities and the healthcare professions keep shifting.

While examining a patient who wanted advice about hormone replacement therapy, a gynaecologist noticed several unsightly skin lesions. He asked the patient whether she would like them removed under a general anaesthetic. She agreed but was not warned about possible scarring. The gynaecologist carried out the procedure but when sutures were removed some of the wounds gaped and steri-strips were applied. No follow-up treatment was offered. The patient developed Keloid scarring and successfully sued the gynaecologist. Following the case, the Medical Protection Society[16] emphasised the importance of doctors acting within their sphere of practice and the importance of referring patients to a colleague in the relevant specialty.

I. A. Evans was struck off the UK nursing register in 2019 for prescribing drugs to patients when he had not taken and passed the required course. A total of 31 patients were involved and his unauthorised prescribing included controlled drugs. He had told his employer and his clinical team that he had taken and passed the course. He had also failed to keep up to date with his Continued Professional Development.[17]

Poor Professional Performance

Dr. Lidia Hristeva qualified in Bulgaria where she trained in paediatrics. She then practised as a middle grade locum in a number of UK hospitals. Concerns were raised by one of her employers about her knowledge, technical competency and communication skills. The GMC asked her to undergo a performance assessment which found her to be of an unacceptable standard in the areas of maintaining good standards of clinical practice, relationships with patients, working with colleagues, attitude and time management skills. Her case was first considered in 2018 and she was granted a limited nine-month licence subject to close supervision. Having reviewed her progress, second and third tribunals granted her two more conditional periods of nine months. In 2020 she was still working with only a strictly conditional licence to practise in the UK.[18]

Dr. Leopold Reinecke qualified in medicine in South Africa and worked as a locum Consultant Oncologist at two NHS Trusts. An inquiry was launched when a patient complained about the treatment and care of his wife. As the inquiry developed, 11 further complaints emerged. The problems identified included an inappropriate interpretation of a CT scan indicating disease progression, inappropriate medication, the absence of proper treatment plans and inappropriate patient communication. His clinical skills were deemed to be below standard as was the organisation of his patient's treatment. Dr. Reinecke's conduct and actions, the tribunal found, caused real harm, pain, suffering and distress to patients and their families. The only proportionate response was his erasure from the medical register.[19]

Misconduct

Issues of misconduct constitute the majority of complaints and concerns presented to licensing bodies, but incompetent clinical practice is one of the most common reasons for being struck off.

Muhammad Siddiq, a radiographer registered by the UK's Health and Care Professions Council, was struck off the register in 2019 after evidence was presented that he had carried out unauthorised and inappropriate CT scans. He did not conduct a patient ID check and had scanned a head when a scan of the pelvis had been requested and then taken steps to cover up his error.[20]

Peters O. Aremu, a biomedical scientist, was struck off after a number of suspensions for failing to follow standard operating procedures with regard to quality management despite reminders to do so. He was the head of a large hospital's cytology screening service. The tribunal said that the main cause of his misconduct involved attitudinal issues.[21]

Three nurses were charged with professional misconduct in Hong Kong following a serious clinical mistake. A patient had undergone surgery that included a permanent tracheotomy to enable him to breath. The gauze over the opening in the throat was taped to the skin on all four sides resulting in the death of the patient. The nurses were found guilty of professional misconduct and had their licences suspended for a month.[22]

A dentist in Australia extracted four healthy teeth in order to commence the straightening the teeth of a 17-year-old patient. The dentist was not an orthodontist. Teeth fragments remained in the patient's mouth causing an infection. The investigation panel judged that the dentist had engaged in unsatisfactory professional performance and placed a condition on the practitioner's registration so that any future orthodontic treatment plans had to be approved, checked and supervised by a registered orthodontist.[23]

Sanctions in this area of clinical competence often include further training for the practitioner.

A patient presented to a licensed chiropractor with multiple neurological symptoms. The chiropractor manipulated the patient's spine after only a minimal examination and took no patient history. After a third consecutive day of treatment, the patient reported pain and tingling in the spine. The practitioner's advice was to rest and to try short walks. The investigating panel found that the practitioner did not perform an adequate neurological examination at any stage during his consultation with patient and made an incorrect diagnosis. A condition was placed on his licence requiring him to complete further education and training within six months to address these concerns, with a progress review in one year.[24]

Some regulators have accepted the arguments for recognising an honest mistake by a healthcare professional provided the individual acknowledges and learns from it.

System Failures

Inappropriate or incompetent clinical practice is almost always the subject of an investigation and is usually reported to the appropriate licensing authority by an employer or other professional. But in some cases, faults in the system are blamed rather than individuals.

In a highly unusual case, **Dr. H. Bawa-Garba** was found guilty of manslaughter by negligence after the death of a child at a hospital in Nottingham, England. She was given a two-year suspended sentence. The Medical Practices Tribunal reviewed her case and suspended her from the medical register for one year. The GMC appealed the decision of its own Tribunal at the High Court and won. As a result, Dr. Bawa-Garba was struck off. Dr. Bawa-Garba then successfully appealed the court decision and returned to her one-year suspension. In 2019 she returned to practise under close supervision. An independent review of gross negligent manslaughter and culpable homicide followed.[25]

At the heart of this case was the assertion that the death of the patient had more to do with systemic faults at the hospital (particularly understaffing) than the doctor concerned. An independent review recommended that the government remove the right of the GMC (and presumably other bodies) to appeal decisions made by their independent tribunals. This case also reopened questions on whether a hospital board, or any other health organisation, could be charged in a criminal court with corporate manslaughter. The issue has rarely been legally tested but it is possible under UK law in the most serious cases.

A man admitted to a UK hospital for a routine knee operation developed a bacterial infection that two doctors failed to diagnose and treat. The patient subsequently died of staphylococcal toxic shock syndrome. The doctors were convicted of gross negligent manslaughter and given suspended prison sentences. The hospital pleaded guilty to an amended charge of failing to adequately manage and supervise the doctors.[26]

Corporate manslaughter is proving difficult to prosecute in many other countries, but as system failure resulting in patient harm becomes more widespread, more successful prosecutions can be expected.[27] System failure due to austerity-induced low staffing levels has never been tested in court, but if it were, it would be the health organisation rather than the politicians that would be charged. Again, this highlights the importance for health and social care providers of either being able to operate their services safely or face closure.

Dishonesty

Dishonesty of various kinds — including cheating in exams, failure to disclose conditions placed on a licence to practise with a new employer and prescription fraud — sometimes leads to practitioners being struck off or having their licence suspended.

> *Dr. Ernest Jangwa was suspended from the medical register in 2019 for nine months for prescribing opioids and other drugs to a patient/person with whom he had a close personal relationship and who was not registered as a patient at the hospital where he worked. He then lied about his actions. He also made a dishonest statement to another NHS Trust when asked if he was currently subject to any fitness-to-practise proceedings. His clinical practice was never called into question.[28]*

> *Dr. Pandeshwar Gururaj was suspended for one year after fraudulently adding his name to an operating theatre list knowing that he would receive financial remuneration to which he was not entitled. The Tribunal considered that his misconduct was at the high end of seriousness.[29]*

> *Isaac Baidoo had trained in Ghana and was licensed to practise as a General Practitioner (GP) in UK. He also worked locum shifts at an urgent care centre. It was alleged that he worked his locum shift whilst off sick from the general practice where he was employed and receiving sick pay from. He lied to NHS England when challenged about his conduct. NHS England concluded that he had deep-seated attitudinal issues with honesty and he was struck off.[30]*

False Research

In a small number of cases, doctors have been stuck off for failing to follow clinical trial protocols or for falsely claiming the authorship of research papers.

> *Dr. Mohammed Shali acted dishonestly in 2017 by claiming to be the lead author of two papers he submitted to an international journal. In so doing he brought the profession into disrepute and was suspended for a year. His case was reviewed in 2018 and he was suspended for a further year. As a consequence of no remediation, he was struck off the UK register in 2019.*[31]

Record Keeping

Failure to maintain proper clinical records has, in extreme cases, been judged as serious misconduct.

> *Sharmila Kale, a registered nurse and manager of a care home, did not ensure that patients had adequate care plans or properly complete 24-hour care charts or risk assessment records. She had failed to make a referral for safeguarding when one patient was making withdrawals from a cash machine for another patient. Medication given to patients was not properly recorded including, on some occasions, controlled drugs. GPs had also not been called when residents were unwell.*
>
> *The panel judged this case to be so serious that Kale was struck off the register in order to protect the public and send a clear message to both the public and the profession about the standard of behaviour required of registered nurses.*[32]

Overworked Doctors

Doctors often practise in other countries with the prime aim of boosting their potential income. Gaining experience and enhancing their skills is often subordinated to this aim. They are often prepared to work very long hours and for more than one employer at the same time — often as locums — and see nothing wrong with this. The employer must therefore share some of the blame when a tired doctor makes mistakes.

> **Daniel Ubani**, *a 67-year-old doctor licensed in Germany, flew into the UK in 2008 to undertake a 12-hour shift for a general practice service provider. He had only had a few hours' sleep when he injected 10 times the recommended level of diamorphine into a patient who later died. The GMC banned him from practising in the UK.*[33]

Inappropriate Sexual Relationships

An inappropriate sexual relationship with a patient is a serious offence for a medical professional — as is possessing pornographic images on a personal computer. In both cases the severity level increases if children are involved. Inappropriate examinations of patients have also led to erasure.

> **Dr. Manish Gupta**, *a consultant obstetrician, was removed from the medical register in 2019 after he had been found guilty of possessing extreme pornography, including prohibited images of children. He was sentenced to 24 months community service.*[34]

> **Dr. Jonathan Bainbridge** *was working as a consultant radiologist in Wales when he was arrested and charged with sexually exploiting a child by asking her to send him indecent images of herself. He was convicted of the offence, sentenced to a community order of 18 months and added to the Register of Sex Offenders. In his oral evidence he accepted that he remained a continuing risk. His name was erased from the Register.*[35]

> **Dr. Chizoba Christopher Uzoh**, *who qualified in medicine in India, was judged to have accessed a patient's record for her contact details whilst working as a locum GP in England and then pursuing her for a personal relationship using phone, text and letters. His actions continued after he was*

asked to desist. He told a Tribunal that he thought she was playing hard to get. He was struck off the register in 2019 for failing to provide any evidence of remediation. He moved to Canada to practise but failed to notify the appropriate authorities of his erasure from the UK register. When this was discovered he was referred to the Disciplinary Committee and charged with disgraceful, dishonourable and unprofessional conduct in another jurisdiction.[36] *His licence to practise was suspended for a year and then again for a further year in 2018. In 2020 he reported that he had started a one-to-one educational course in professional boundaries, ethics and self-regulation with a consultant. His licence application will be reviewed in 2021.*

Dr. Dilip Dhillon, a GP from Victoria, Australia, was disqualified for applying for registration three years and ten months after he was convicted of two counts of wilfully committing an indecent act with a child under the age of 16, and for failing to comply with the chaperone conditions that had been applied to his licence when first charged with these offences. He was also found to have engaged in inappropriate billing practices. This behaviour represented professional misconduct.[37]

Dr. Manish Shah, a London GP, was convicted in 2019 of sex crimes against 23 women and girls and sentenced to life imprisonment. His interim suspension from practice will no doubt be converted to removal from the register in due course. He had convinced his patients to have unnecessary invasive examinations by citing high-profile celebrity cases. The examinations were not in interests of his patients but for his own sexual gratification. Some of his victims were particularly vulnerable because of their young age. He breached guidelines on the use of chaperones and on occasion did not wear examination gloves. He had previous convictions for sex offences.[38]

There are, however, grey areas in how sexual conduct is perceived.

In an Australian case, a doctor and a patient had been friends in the early 1990s. In 2000 she presented to the doctor for treatment. Eight years after the clinical relationship was established, they had sex together. This was deemed

> *to be unprofessional conduct (rather than professional misconduct). The doctor was reprimanded for failing to maintain professional boundaries and cautioned against repeating such conduct in the future. Conditions were imposed on the doctor's licence to practise, requiring him to complete an educational programme on professional boundaries.*[39]

Many licensing authorities are reporting incidents of online professional violations, including substance misuse, sexual misconduct and abuses of prescribing privileges.[40]

Harassment

The persistent harassment of a colleague has been a cause of erasure, particularly when it has a sexual connotation. Good medical practice includes the obligation to work collaboratively with colleagues respecting their skills and contributions.

> *Dr. Serban Gheorghiu was working as a Consultant in an Endoscopy Unit in Yorkshire when he was found to have acted inappropriately on a number of occasions. He had constantly asked colleagues about their sex lives and swore in front of patients. He had been warned on multiple occasions about his behaviour by his employer and given a number of written warnings. He had also received a warning from the GMC. The Tribunal judged that he had limited insight into his pattern of unacceptable behaviour and, as a result, was suspended from the UK register for nine months with a review to be undertaken at the end of this period. With no evidence of remediation, he was struck off in 2019.*[41]

Mental Health

In some cases, inappropriate behaviour is connected to an underlying mental health condition; a situation that can present licensing authorities with difficult and sensitive decisions.

Dr. LC trained in Michigan and became certified in psychiatry and neurology. He provided psychiatric treatment to a patient between 2008 and 2014 but in the final year of this treatment engaged in sexual activity with her. In addition to this violation of professional boundaries, he departed from the standard of care with regard to the prescription of hypnotic agents and failed to document any assessment of the patient for substance abuse or dependence. In January 2015, Dr. LC completed a comprehensive psychosexual evaluation and was deemed unsafe to practise. He was admitted for inpatient treatment shortly after this judgement and diagnosed with personality disorder unspecified with prominent narcissistic traits and histrionic and compulsive anti-social features, including obsessive compulsive disorder (sexual compulsivity) and general anxiety disorder. He also had drug and alcohol dependency problems. He was discharged from the hospital programme for a violation of the confidentiality of a fellow patient. In June 2014, the Arizona Medical Board issued an order for the surrender of his licence.

After extensive treatment he applied for the return of his licence in 2019 and produced a number of referees to vouch for his reformed character. His request was granted for a five-year probationary period, but with strict conditions. His clinical practice had to be monitored, at his expense, by a Board-nominated clinician. He was required to completely abstain from taking non-prescribed drugs and alcohol. Any positive test would lead to the immediate suspension of his licence to practise. He was also required to use a third-party chaperone when treating female patients and to attend therapy groups for the whole of his probationary period. Finally, he was ordered to inform any employer of the restrictions on his licence. Solo practice was banned.

Health and Misconduct

Problems related to health are usually separated from misconduct cases and often lead to voluntary interim suspensions whilst the practitioner seeks treatment. Specialist physician healthcare services are now slowly developing. The NHS in the UK provides one of the largest publicly funded comprehensive physician healthcare services in the world.[42]

Dr. Richard Cunningham was an alcoholic under treatment with a physicians health programme when the Director of the programme reported him to the State Medical Board on the grounds that he had started drinking again and was exhibiting increasingly uncontrolled behaviour. He was charged with professional misconduct, but a month later, the charges were placed in abeyance because Cunningham had allowed his licence to lapse. He moved from Canada to the US but had his licence revoked in Alabama. He never disguised his alcoholism when applying for licences. He moved to other US states but eventually relocated to the Northwest Territories of Canada, where he was sent to jail for threatening to kill his wife. He later moved to Alberta with conditions on his licence that required him to blow into a breathalyser each day. He relapsed again in 2017 but returned to practice three months later. He told a local newspaper that: 'I'm open about the fact that I am an alcoholic, but I am in recovery. The public does not have a right to know about my past'.[43]

Mitchell Dean Feller, who qualified in the US, was charged in New Zealand with giving his patients the drug TeKiriGold without disclosing his financial interest in the product. He conducted clinical trials on patients — including those that were vulnerable or suffering from terminal conditions — without their informed consent. His licence to practise was revoked and his conduct reported to the American licensing authorities.[44]

Illegal Prescription of Drugs

The illegal prescription of drugs is proving to be a major problem in most jurisdictions. The so-called opioid crisis in US is partly fuelled by inappropriate clinical behaviour. The Medical Board in California undertook a review of death records where the death involved a prescription drug. In 2019 it reported that 23% of the cases examined have resulted in the filing of an accusation or disciplinary action against a physician (including cases where action had already been taken) for inappropriate prescribing issues.[45]

Robert Delagente, a *registered doctor from New Jersey, described as the 'El Chapo' of opioids, was indicted in 2019 of prescribing vast numbers of highly addictive prescribed controlled substances outside the ordinary course of professional practice and without a legitimate medical purpose. According to the statements made in court he had allowed patients, who he had not seen, to name their own dose. He had admitted in another action that he had also committed healthcare claims fraud for which a prison sentence was imposed. His licence was suspended.*[46]

Majid Mustafa, a *dentist registered in UK, encouraged Patient A to obtain GBH on his behalf from drug dealers in Poland with the intention of administering it unlawfully and without consent to his wife. He was judged to have failed to maintain adequate professional boundaries with Patient A and this was deemed to be unprofessional and lacking in integrity. He had also committed an illegal act. His name was erased from the register.*[47]

Complaint Resolutions

The Canadian disciplinary system is organised at the state level and often uses a consensual complaint resolution system. This is a legal agreement between a registrant and the licensing body that outlines the action the registrant will take to address the issues identified during the investigation process. It seems to work.

Gary Dromarsky, a *licensed nurse, visited a client at home to provide private foot care services. He put his hand under his client's underwear in an extremely inappropriate manner. The client complained to the police and to the licensing body, the College of Registered Nurses. While the investigation was ongoing, Dromarsky signed an interim undertaking to cease all private nursing care, remain in the sole employment of his current employer and to see female patients only with a chaperone. Shortly after signing this order, Dromarsky broke it by providing foot care to two patients in their*

> *homes. This was reported and he was required to sign a second undertaking to cease all nursing practice until the investigations were completed. The Inquiry Committee concluded that the cancellation of Dromarsky's registration was the only appropriate outcome to protect the public. He agreed not to apply for the reinstatement of his registration for five years.*[48]

Forgery

Forgery is a common cause of disciplinary action against medical professionals under supervision, usually manifested either by presenting false evidence of educational attainment in order to obtain certification or by dishonest reporting to employers.

> ***Dr. Justine McIntyre*** *was suspended from the UK medical register in 2019 for forging a postgraduate diploma in surgical anatomy from the University of Otago in New Zealand. She admitted the offence and was suspended for six months. This was later extended to nine months to allow a hearing of the New Zealand Licensing Board to consider the same charges.[49] The New Zealand Medical Board permitted her to practise under supervision until August 2020 when her case would be reviewed.*

> ***T. J. Watson,*** *a school nurse, told her employers and colleagues that she had cancer and took sick leave for treatment. This was untrue and evidence was presented to show that she had forged a letter from a cancer specialist as evidence of her claim. She was dismissed, but later lied to a potential new employer by not mentioning the incident and claiming that her motives in applying for the new position were to enhance her career.[50]*

Assault on a Patient

Any assault on a patient — for whatever reason — is always subject to an investigation, and this includes unreasonable restraint. We will look at many more instances of unreasonable restraint in Chapter Six.

At the Royal Darwin Hospital, Australia, in 2012, a nurse yelled at a disabled patient to 'hurry up' and pushed him in the chest, causing him to fall. She later talked about the incident on social media and included inappropriate comments about the patient. The nurse was reprimanded, required to visit a psychologist and attend a course in legal and ethical nursing practice. The panel agreed to review the decision after 12 months.[51]

B. Smith, a registered nurse, was reprimanded in May 2017 by the State Administrative Tribunal of Western Australia and disqualified from applying for registration for one year. On a mental health unit, he had used excessive restraint on a patient, placed his finger in his eye and restricted the patient's airway with his hands around the patient's neck.[52]

Language Problems

The requirements for professional registration have changed over time and often include a language requirement so that professionals can communicate properly with patients and colleagues. In the nursing profession, failures to pass the language test are increasingly common as more nurses are recruited from other countries. This has proven to be a particular problem with the recruitment of nurses trained in countries within the EU who expect to obtain speedy licences to practise anywhere in Europe.

Clodualdo Cabia, a registered nurse, had first been suspended in 2018 as he did not have the necessary knowledge of English to practise safely and efficiently. He was required to take an English language test but not obtain a satisfactory result and at a hearing in December 2019 he was suspended for a further year and a year later in 2020 struck off.[53]

Pharmacists and Other Healthcare Professionals

Pharmacists and other healthcare professionals are all required to obtain a licence to practise in most countries. This increasingly includes assistants who work for professional staff. As new professions emerge, such as paramedics, they also require registration, as do the schools where they secure their basic qualification. In the UK, the General Pharmaceutical Council also inspects pharmacies and grants them a licence to provide services.

> *In a routine inspection in 2019, an inspector found that **Vincent Kwadzo Torku**, a registered pharmacist and the owner of a pharmacy had, over a period of four years, failed to ensure that he had appropriate indemnity insurance and had made false declarations to the General Pharmaceutical Council. His licence was suspended for three months. The panel had considered an order of removal but as there were no concerns about his clinical skills, his insights, regret and personal remediation they concluded that a short suspension was adequate.*[54]

> ***Nicholas Bawden**, a registered pharmacist, was convicted in September 2019 of attempting to engage in sexual communications with a child. He pleaded guilty. At his tribunal hearing he claimed: 'I can still do my job, it hasn't affected the way I work or my work ethic towards pharmacy, but you are going off ifs and buts and not facts that the public would be shocked. I'm happy in my dispensing role currently and am trusted and valued at my pharmacy'. He was struck off the register.*[55]

This case raises the question as to when a criminal conviction, not related to clinical practice, lowers the faith of the public in the profession and therefore deserves a sanction. A simple speeding offence would, for example, appear to be immaterial in this regard, but driving under the influence of drugs or alcohol clearly would be, particularly if it resulted in injury to another. In this area, we can expect some variation in judgement between the different licensing bodies.

Deliberate Harm

In one particularly nasty case, Ian Paterson, a breast surgeon in the UK, was found guilty of wounding with intent many of his patients and sentenced to 15 years in prison. He had carried out hundreds of unnecessary operations on both NHS and private patients. He had also been using a technique called cleavage-sparing mastectomy that did not conform to recognised practice. In 2017 his sentence was extended to 20 years after the Attorney General referred his first sentence to the Court of Appeal on the grounds that it was too lenient. According to the Solicitor General, Robert Buckland: 'His victims had been left feeling violated and vulnerable and lost their faith in others, particularly some medical professionals'.

After his conviction his case came before the GMC and he was unsurprisingly struck off the register. He had deceived patients and fellow professionals by falsely claiming that the patients were at risk of cancer and needed to undergo operations. He then undertook and charged for these procedures, none of which were necessary. Many legal claims against Paterson and the hospitals where he worked resulted. An independent Inquiry reported in 2020.[56]

This case produced an important comment from the Chief Executive of the GMC: 'His terrible actions went unchecked for too long because managers and colleagues had their concerns but did not speak up. It took brave patients to bring these issues to our attention whereupon we took action to suspend him and refer the matter to the police'.

The independent inquiry led by Bishop Graham James took an even tougher line: 'this is a story about a healthcare system which proved itself dysfunctional at almost every level when it came to keeping patients safe'. The NHS Trust and private hospitals where Paterson worked were criticised for failing to supervise him appropriately and did not respond correctly to well-evidenced complaints about his practice. There was a culture of avoidance and denial.

According to the report: 'The capacity for wilful blindness is illustrated by the way in which Paterson's behaviour and aberrant clinical practice was excused or even favoured'. Five of Paterson's former colleagues were reported to their licensing body for their conduct in the affair. One was reported to the police.

The Paterson case was not the first to expose the reluctance of colleagues and managers to act. Earlier, Raymond Ledward had been struck off the medical register for gross professional misconduct in 1998. His actions must have been evident to those who worked with him but they were reluctant to speak out.

Rodney Ledward was greeted as a breath of fresh air when he arrived at the William Harvey Hospital in Kent, England, in January 1980. A flamboyant figure with an impeccable record, he often gave his patients carnations and arrived at clinics in riding boots and jodhpurs. He claimed to be the fastest gynaecologist in the southeast of England after he performed seven hysterectomies in three hours and 40 minutes. In addition to his position in the NHS, he had a lucrative private practice. In 1996 his colleagues finally reported his conduct and performance to the local NHS Trust and the GMC. The complaints against him included brutality in internal examinations — some undertaken without gloves and with the routine belittling of patients. His surgery was judged to be incompetent with repeated mistakes, numerous unnecessary operations and damage to his patients' bladders, kidneys and livers (the details of which were never communicated to them).

A later independent inquiry, chaired by Jean Ritchie QC, reported that there had been ample evidence that something was wrong with his work but junior staff and nurses were reluctant to speak out. Concerned GPs 'buried their heads in the sand'. Everybody hoped that someone else would deal with Mr Ledward.[57]

Legal Damages

Misconduct or incompetence cases that lead to patient injuries often end up with a claim for damages. NHS Resolution (formerly the NHS Litigation Authority) handles such claims on behalf of the NHS. It dealt with over 10,000 claims in 2017–2018, resulting in mostly out-of-court settlements amounting to £1.6 billion.[58]

In Australia, it is thought that about 18,000 patients have died each year as a consequence of clinical malpractice. A further 80,000 people a year are hospitalised as a result of medication errors. Medical negligence is now a significant part of legal practice in most countries.[59] This topic is considered in more detail in Chapter Five.

Appeals

None of the licensing, registration or tribunal services are above the civil or criminal law and this leads to occasional and sometimes drawn out cases with multiple appeals.

*The Court of Appeal in Western Australia dismissed an appeal lodged by a specialist physician **Anish Singh**. He had been disqualified from applying for registration for 10 years after engaging in professional misconduct in the treatment of his patients. On multiple occasions he had inappropriately prescribed drugs, including anabolic steroids, human growth hormone, testosterone and other treatments to patients for whom there was no proper therapeutic basis for use and, as a result, put patients at risk of adverse side effects. The Court decided that the Tribunal that had imposed the sanction had acted within the law and that the period of disqualification was within a sound exercise of discretion.*[60]

In Denmark, a junior doctor who had been convicted of negligence was allowed to be retried at Denmark's Supreme Court. The original conviction followed the death of a patient with diabetes in 2013. After seeing the patient, complaining of stomach pain at his hospital's Accident and Emergency Department, the doctor, having seen from the patient records that he was a diabetic, ordered a blood sugar test. This instruction was given verbally, and not on paper, to a nurse but was never carried out. The patient was then started on a fasting process in preparation for a CT scan. Later, the patient was found unconscious and died four weeks later, most likely as a result of low-blood-sugar-related brain damage. Although the doctor was acquitted in the lower court, a higher court reversed this decision and fined the doctor 5000 Danish kroner plus costs. In their view, the doctor should have checked that his verbal instruction had been acted upon. A major social media campaign was launched by medical organisations under the banner 'it could have been me' and this eventually led to the referral to the Supreme Court where the doctor was ultimately acquitted by a majority of four to three.[61]

Regulators Under Fire

From time to time, the regulators themselves have come under fire. The independent Inquiry into the mass murderer Harold Shipman (see Chapter Two) was very critical of the UK's GMC and led to the introduction of Independent Tribunals to hear serious misconduct cases in all registration bodies in the UK.

Investigations are clearly very challenging and stressful for professionals whose conduct is under review. An anonymous 2015 UK survey showed that doctors under investigation were significantly more likely to suffer anxiety, depression and have thoughts of self-harm. There have also been a number of reports into the number of suicides amongst healthcare professionals under investigation. The GMC in the UK is testing a new approach for doctors who have made a one-off clinical mistake. If it can be demonstrated that the practitioner understands what went wrong and has taken steps to ensure it will not happen again, then a full investigation will not be required.[62]

The UK's NMC was heavily criticised by the Professional Standards Authority for its handling of complaints about midwives at Furness General Hospital in Cumbria (see Chapter Three). The NMC had received its first complaint about potential problems in 2009 but it was not until 2017 that its last misconduct review was concluded.[63] Its disciplinary processes were not, it was ultimately agreed, fit for purpose and required change.

The Medical Board of Australia also faced much criticism, when, facing concerns about the quality of practice in rural and regional areas, it imposed a clinical examination on overseas doctors. Historically, doctors had not been required to immediately sit any local exams before they were placed in 'areas of need' and had up to three years to pass the examination. Under the new system, many failed the exam and lost their licences, to the dismay of their local communities. As the Chair of the Medical Board explained: 'The Board has a set of standards which are now being very deliberately implemented. For some people that raises the bar that they have to cross, to be able either to get into the workplace in the first place or remain in the workplace'. Ministers refused to intervene. Dr. Gerard Ingham, who had been supervising international doctors for 25 years, said the crackdown was long overdue. It was, he said, a mistake of previous policy that doctors could practise in rural areas without proving their competence and that the policy of 'any doctor is better than no doctor' was unacceptable.[64]

> *Dr. Maurice Haddad was an orthopaedic surgeon in Argentina for 30 years before bringing his wife and three sons to Australia. He worked as a GP in the small town of Wonthaggi. He became the only doctor in the region to deliver the methadone programme to drug-dependent patients. His surgical experience meant that he could treat patients with skin diseases and save rural patients the long drive to Melbourne. He had received an award for an outstanding contribution to rural communities. He failed the clinical examination and was deregistered.[65]*

The Medical Boards in the US have been under almost constant pressure since the Inspector General at the US Department of Health and Human Services reported in 1986 that their structure — typically comprised of doctors with only a small number of lay people — imposed strikingly few disciplinary actions for physician misconduct. However, his review of individual state performance was ended when the Justice Department declared that he had no jurisdiction over State Medical Boards, not funded or regulated by the Federal Government. The Federation of State Medical Boards has since stopped issuing enforcement data and instead now only publishes anonymised annual trends. These show that the number of physicians investigated in 2018 was less than in 2008 and the total number of licences revoked was only 248 — a very low number.

The Obama Administration provided federal funding to design and implement approaches that enhanced the portability of licences across States. The Trump Administration has recently highlighted the fact that such occupational licences still make it more difficult to move to another State where there are available jobs (though these economic arguments usually exclude occupational licences for medicine). Some US States have exploited their licensing powers to shockingly reinstate doctors previously struck off to provide healthcare for their burgeoning prison populations.[66]

In Canada, Medical Boards have come under pressure for their alleged endemic secrecy. Some Boards claim that privacy laws make it impossible for them to release investigative reports or complaints that result in disciplinary action. The Yukon Medical Council makes no disclosures at all, not even the dates when hearings will be held. As their Chairman put it: 'our policy is not to disclose. It's a confidential process'. However, many Canadian doctors also have licences to practice in the US, many of whose medical boards are much more willing to publish information about disciplinary events. Canadian citizens can and do access these US sites. The Ontario College of Physicians and Surgeons now publishes information about disciplinary hearings, but these are only available for two months. The register of individual doctors, which is open to the public, will, however, contain a note on any sanctions that have been imposed (but not include the circumstances).

Creating single boards to license the training and regulation of all healthcare professionals has always proven problematic. The merger of the medical and nursing boards in England has been suggested from time to time but nothing has happened. The Australian government proposed a single authority in a review they initiated after a Productivity Commission was highly critical of the inefficiency of the 90 professional boards in operation across the country. The Medical organisations objected, and the government withdrew the proposal and adopted a less fundamental reform of the system.

Regulation of Managers

It has been suggested from time to time that healthcare service managers should be regulated, but given the range of disciplines, filling such posts it has proven almost impossible. Who, other than an employer, can judge the professional merits of a Chief Executive? Who, other than an employer, could judge the performance of the head of a service department such as medical records? The conduct of one NHS Chief Executive accused of mismanagement was reviewed by the Institute of Health Services Management who decided he had no case to answer. He may have been wrong but he was not unprofessional. The only sanction in this case would have been the removal of his membership that was not essential for another post. Treasurers who have admitted mistakes in financial reporting have been sacked by their employers but not struck off a professional register unless their conduct was corrupt in some way. Those who want regulation are searching for a means of ensuring that a manager dismissed by one employer can never work for another health organisation. Some managers who have been sacked are perfectly capable of performing well in a different situation or at a lower grade level.

Regulation for managers is therefore not a practical idea, but employers should be just as careful in making managerial appointments as they are with clinical posts.

Lessons for the Future

Can the principle of self-regulation be sustained for much longer in the complex world of modern medicine? Can the healthcare professions be trusted to protect the public from practitioners who harm patients, or is their primary focus always going to be the protection of their professions? There are some who think that many professional oversight systems are slow to act, fast to find excuses for problems and fail in their duty to protect the public. Some of the cases in this chapter would support such a view. But would a State or national government run system, or independent boards, dominated by patient interests and politics work any better? Would it turn the regulator, in the eyes of the professions, into an enemy who must be fought at every turn? Self-regulation, it can be argued, binds the professions into conduct and standards that they have established and, as a result, they respect and comply with. In some jurisdictions, governments have moved to deal with this problem by changing the balance between professional and lay members on licensing boards. There do, however, remain worries that the licensing bodies are too lenient in letting practitioners return to the register after a period of suspension. The NMC in the UK has in past reinstated or just cautioned practitioners found guilty of major criminal offences, including smuggling heroin and sexual assault.

The current systems of licensing are very expensive. The combined cost of the healthcare regulatory bodies in the UK is £300 million a year, a cost that is primarily met by the practitioners who are being licensed to practise. The Australian Regulator has 744,437 registrants. In the UK, there are 1.5 million. These are huge businesses. The economic evidence that there is a link between licensing and service quality is, according to some economists, tenuous at best.[67] The Trump Administration rolled back on occupational licensing although, to be clear, they probably had florists, beauticians and dog walkers in mind. However, assistants such as nursing associates are increasingly being drawn into the licensing net.

Regulators are now increasingly demanding that some form of revalidation be considered. Many have taken the view that a licence to practise should not be for life. A UK government review in 2007 advised that revalidation was necessary for the healthcare professions, but its intensity and frequency needed to be proportionate to the risks inherent in the work in which each practitioner is involved.

Doctors in the UK now have to revalidate every five years and go through an annual appraisal with a responsible officer (usually a senior doctor in a healthcare organisation) or submit annual returns and use an assessment tool. Nurses go through a similar process every three years and have to demonstrate that they have completed sufficient hours of practice and programmes of continued professional development, sought practice-based feedback and had this confirmed by a line manager or other registered nurse or midwife. Australian nurses go through a similar process.

In the US, the process varies from State to State with some, but not all, requiring evidence of continuing education and professional development as one of their renewal requirements. The Canadian Code of Ethics requires doctors to engage in lifelong learning but there is no traditional revalidation in most Canadian provinces. However, regulatory bodies do undertake random assessments of clinical performance and insist on review for any practitioner over the age of 70 years.

Australian doctors decided not to follow the revalidation route. Instead they plan to develop a Professional Performance Framework to support doctors to take responsibility for their own performance. The Health Professions Council in England has also concluded that revalidation is not appropriate for the professions that it regulates. The Pharmaceutical Council has an online validation system that allows practitioners to record their continuing professional development events and every three years submit a reflective account focussed on communication skills, behaving professionally or leadership.[68]

Underlying the concerns about revalidation is the complexity of reaching a judgement about clinical competence. Dr. Harold Shipman, who murdered many of his patients, would have scored highly on some aspects of an appraisal. Until he was convicted, he was highly regarded by many of his patients. No clear evidence has yet emerged about the link between revalidation and safety and quality, but some commentators have pointed out that it does strengthen organisational accountability, particularly in hospitals.[69]

Overall, doctors are not of the view that revalidation improves healthcare. The processes are complex and burdensome, and in the view of some, are driving many doctors to leave the profession prematurely. Since revalidation was introduced in the UK in 2012, the number of doctors who have given up their licence to practise has increased sharply.[70] Niall Dickson, the then Chief Executive of the GMC thought that the concept of revalidation was sound but the Chairman of the British Medical Association saw it as an administrative burden with little evidence to show that it could produce positive changes in clinical practice.[71]

Another recent trend has been to enforce a distinction between those who investigate complaints and concerns and those who decide on the outcomes. The argument is that the regulatory bodies should not be both the judge and the jury when decisions are being made about a licence to practise. Most regulatory bodies handle the first stages of any investigation themselves and then decide whether to proceed to the next stage. The majority of cases are resolved at this stage if the practitioner acknowledges that an error has been made and has taken steps to prevent a reoccurrence. A warning, reprimand or undertaking to remediate is often enough. Sometimes, a programme of remediation is set out in a legal agreement.

However, more serious cases of alleged misconduct are increasingly being referred to independent tribunals such as the Medical Practitioners Tribunal in the UK that have a strong legal foundation.[72] Some cases also lead to claims of negligence, which are explored in depth in Chapter Five.

There have also been concerns raised about evidence that practitioners undergoing investigation by the GMC and other regulators are significantly more likely to suffer anxiety, depression and have thoughts of self-harm. According to Clare Gerada, a former President of the Royal College of General Practice, doctors live in fear of receiving a legalistic accusatory sounding letter from the GMC. All professionals, she argues, should be regarded as being at risk of self-harm once investigations have been launched.

Hypervigilance might also produce defensive medicine and block innovation. Doctors and patients are often as frustrated as each other by the time it takes to deal with disciplinary matters.

But does the safety of the public require all of these expensive regulatory bodies, and do they work for the people they are meant to protect? Is there an alternative way of protecting the public? Do medical and other schools really need a licence to operate and regular inspection? Could we be persuaded that the medical, nursing, pharmacy and other schools could produce competent professionals ready to start practice on qualification and trust the professionals to keep themselves up to date? There might be a need for mandatory refreshers every five years to take account of the rapidly changing face of medicine. Some employers already insist on regular training and continual assessment for their staff. Should the licensing bodies duplicate this? Misconduct and health reviews could be undertaken by quasi-legal organisations such as the Medical Practitioners Tribunal service. Given that teamwork is fundamental to modern medicine, a single organisation could deal with all professions in most provinces, States or countries. This approach seems to work in New York. Such a step would also consolidate codes of conduct and ethics for healthcare professionals who work together in teams.

Some licensing bodies have been corrupted by bribery and kickbacks that devalue not only local professional standards but also international reputation.[73]

Given increases in the migration of healthcare professionals, it needs to be easier to establish the international validity of basic qualifications and track decisions about misconduct. An international licensing passport, kept up to date by the licensing bodies concerned, is certainly worthy of discussion.

This is an area of public policy where change is slow. The current systems have obvious flaws, are expensive, and the evidence to show that they really protect the public is weak.

Chapter Five
Medical Negligence

As we saw in Chapter Three, there are occasions when patients are hurt or lose their lives whilst being treated or cared for. For the most part, such injuries result from simple unavoidable accidents, but on occasion, they are a consequence of malpractice amounting to negligence. Sometimes, an individual healthcare professional is to blame, but it is also possible that the harm caused is more appropriately and fairly attributed to the failure of a healthcare system.

Medical negligence is normally defined as the inadequate treatment of a patient by a healthcare professional, which leads to injury, pain, trauma or the worsening of an existing medical condition. A more legalistic definition would explain professional negligence as an act or omission by a healthcare professional in which treatment falls below the accepted standard of practice in the medical community and causes injury or death to a patient. All health and social care professionals understand negligence in similar ways.

In some countries, such as the UK or the US, patients affected by negligence have to pursue their claims through a court of law, often on a no-win-no-fee basis. Other countries, however, have developed compensation systems that do not require proof of negligence, but only proof of damage. Examples from eight countries are discussed below.

The Swedish system for the compensation of patient injuries dates back to 1975 and was originally based on a voluntary patient insurance solution. In 1997, the Patient Insurance Act required healthcare providers to carry patient insurance that covered compensation for injuries. In Sweden, county councils are responsible for most medical services and are therefore the target of most claims. They use a common insurer. A Patient Claims Panel issues advisory opinions on cases referred to it by patients, care providers or insurers. Although these are classed as advisory opinions, there is a high level of acceptance of the conclusions reached.

The main types of compensable injuries are diagnostic, treatment and infection related. A causal relationship must be established between the injury and the medical care received and it must be demonstrated that the injury could have been avoided. The key test is whether there is a substantial likelihood that the injury was caused by defects in medical equipment, incorrect or delayed diagnosis, infection, accidents whilst in care, prescribing problems, risky care without consent and other reasons. A claim is only compensated if the injuries to the patient would not have occurred in the hands of an excellent healthcare practitioner: 'the experienced specialist rule'. Thus, the benchmark is set at excellent care, rather than acceptable care. In 2018, there were 1801 claimant cases heard of which about 10% received compensation. There is a financial limit to claims. The processes used in the compensation system are highly digitalised.[1]

It is asserted that a key benefit of this system is that it supports a no-blame culture for doctors. Claimants do not have to prove that the doctor was guilty of negligence or made an error or omission. There is no risk for the doctor as employers pay the insurance premiums.[2] Nor is there a risk of disciplinary action, as insurance companies never share the outcomes with other organisations. It is also argued that the system facilitates a higher rate of adverse event and near miss reporting.

Poland adopted a similar system, with rather less success, as the Supreme Audit Office reported in 2018: 'the extrajudicial system of adjudication on medical events by the district committees does not provide patients with an effective route for quickly obtaining compensation and has not become an alternative to the judiciary'. Poland does not have the same level of compliance with panel (district committee) opinions. Reform of the system was under active debate in 2020.[3]

New Zealand has a national system of accidental injury compensation funded by taxpayers. Injured patients receive government-funded compensation but relinquish the right to sue for damages except in rare cases involving reckless conduct. Patients can file a claim without the support of a lawyer. Healthcare professionals can still be held to account (and punished) through separate accountability processes. Doctors are free to participate in the compensation claims process without fear of punishment. The focus of the compensation scheme is to provide assistance with treatment and rehabilitation rather than proving negligence. Patients cannot sue for medical negligence. However, the New Zealand system has its critics and the following two cases have been used to illustrate some of the problems.

When Vicky Gibson took her eight-year-old son Kaya to an ophthalmologist for the second time in 10 weeks, she knew something was seriously wrong. Kaya was nearly blind. He could not see food on his plate and used his feet to find things in front of him. The ophthalmologist did not seem overly concerned and thought his symptoms were functional i.e. he was making them up. He made a semi-acute referral to a paediatrician to rule out a neurological condition. In fact, Kaya was terminally ill with a metabolic brain disease. Had the ophthalmologist referred him to another specialist when he was first seen, his life might have been saved with a bone marrow transplant. Mrs. Gibson complained to the Health and Disability Commissioner, who decided to take no action. Expert advice had determined that the ophthalmologist's care had been reasonable and consistent with expected standards.

In a second case involving the same Commissioner, an optometrist failed to diagnose a brain tumour as the cause of vision and eye problems in a six-year-old child. His diagnosis was lazy eye and exotropia (outward turning eye). He failed to refer the child for further testing. Although the optometrist breached the patient's code of rights, he was not referred for disciplinary action.

Professor Jo Manning, an expert in health law has pointed out the glaring inconsistency in these two cases. 'Patients who cannot sue for medical negligence because of our Accident Compensation

Corporation laws are being denied justice', she said. She recommended that decisions by the Commissioner be subject either to expert review or appeal.[4] There is little evidence that the no-fault system has markedly improved patient safety.[5]

> *The Danish compensation system provides information and compensation to patients regardless of whether negligence is involved. There is no cost to a claimant for filing a claim. The hospital or clinician is required to file a detailed response to a claim and patients have access to their medical records and a detailed description of the medical reviewer's conclusions. A case worker is assigned to each patient to help them through the process. The compensation is awarded if reviewers determine that the care could have been better, or if the patient experienced a rare and severe complication that was more extensive than the patient should reasonably have to endure. The average claim paid was US$30,000.[6]*

The law in France changed in 2002 with the introduction of a National Compensation Medical Office (Public Guarantee Fund) to compensate certain patient injuries when no party is found to be legally liable as well as accelerate and guarantee payment when liability exists. It ended professional liability for wrongful birth and a government decree subsidised liability insurance for obstetricians by having social security pay a portion of their premiums. In a second reform, an Alternative Dispute Procedure was instituted as an alternative to using the courts for certain grave medical injuries, using Conciliation Commissions.

Germany has strengthened patients' rights to the extent that a physician must inform the patient of any treatment error if it becomes recognisable to the physician, and this information must be provided either on the request of the patient or when it is necessary to avert injurious consequences. The information can be used in criminal proceedings only with the consent of the physician. This is in line with a long-standing principle of no self-incrimination. The information can, however, be used in civil cases. Most of the mistakes lead to only temporary side effects but in a few cases, the consequences are more serious — around 1% died. Most of the complaints involved surgery on the knee or hip joint followed by a lack of treatment for broken legs, arms or ankles.

In England, all claims are made to a single organisation: NHS Resolution, which is largely funded by NHS organisations, thereby creating a large risk pool. Similar fault-based schemes operate in the rest of the UK. Scotland has considered a move to a no-fault scheme, but no action has yet been taken.

In Australia, medical malpractice laws vary from State to State, but usually three things must be established in order to make a claim. The treatment must meet Australian standards, result in suffering or injury, and the harm has to be as a direct result of the negligence.

In the US, claims start at State level, with failure to correctly diagnose comprising the largest percentage of cases. In some States, punitive damages can be awarded.

The costs involved in compensating patients are enormous. In England, the bill in 2017–2018 was £1.63 billion. The provision for claims that may turn into liabilities was £83 billion as of the end of March 2019.[7] In the US, it is estimated that the total annual cost of the medical liability system, including 'defensive medicine' was about 2.4% of total healthcare spending.[8]

Many healthcare professionals insure themselves against legal claims, and this adds to the overall cost of healthcare. A surgeon in the US might have to pay up to US$50,000 a year or more for adequate coverage. Some US States insist on physicians having malpractice insurance, though others do not. In many countries, healthcare professionals obtain such cover through their employer. The insurance market is volatile with regular withdrawals by providers.[9] Texas and many other States have introduced financial limits to non-economic damage (i.e. pain and suffering).[10]

Of course, all such systems are open to patient abuse. Some claimants have attempted to defraud the systems by exaggerating their injuries, but they are often caught.

Leslie Elder was sentenced to five months in prison and fined for contempt of court after fraudulently exaggerating her injuries in order to seek £2.5m damages. She had undergone a vaginal mesh operation in 2010 that she alleged had left her in constant pain and with restricted mobility. She claimed to have to walk with a stick, using crutches on occasion and sometimes a wheelchair. Elder also claimed that she was unable to work. It later emerged that the operation had not been necessary at all because she had been misdiagnosed. The hospital admitted liability but appealed the amount of damages awarded. Surveillance of Elder in 2016 showed her walking unaided. She had also been to Spain for a hen party for her daughter. She received some damages but the judge hearing her case found that she had grossly, dishonestly and repeatedly exaggerated her symptoms.[11]

It is not just healthcare professionals that owe a duty of care to patients. In England, this responsibility extends to receptionists in emergency departments.

Following a head injury, a patient attended a hospital in South London with a friend. The receptionist advised him that the waiting time was four or five hours. He was not told that he would be triaged within 30 minutes of his arrival. He waited for 19 minutes and then left without telling anyone. After arriving home, the patient deteriorated and suffered a significant lasting injury. When the case was first heard, the Hospital Trust argued that the fault lay with the patient for leaving the hospital. However, the Supreme Court overruled this decision and decided that as soon as the patient presented at the hospital a duty of care had been established. The patient should have been clearly told about the triage policy.[12]

There are many case studies of negligence claims, but the following examples allow readers to distil some practical ways of preventing recurrences.

Mrs. D had suffered from back problems and agreed to undergo a spinal operation in order to regain the degree of mobility and flexibility she had enjoyed before her affliction. She had young children. She had agreed to a discectomy, an operation that would either remove the section of a disc that was pressing on a nerve or the spinal cord or have it replaced altogether; whichever was more likely to achieve the outcome she wanted. However, during the operation, the surgeon, finding himself without the right equipment for a discectomy had to perform a fusion operation instead. The patient was in considerable pain after the operation and has been left with permanent debilitating back and leg pain. The hospital admitted a breach of duty, but not negligence, and Mrs. D received a large financial settlement.[13]

Mr. I was supposed to have a back surgery that involved inserting titanium surgical rods into his spine. His surgeon could not find the rods that were supposed to be inserted. Instead he removed the handle from a screwdriver and inserted it into Mr. I's back. Within a few days it broke, causing serious pain and a complete lack of stability in the patient's spine. The patient underwent several more operations but died two years later. His estate was awarded substantial damages.[14]

In both of these cases, a check that everything required was available prior to surgery would have pre-empted the problem. The prime responsibility lies with the surgeon, but other theatre staff should have double-checked. This should have been a routine way of working, as it is in most operating theatres. Failure to follow standard operating procedures is a common cause of medical accidents.

The following examples illustrate errors that can be classified as 'Never' events, which were also discussed in Chapter Three.

In 2003, a heart and lung transplant at Duke University Hospital in the US was performed on 17-year-old Jesica Santilian, who suffered from congenital restrictive cardiomyopathy. The family were illegal immigrants from Mexico. They lived in a trailer home and begged on the streets for money to pay for her transplant. She was placed on a waiting list for three years until a donor was found. The surgeon had almost completed the transplants when he learned that the organs came from a donor with type A blood, incompatible with Jesica's type O. Jesica was kept on life support systems until, astonishingly, another donor was found. However, despite the second transplant, Jesica died. The surgeon took responsibility for the error. Not one of the more than a dozen people working at Duke Hospital and the two organisations responsible for sourcing the new heart and lungs for Jesica ever cross-checked her blood group before surgery to see if it was a match with the blood type of the donor. After this tragic event, double-checking was introduced for all transplant procedures. The New England Journal of Medicine commented: 'When a medical mistake receives this much attention it affects the medical profession and even public policy'.[15]

A patient brought a dental negligence claim against a dental surgeon on the grounds that he had performed unnecessary fillings and root canal work, as well as prescribing antibiotics for the pain she was suffering from, rather than investigating its cause, She was later seen by a locum dentist who immediately identified mouth cancer and referred to a local hospital where she underwent surgery for squamous cell carcinoma. She was awarded a four-figure sum in damages but also reported the dentist to his regulator who placed restrictions on his practice.[16]

In 2014, an Air Force veteran went for treatment at a VA medical centre in Los Angeles for a possible cancer in his left testicle. The surgeons removed the healthy testicle by mistake. The mistake was traced back to the patient's record where the surgeon had failed to mark the correct side before the operation.[17]

As part of her treatment for breast cancer, a patient needed to have a lymph node removed from her armpit, but the surgery was performed on the wrong side. The surgeon wrote down the wrong side during a busy multidisciplinary team meeting when the laboratory results for both sides were discussed. The surgeon's notes, including the error, were typed up by the administrator, put into the medical notes and fed into the operating theatre list session. The patient had a benign lump on the opposite side to where the surgery was intended. When the patient was examined prior to surgery the surgeon felt the lump on the wrong side. The WHO Safe Surgery Checklist was undertaken pre-procedure, but the imaging and histology results were not reviewed, only the patient's record. The error was found when the results of the test on the node that had been removed came back as benign. The patient was readmitted, and the correct procedure undertaken.[18]

Willie King, a heavy equipment operator with a diabetes-related circulatory disease, was due to have his right leg cut off below the knee. Instead, the left leg was amputated in error following a series of mistakes. The incorrect leg was listed in various places including on the board in the operating room, the hospital computer system, and the operating room schedule. Staff had sterilised and prepped the wrong leg for surgery. The patient's other leg was later amputated at another hospital. He now walks with artificial legs. King was awarded damages of US$1.15 million. The surgeon lost his licence to practise for six months.[19]

Surgical errors such as these, are widely reported but represent an exceedingly small proportion of all the surgery performed. Surgery remains a highly skilled procedure and it is impossible to remove all danger and risk for the patient. Informing patients of the risks involved and the chances of the success of a particular procedure has been the cause of much litigation. Surgeons must provide patients with full, frank and transparent information in a way that they can understand.

A patient in their mid-70s with a history of heart disease presented with continuing problems re-presented with recurrent early prosthetic aortic valve endocarditis, haemolysis, because of a leak around the aortic valve, and moderate recurrent mitral regurgitation. The indication for

> *the operation appeared to be haemolysis related to the aortic valve rather than mitral regurgitation, and the patient was consented for redo AVR +/– mitral valve surgery. The quoted risk of death for this procedure was 10%–15%, but EuroSCORE II[20] was calculated to be 33.7%. The patient underwent urgent redo mitral valve replacement (only) and died three days later from liver failure. The Panel judged that the operative decision-making was unclear, the patient received a different operation from that they had consented to and the actual risk of surgery was significantly higher than the risk that had been quoted.[21]*

Anaesthetic mistakes have resulted in a number of malpractice cases. When patients are placed under general anaesthetic during surgery, they usually receive two types of anaesthesia. One is a paralytic to prevent movement and the other is inhalation anaesthesia to cause loss of consciousness. Studies show that 0.1%–0.2% of patients are partially awake during surgery. This is termed Intraoperative Awareness (IOA).

> *In 2006, Sherman Sizemore, a Baptist minister, underwent an exploratory laparotomy. Whilst the paralytic was properly administered, inhalational anaesthesia was never turned on. This meant that the patient was awake throughout the surgery, could feel everything, but was paralysed and could not move or speak. Sixteen minutes into surgery, the medical team realised this and acted. They also gave him a drug to induce amnesia of the event. The patient was never informed of what had taken place and subsequently suffered insomnia and nightmares. He committed suicide a few weeks later. The case was settled on a confidential basis in 2008.[22]*

Diagnostic results are normally very reliable, but mistakes do happen, often involving identity errors. Diagnostic errors are involved in over 30% of malpractice claims.

> *Darrie Eason, aged 35 years, was told she had an invasive form of breast cancer and went into hospital in 2007 for a double mastectomy on her doctor's advice. She sought a second opinion that confirmed the advice.*

> *After her surgery, she learned that the laboratory had mislabelled her biopsy results and she did not have breast cancer at all. Her case against the hospital was settled for US$2.5 million and she went on national television to warn other women. 'A second opinion is good, but a second biopsy is better', she said. It was only after the Eason error came to light that the other woman involved in the mix-up was told that her biopsy report had also been wrong; she had breast cancer.[23]*

Nursing home care is of variable quality in many jurisdictions and has produced a number of malpractice claims against the owners.

> *An elderly woman with early onset dementia was neglected so severely in a Florida nursing home that she fell and struck her head on a number of occasions, finally causing a subdural hematoma. Relatives brought a legal suit alleging that staffing was inadequate and treatment negligent. On the day of the final fall, only half of the required staff were on duty. It transpired that the nursing staff had asked the administrators for more staff without success. Staff had been shifted by the owners from one facility to another when regulators performed inspections to make it appear that they had more staff than were actually on the payroll. The final settlement in the case was US$1 million, the full extent of the nursing home's insurance policy limit.[24]*

Maternity care results in some of the most expensive malpractice claims as these can involve the costs of rearing both injured and healthy children. Such cases represent 50% of the total value of claims in England.

> *In Australia, K. A. Melchior asked gynaecologist Dr. A. Cattanach for a tubal ligation to be performed on her, citing her financial inability to support a third child. She recalled having one ovary removed as a teenager and that her fallopian tube had also been removed. Cattanach, seeing no evidence of a fallopian tube, assumed that Mrs. Melchior's recollection was correct. Sometime later, she became pregnant and sued her doctor. The*

> *Supreme Court of Queensland held that the failure of Mr. Cattanach to warn the Melchior's of their capacity to conceive and his negligent advice caused them to become parents of an unplanned child and awarded the couple substantial damages, including a sum for the cost of raising and maintaining a child. A subsequent appeal by Mr. Cattanach and the State of Queensland who were vicariously liable for his actions failed.[25] However, a few months later the Queensland Parliament passed a law that prevented courts awarding damages for financial loss suffered in rearing a healthy child.*

In Chapter Three, the serious problems with maternity services in Shrewsbury, England, were discussed. There is a possibility that this scandal may lead to hundreds of claims for damages by bereaved parents and relatives.

> *The claimant's mother opted for VBAC.[26] There had been an interval of 16 months between the previous caesarean and the expected due date for her new baby. The mode of delivery was discussed at 16 weeks with the consultant and a maternal preference for vaginal delivery was noted. The mother attended hospital at 41 weeks gestation, having noticed occasional tightening, but she was not in labour. Prostin E2 3mg was inserted and IV Syntocinon was commenced 24 hours later, with three increases in the rate of infusion in the next three hours up to 36 lml/hour. Ultimately, a forceps delivery was performed, following a delay in the second stage, in the presence of fetal bradycardia. Blood and mucus needed to be removed from the claimant's trachea before intubation and successful re-establishment of the circulation. When the claimant's mother was taken to theatre post-delivery, when the placenta did not deliver, a gaping hole was discovered in the lower segment of the uterus. The claimant, as a result of this, has cerebral palsy. The principal allegations were: (1) that in breach of the Trust's own guidelines, medical induction was carried out despite the fact that these guidelines stipulate that there should be no such induction in women with a previous caesarean section scar and; (2) that the Claimant's mother was not advised antenataly, or following her admission to hospital, of the increased risk of uterine rupture associated with induction of labour.*

> *Liability was admitted. The Trust's guidelines on use of prostaglandins for induction in a VBAC case were inconsistent with the Royal College of Obstetricians and Gynaecologist's guidelines and it was accepted that there had been a failure to consult the claimant's mother about the increased risk of uterine rupture with induction of labour in a VBAC case. The claim resolved on the basis of an order for periodic payments with a conventional lump sum value of £6.1 million.*[27]

Operating theatres are extremely complicated environments in which to work, and as technological advances continue to accelerate, sometimes the sophisticated equipment utilised can be operated incorrectly or go wrong.

> *Lisa Smart, the wife of a New York policeman, was admitted to Beth Israel hospital for the removal of a benign tumour on her uterus. What she did not know was that her two surgeons were using a new piece of equipment supplied by Johnson & Johnson for the first time and that the salesman would be present in the theatre. The machine pumped too much saline into Mrs. Smart's body, causing her to die of a cardiac arrest some hours later. The hospital was fined but no charges were brought against the doctors. Her husband, in evidence to a Committee of Congress, claimed that she would have been alive today if she had been allowed access to the National Practitioner Data Bank that would have disclosed that one of the surgeons was on probation for misconduct.*[28]

The problem of foreign bodies being left inside patients after surgery still happens despite many attempts to introduce procedures to prevent it. It has been estimated that it occurs in between 0.3 and 1 per 1000 abdominal operations. Sponges are the most common foreign body, followed by surgical instruments and clamps. Before every operation, a scrub nurse or operating department practitioner counts the number of operating instruments and swabs and then repeats this when the operation is complete. Evidently, these should tally. One of the most harrowing and drawn out cases of the consequences of leaving a foreign body inside a patient began in 2009.

Kapka Petrov, then 33 years old, was working as a vocational rehabilitation consultant, handling disability management claims for an Ontario government institution. She awoke one morning with abdominal pain so severe she had trouble walking. At the hospital, after initial tests seemed to rule out gallstones, she was given morphine and sent home with dietary restrictions to calm a suspected inflammation of her pancreas. However, she grew sicker and the pain more intense and so she returned to hospital. Within a week she underwent surgery to have her gallbladder removed.

But something was still not right.

'I paid attention that when I came out from the surgery the other patients that were with me in the room for recovery were able to stand up, to walk around, to move, and to eventually go home with the help of their family members', Petrov recalls. 'I could not move. Something was very heavy and pulling wherever the surgery was on the right upper abdominal side.'

In what was to become a numbingly familiar refrain in the months ahead, the nurses assured her that some post-operative pain was to be expected and could be managed with appropriate medication. The next day, her surgeon informed her that the gallbladder had been full of stones and so inflamed that in removing it he had caused a minor haemorrhage of the liver. He assured her that everything should be fine, though, and she should just stay home and take her painkillers. After a few days of escalating discomfort and vomiting, Petrov and her husband, fretful and confused, returned to the hospital to appeal for help. She underwent more surgery, this time an ERCP liver procedure and a sphincterotomy to release any remaining stones that might be causing the trouble. She was discharged from hospital and sent home with a jar of morphine.

In the ensuing months, the pain and gastro problems persisted. Her original doctor insisted it was not a surgical issue and instructed her not to bother calling again. Her gastroenterologist filed a report stating that she was much improved. She and her husband tried another hospital, hoping for a second surgical opinion. After more tests, Petrov was administered a cancer medication for nausea to go along with the continuing morphine. After several visits, she was again told that her problem was a pain management issue. The implications were clear. This was mostly in her head.

Still, Petrov and her husband pressed for answers. A new MRI, like the previous ones, seemed to indicate everything was fine. Yet she was now so weak she needed help to dress, shower and eat. Her husband almost lost his job because of all the time he spent attending to her needs. Her 12-year-old daughter was an emotional wreck, convinced she was about to lose her mother.

Her parents, back home in Bulgaria, were certain that she was dying. They urged her to fly there and seek treatment. She spent several weeks at a hospital in Sofia, seeing several specialists, before undergoing another round of surgery. This operation took place on March 19, 2010, almost a year from the day of her first surgery back in Toronto. The Bulgarian doctor discovered a surgical metal clip deep inside Petrov's abdomen, inadvertently left behind during her original Toronto operation and not visible through standard testing. That clip had been clenching the main nerve of the liver, along with an artery, the ganglion and a 3.5 cm remnant cystic duct.

The main nerve of the liver had become so deformed it had to be extracted completely, along with peripheral nerves on the gastro tract that had also been damaged. That had been the cause of months of debilitating pain and frustration.

Two years later, during her slow, continuing recovery, Petrov suddenly fell ill again and required an emergency hysterectomy. Once again, she was wracked with severe pains, this time in the pelvic and rectal regions. Her doctors prescribed painkillers and suggested anti-depressants. Six months later, a surgeon concluded Petrov was suffering from damage to the pudendal nerve and gave her a nerve block injection, which led to partial paralysis on her left side.

Petrov felt herself sliding into the same trauma she had endured earlier. She returned to Bulgaria to search for a solution. There, surgeons found a huge endometrial nest in her left ovary, as well as severe burns to the sigmoid colon and urinary tract from the laparoscopic hysterectomy.

'It's obvious, mistakes happen in the medical community', she says. 'My expectation as a patient is that you don't run away, that as a doctor you come back, and you help me to get better instead of closing yourself in your own insecurity shell.'

Petrov has drawn deeply from her own misfortunes in lobbying for the importance of the patient's voice. As a member of Patients for Patient Safety Canada, she has tapped into an enriching reserve of empathy and support.[29]

Emergency departments are high-pressure settings within a hospital and, perhaps unsurprisingly, are often the scene of medical mistakes.

> *The plaintiff, who was 48 years old, suffered a fall at her home and was taken to the Accident and Emergency department at a large Dublin Hospital. She was complaining of pain in her right arm and an X-ray of her wrist confirmed that she had suffered from a right Colles' fracture. No examination was made of her elbow despite her complaints of pain. She was admitted and had an open reduction to the fracture of her right wrist. She was discharged with a plaster and seen at a follow-up clinic on two occasions over the next six weeks. At no point was an injury to her elbow investigated. After a routine scan of her wrist she asked the radiographer to scan her elbow. The scan confirmed a dislocation that was then treated. Due to the delay, the joint had been irreparably damaged, and the patient lost a significant range of motion in her arm. The hospital admitted liability and the case was settled for Euro 250,000.*[30]

However, deciding on when injuries actually occurred can be complicated, as the following case illustrates.

> *A young woman was a rear-seat passenger in a vehicle that was involved in a road accident and suffered severe spinal injuries. On arrival at hospital at 10.15am, the patient was able to assist the nurse in removing her trousers and to push her feet against the nurse's hand. However, an hour later she could no longer move her legs. A scan at 3.00pm revealed a fracture of the spine and she was referred to another hospital for surgery.*
>
> *The insurers of the negligent motorist settled the claim for £3m but started contribution proceedings against the hospital on the grounds that insufficient precautions had been taken in the emergency room. Expert witnesses demonstrated that the fracture dislocation almost certainly occurred at the accident rather than at the hospital.*[31]

One surgical practice, until recently a well-kept secret, was for some surgeons to carve their initials on patients and their organs during operations.

> *Simon Bramhall, a distinguished liver surgeon, used an argon beam machine to write his initials on the organs of anaesthetised patients in 2013 whilst working at Birmingham's Queen Elizabeth Hospital. After one of his operations failed (for reasons unconnected with his actions) another surgeon spotted his initials on the organ. He was fined and given a community sentence followed by a formal warning by the General Medical Council. His conduct was, the Judge said, 'conduct born of professional arrogance of such magnitude that it strayed into criminal behaviour'.[32]*

> *In 2000, Liana Gedz, a Russian-born dentist, gave birth by caesarean section to a healthy girl at Beth Israel Hospital in New York. A day or two later she discovered that her doctor had carved his initials 'AZ' into her abdomen. Gedz commented: 'I feel like a branded animal'. The doctor resigned but continued to practise at another centre for five months. He was later found guilty of assault, sentenced to probation and barred from practising medicine for five years. A financial settlement was agreed for US$1.75 million. Beth Israel Hospital was also fined and told to improve its oversight of doctors.[33] Mrs. Getz later gave evidence to a committee of the US Congress arguing for public access to the National Practitioner Data Bank.*

Medical Manslaughter

On occasion, a negligent act leads to criminal charges as happened in both of the surgeon branding case studies. Medical manslaughter is involuntary manslaughter where the patient's death has resulted from a grossly negligent (but otherwise lawful) act or omission. Such cases are rare but on the increase. In England, 11 doctors were charged with medical manslaughter between 2006 and 2013. Six were convicted and three given custodial sentences. In Australia, there were cases in 2000 and 2006, and in the US, just 14 cases have resulted in convictions in the past 30 years.[34,35]

In 1994, a case reached the House of Lords in England.

Dr. Adomako was the anaesthetist in charge of a patient during an eye operation. During the operation, an oxygen pipe became disconnected from the ventilator. Adomako failed to notice the disconnection for six minutes, and as a result, the patient died. The anaesthetist was convicted of manslaughter. His gross negligence had been enough to amount to criminal liability.[36] The House of Lords confirmed the conviction but defined a four-stage test for gross negligent manslaughter that became known as the Adomako Test. The defendant must owe the victim a duty of care and breach that care. The breach must cause or significantly contribute to the victim's death and the breach must be grossly negligent.[37]

In 2000, Dr. Margaret Joy Pearce, a Brisbane GP, injected a baby with morphine to stop her struggling whilst she examined her burnt hand. The dose was 15 mg — about 10 times the required amount. The baby died overnight. The Court sentenced Dr. Pearce to five years in jail suspended after six months. Dr. Pearce's registration was reinstated three years later.[38]

In 2008, Dr. Arthur Garry Gow inappropriately prescribed morphine tartrate for unsupervised use to a patient with lower back pain. The prescription was grossly excessive and did not include adequate directions for use. The drug is normally only prescribed for patients in the terminal stages of cancer. The patient died of an overdose. Gow admitted his guilt and was sentenced to a term of imprisonment that was suspended. Justifying his decision to suspend the sentence, the Judge explained: 'system failure had contributed to the death and professional people do make mistakes'.[39]

Other judges in Australia have been reluctant to associate negligence with medical manslaughter as the following case demonstrates.

In 2011, a baby named Tully Oliver Kavanagh died from hypoxic-ischaemic encephalopathy in Adelaide. The baby boy was a twin. His mother, against her doctor's advice, had opted for a planned home birth where the only supervision was provided by a former midwife and home-birth campaigner Lisa Barrett.

The first twin was born healthy, but Tully's heart rate dropped and his mother noticed a large blood clot so they raced him to hospital. Clinicians managed to resuscitate him but diagnosed brain damage that was, in the words of the local coroner: 'incompatible with life'. Life support was turned off. The police charged Lisa Barrett with manslaughter deciding that her care of Tully's mother was so negligent that it required a criminal punishment. The case eventually ended up in the Australian Supreme Court, where the judge decided that whilst Lisa Barrett's conduct was less than competent, she was not satisfied that her conduct merited a criminal sanction.[40]

The first manslaughter case in Hong Kong involved the use of sedative drugs during an illegal abortion in 2003 and a small number of further cases have followed.[41]

The UK has seen a steadily increasing number of cases and some of the most notable are presented below.

In 2003, a teenage patient died after a toxic cancer drug was wrongly injected into his spinal fluid at a Nottingham hospital. It should have been injected into a vein. He was undergoing treatment for leukaemia, from which he was in remission, when the mistake happened. The doctor who ordered the wrong drug, Feda Mulhem, had only been working at the hospital for two days when the error occurred. He was charged and convicted of manslaughter and later sentenced to eight months in prison. The General Medical Council later withdrew his licence for a year. An independent report later criticised the hospital for poor procedures and highlighted design faults with the syringes.[42]

Dr. Bala Kovvali had qualified as a doctor in India, but worked as a GP in Sheffield for some years before returning to India but coming back to the UK every summer for two or three months to work for a deputising service. In June 2009, he was called to see a patient who had been reported as 'very mumbling and muddled with erratic breathing, thirst, sunken eyes and a breath that smelt of pear drops'. Dr. Kovvali said the patient was depressed and should visit his GP the following day for his medication to be reviewed.

> *The patient did have a history of anxiety and depression, but died in bed that evening. The court heard that the patient had run out of insulin in his body and switched to burning fatty acids and producing acidic ketones. When ketones are produced in excess, the blood becomes more acidic and blood sugar levels rise, leading to a coma. In the view of one expert witness, Dr. Kovvali could and should have checked the patients sugar levels and referred the patient to hospital. He was sentenced to two and a half years in jail.*[43]

In another English case, the reluctance of judges to use the criminal sanction to its full effect is quite evident.

> *In 1995, a patient in her mid-70s suffered catastrophic blood loss and died during an operation to remove a liver tumour. The procedure should only have been attempted by a specialist liver unit as the tumour was found to be double the expected size and close to key blood vessels. The surgeon involved, Steven Walker, was suspended from duty at Blackpool Victoria Hospital, after all 16 anaesthetists refused to work with him. The General Medical Council reviewed his conduct and decided that he had displayed 'serious incompetence and clinical misjudgement' in the treatment of 10 patients, four of them had died, and struck him off the medical register. The Blackpool Coroner then initiated a police investigation that eventually led to a trial at the Old Bailey in London. Walker admitted manslaughter by gross negligence, but the judge gave him a suspended sentence while criticising the astonishing delay in mounting an investigation and stating that there had been a 'lamentable systemic failure at the hospital'. Walker was, he said: 'a decent man with an inability to recognise his limitations'.*[44]

Medical malpractice lawsuits remain on the rise in most countries although there is a noticeable trend towards mediation and settlement prior to trial.

> *The claimant underwent treatment for ulcerative colitis. It was alleged that there had been a delay in the treatment provided by an NHS hospital that caused the claimant to sustain avoidable pain and suffering, the*

worsening of her condition and the loss of her unborn baby. The hospital made a partial admission of liability, but the extent of the claimants' injuries and the value of the claim was disputed. The parties agreed to move to mediation. Settlement was agreed at this stage to avoid further legal process and the emotional distress this would have caused the claimant and her family. In addition, a representative from the hospital spent time with the claimant and offered an apology and a reassurance that lessons had been learned and action would follow.[45]

In May 2015, Baby AF died at just seven hours old in Watford General Hospital in England. A subsequent independent review identified multiple problems in the hours prior to the birth, in the delivery and then in the treatment the baby received once born. There were failures in resuscitation and stabilisation attempts and delays in referral to a tertiary centre. The Coroner determined that these faults had contributed to the baby's death. AF's mother was an NHS nurse. Despite the circumstances, the family and clinicians kept open their lines of communication and this led to a mediated settlement prior to the issue of proceedings.[46]

Mr. L had suffered from ulcerative colitis throughout the 1990s and underwent bowel surgery to relive his symptoms. The bowel surgeon created a pouch in place of his rectum so that he would not need an ileostomy. The surgery was not successful and so a year later Mr. L returned to the hospital to have the pouch removed and an ileostomy was performed. For the next 12 years, the patient wore incontinence pads and was unable to work. In 2012 it was discovered that the pouch had never been removed. The hospital admitted liability and Mr. L received substantial damages.[47] This was another case settled by mediation. A representative of the Trust had spoken to the claimant at length and provided an apology, reassurance that lessons had been learned and set up a meeting with clinicians involved.

As one German legal firm put it: 'Don't declare all-out war on a hospital or physicians because if you do, they will close ranks, shut up, inform their liability insurer, lawyer up and stall proceedings'.[48]

Lessons for the Future

One obvious lesson from these cases is that it is always better to acknowledge mistakes immediately and inform the patient. Healthcare professionals are required by an ethical duty of candour to be open and honest with patients, colleagues, employers and other relevant organisations but in England this is now also a statutory requirement. A full explanation and demonstrable evidence of learning from mistakes that have been made will often prevent a subsequent legal claim. Healthcare professionals and organisations have an obligation to stay close to patients who they know have been injured and offer whatever support they can. In one of the case studies mentioned above, this approach enabled a speedy mediated settlement.

No-fault systems that in theory offer a blame-free environment for dealing with errors have their strengths but are also very culture-specific and have their drawbacks. In the long run, patients are safest in open organisations that positively seek out problems and errors so that they can make sure they do not happen again.

Clinical protocols that exist to minimise mistakes must be observed in all but the most exceptional circumstances. Exceptions need to be carefully recorded. There is a particular challenge with new staff and locums who require full, proper and comprehensive briefing before they treat patients. The 'how we do things here' culture should never be seen as an affront to professional independence. Safety checklists, such as the WHO Surgical Safety Checklist for operating theatres, must operate rather like safety briefings in aeroplanes: boring, repetitive but essential. Of course, checklists can always be improved: it is possible to design systems that make it harder for people to do the wrong things. Teamwork in areas where the risks are the greatest, such as in operating theatres, must allow even the most junior of staff to call out errors or mistakes if they spot something unusual or unexpected.

There are particular problems and heightened risks for patients when toxic relationships develop between senior staff. In some countries, like the UK, external mediation is available to resolve disputes, but for the most part solutions are highly dependent on strong and professional leadership. Such problems can become particularly acute when the offending physicians are crucial to the survival of the organisation. The process of revalidation for professional competency might be helpful in this regard, but all too often the problems are too sensitive to be properly recorded. Inspecting bodies should always regard unresolved poor interpersonal relationships as a significant sign of organisational distress.

Hazard warning systems need constant refreshment and follow up to ensure that action has been taken and the reporting of such efforts should be made mandatory.

Adverse and 'Never' events must always be reviewed using, whenever appropriate, root cause analysis. Near misses are equally useful to focus on but reporting is currently patchy. Nevertheless, improvements to such reporting systems should be encouraged.

The emerging worldwide research into patient safety explored in Chapter Three will produce new safety ideas and the evidence required to justify investing in them. Patient safety makes economic as well as moral sense. There is a clear rationale to reduce the huge amounts of money being spent on patient claims.

Finally, whether you are a claimant or defendant, employ an experienced lawyer who you can trust. Corporate lawyers working for insurers or hospitals have in the past adopted tactics to obstruct settlements. Such tactics are wrong and not serving the best long-term interests of their clients. There is a moral and ethical duty to achieve justice for patients who have been harmed.

Chapter Six
Mental Health

The huge advances in medical science in recent years have been slow to impact on mental illness. New drugs have become available that lift depression and anxiety, but some patients have found them to be very addictive. Schizophrenia has proven more intractable to treat and can be very disabling for patients and disruptive for families. As populations age, so does the incidence of dementia in its various forms. Recent research, finding links to gene variants, may offer better treatment options in the long term, but in the short term, psychological treatments like CBT[1] will be used more extensively to help patients cope with their illnesses and resume something approaching a normal life. There are special problems for patients who commit serious crimes whilst suffering from a mental illness. People who have learning disabilities[2] have increasingly sought to separate themselves from mainstream mental health services although some do also suffer from mental health problems. Autism remains an unresolved scientific mystery of considerable complexity.

Patient Story: Schizophrenia

Myles was a 20-year-old who was brought to the emergency room by the campus police of a college from which he had been suspended several months earlier. A professor had called and reported that Myles had walked into his classroom, accused him of taking his tuition money and refused to leave. Although Myles had much academic success as a teenager, his behaviour became increasingly erratic. He stopped seeing his friends and no longer

---

seemed to care about his appearance or social pursuits. He began wearing the same clothes each day and seldom bathed. He lived with several family members but rarely talked to them. When he did talk he said that he had found evidence that his college was a front for organised crime. His sister said she had often seen him mumbling to himself and at times seemed to be talking to people who were not there. His family had never seen him take drugs or alcohol and his drug screening results were negative. There was some family history of poor mental health. He agreed to be admitted to a psychiatric unit where he was found to have persecutory delusions, auditory hallucinations and negative symptoms that fitted a diagnosis of Schizophrenia.[3]

The abyss of despair

The depression insidiously took hold over several months. It happened so slowly that I didn't realise for a long time what was going on. The signs were all there: lack of sleep; loss of appetite; apathy; and withdrawal from friends and family. In my mind depression was something that afflicted people who had weak temperaments, people who were unable to cope with the daily struggles and difficulties of life. I believed I had a strong disposition and could take the knocks that life threw my way. How wrong I was. The depression tainted my personality as I fell deeper and deeper into the abyss of despair. It was a friend who told that I was depressed but I ignored her advice and wallowed in self-pity. Eventually, I went to see my GP and eventually I climbed out of the abyss.[4]

Mental health has traditionally been the 'Cinderella' of healthcare with lower investment than other specialties in the acute sector. The World Health Organization (WHO) notes that mental illness accounts for 13% of the world's health burden yet most countries still underinvest despite the huge social and economic costs of such afflictions. The Royal College of Psychiatrists in the UK reports that mental illness is the single largest cost to the NHS and the largest single source of burden of disease. No other health condition matches mental illness in terms of the extent of its prevalence, persistence and breadth of impact. Mental illness is consistently associated with deprivation, low income, unemployment, poor education, poorer physical health and increased risk behaviour. In countries with insurance-based health systems, people with mental health problems are often uninsured. In the US, over a million prisoners have mental health problems.

The international variations with regard to investment differ enormously. Developing countries invest on average only 0.5% of their total health spending on mental health while in developed nations, 5% is a typical norm with spending rising as high as 10% in some countries. Canada, one of the richest countries in the world, invests only 7% of its total health spend, while in Australia the total spend is only 6.5%. In the UK, the spending is just under 11%, but in recent years its growth rate has been slowed by the need to cover overspending in the acute sector. This lack of adequate investment may be due to a process of structural stigmatisation where investment in mental health is deemed less worthy. The absence of clear interventions that will cure the most severe mental illnesses, often available in other disease areas, does not help.

> *In Ontario, Canada, most psychiatric beds were lost in the decade between 1959 and 1969. By 1979, the mental health's share of total health spend was 11.3%. Forty years later, it had dropped to 7%. New targets are for 9% of total health spending to be devoted to mental health, along with 2% of health spending directed to housing, employment and income support for those suffering from mental illnesses.[5]*

Poverty

Mental health and poverty are closely linked and interact in a complex negative cycle. Common mental health disorders are twice as likely to occur amongst the poor as compared to the rich. People experiencing hunger or facing debt are understandably more likely to suffer mental ill-health issues. The same is true of poor and overcrowded housing. People with the lowest socioeconomic status have eight times more relative risk for schizophrenia. Poverty increases the risk of mental disorder and a mental disorder increases the likelihood of a descent into poverty.[6]

Radical Thinkers

Psychiatry has always had its radical thinkers who challenge existing orthodoxies. Thomas Szasz, a Professor of Psychiatry in New York asked: 'Is psychiatry a medical enterprise concerned with treating disease or a humanistic enterprise concerned with helping persons with their personal problems. Psychiatry could be either — but it cannot — despite the pretentions and protestations of psychiatrists — be both'.[7] Peter Breggin, another American psychiatrist, argued that: 'drugs are spreading an epidemic of long term brain damage. Therapy, empathy and love must replace drugs, electroshock and biochemical theories'.[8] Neither reflect the views of mainstream psychiatric thinking, but for some patients, it is clear that thoughts about well-being do appear to have a positive effect.

Asylums

Until recent times, patients with any mental illness — as well as those with a learning disability — were cared for in large closed institutions separate from other parts of the health system. In England, from 1845, all County Councils were required to have asylum facilities for 'lunatics' and this period saw them develop in a similar manner in other parts of the world. Asylums have an extremely poor reputation, but they were and are staffed in the main by physicians and nurses who care for their patients. They offered a safe place for patients who could not survive in an unwelcoming wider world. Sadly, they also housed patients who had been locked away for wholly inappropriate reasons such as minor theft, sexual promiscuity or ideas that did not fit mainstream thinking. Increasingly, from the 1960s, the asylums abandoned their locked door regimes, but many patients that had been inside them for many years living very regimented lives had become institutionalised. Asylums are also often associated with patient abuse. Certainly, some recruited staff that abused patients in their care. Over the years, inquiry after inquiry exposed inadequate regimes rife with poor care that stimulated governments to act.

As new drugs such as chlorpromazine became available from the 1950s to control the worst symptoms of severe mental ill health, countries like Italy, the UK, Australia, Canada and the US first started to make hospitalisation voluntary and later began to think about closing their asylums altogether. In the UK, these developments led to asylum closures all over the country in the 1980s. Funds were urgently redirected to community care, although, with hindsight these investments were woefully inadequate.[9]

Other countries were slower to take this path and retained some of their asylums as an integral part of their mental health systems. In 2015, Belgium, Germany and Norway had the largest number of psychiatric inpatient beds per 100,000 population, with Mexico, Italy, Chile and the US with the lowest numbers.[10]

Ely Hospital, Wales

Geoffrey Howe QC conducted one of the earliest inquiries into allegations of the ill treatment of mental health patients in 1968.[11] A newspaper had reported alleged abuses at the Ely hospital in Wales. The allegations included examples of patients who had been handled roughly or injured whilst being restrained. It was also alleged that an elderly patient had been placed in seclusion behind a locked door for unreasonably long periods. There were also allegations of pilfering by staff. An overcrowded children's ward with 50 patients provided a poor environment for the care of children. The inquiry found that most of the allegations were well founded. The nursing care was lax and old-fashioned. The hospital was poorly led and its management poor. The Inquiry demanded that the government introduce a national inspection system for such facilities, which they did.[12] However, despite accepting the findings of the Howe report, the government insisted that Ely was an exceptional case. It was not.

Normansfield Hospital was founded in London in 1868 as a facility for mentally ill children by John Langdon Down (after whom Down Syndrome is named). In 1976, as a part of the NHS, it was impacted when nursing staff went on strike in protest at the reluctance of health authorities to suspend and investigate the conduct of Dr. Terrence Lawlor, a consultant psychiatrist. Two subsequent inquiries found that Dr. Lawlor's style was intolerant, abusive and tyrannical. The second inquiry recommended that his contract be terminated, and that a number of nurses and an administrator be sacked.[13,14]

> *Kingseat Hospital in New Zealand was opened in 1932 and operated as a psychiatric hospital until it was closed in 1999 during sweeping changes to New Zealand's mental health services. At its peak, in 1947, it had 800 beds. It had a very chequered history, with former patients claiming to have been physically and sexually abused. They also alleged that drugs were injected as punishments and that patients were locked in seclusion in straightjackets for hours at a time.*[15]

Reform in Italy

Italy took some of the most decisive and radical steps to reform their mental health system and is internationally recognised as being a pioneer in this field. All new admissions to psychiatric hospitals were stopped in 1978 and, as a consequence, the number of patients had sharply declined until, by 2000, no places at all were available. From 2008 this policy also included forensic hospitals. Mental healthcare was functioning wholly in the community with limited inpatient capacity in general hospitals and other beds available in community residential facilities. This was, according to some commentators, a decisive step forward in the humanisation of society.

> *Summary of the main elements of the 1978 Italian psychiatric reform*[16]
>
> *The main principle of Law 180 is that patients with mental disorders have the right to be treated the same way as patients with other diseases, which means the following:*
> - *Acute mental health conditions have to be managed in psychiatric wards located in general hospitals. These wards cannot exceed 15 beds.*
> - *Treatments should be provided on a voluntary basis, with compulsory admissions reserved for the following specific circumstances: (1) an emergency intervention is needed; (2) the patient refuses treatment; (3) alternative community treatment is impossible.*
> - *Compulsory admissions need to be formally authorised by the Mayor and can only be undertaken in general hospital psychiatric wards.*
> - *New community-based services were to be established to provide mental healthcare to the population of a given catchment area.*
> - *Gradual closure of public mental hospitals by blocking all new admissions.*

Community Care

In more recent times, evidence has emerged of poor, and at times even abusive care in community settings.

Winterbourne View Care Home

Winterbourne View was a private-sector care home located in Gloucestershire, England. In 2011, a whistleblower talked to a television programme who filmed staff slapping extremely vulnerable patients, soaking them with water, trapping them under chairs, taunting and swearing at them, pulling their hair and poking their eyes. On one occasion, a female patient was restrained whilst a paracetamol tablet was forced into her mouth. In 2012, six staff were jailed and five given suspended sentences for offences committed. Lawyers representing the staff apologised on behalf of their clients but also argued that the poor culture in the company that owned the home was a disease, a cancer and a fog that had engulfed the care home. An inquiry into the affair had described a closed and punitive culture. The judge condemned the owners: 'It is common ground in this case that that the hospital was run for profit and with a scandalous lack of regard to the interests of its clients and staff'.[17]

Of course, community care, when properly managed, is more than supported housing. It includes multi-disciplinary teams working to provide constant support for their group of patients; monitoring their condition; checking on their medication; helping them secure whatever state benefits they may be entitled to and acting as a first contact when things go wrong. Such specialist teams also support children.

Problems with organisational culture and professional isolation will feature in almost all of the case studies in this chapter. Negative attitudes to patients can fester unless there is a strong organisational culture that makes such an attitude unacceptable.

Mental Health Crisis in Australia

Mental health services in Australia have also been changing. In 1988 a Royal Commission[18] was appointed to review complaints about the

NSW Neuropsychiatric Institute concerning the use of psychosurgery and deep sleep therapy. A cocktail of drugs put patients into a coma lasting up to 39 days whilst electro-convulsive therapy (ECT) was administered. A total of 24 patients died at the facility after being admitted for non-serious medical conditions. Partly as a result of this commission, doctors were empowered to report serious misconduct by colleagues. The commission exposed the managerial bureaucracy and lack of scrutiny of the mental health profession. Recent research has also exposed the historical use of chemical restraint at hospitals including Callan Park Hospital for the Insane in Sydney.[19]

Problems in New Zealand

New Zealand has had a series of inquiries on mental health, usually prompted by a death of a patient or an innocent bystander.

> *John Papalii had a 20-year-history of mental illness and was in serious distress in June 1987. The day prior to an application being made to have him committed to a hospital under the Mental Health Act, he took a carving knife from the boarding house in Auckland where he was staying and stabbed a man waiting at a bus stop. He then fatally stabbed another boarder and severely wounded two others.[20]*

The Auckland Health Board was heavily criticised in the Inquiry that followed. Judge K. Mason said that they had 'disgraced psychiatry'.[21] There followed a heated and public discussion about the management and placement of mentally ill patients who had offended that would be replicated all over the world. Were these individuals mad or bad? An earlier New Zealand Inquiry[22] had been firm in its advice: 'We do not believe that a hospital is compatible with a prison. Prisoners requiring psychiatric treatment should receive it in a psychiatric hospital where security, though effective, is subordinate to therapy'. However, this was easier said than done. A number of hospitals banned the admission of patients from prisons on the grounds that they did not have sufficient security. A country-wide network of regional secure mental health units emerged to handle these patients.[23] The second Mason Inquiry, in 1996, reported that the mental health system still had major problems and recommended that services should be managed by a special commission, but the government opted to leave the services in the mainstream of health provision.

> *In 1994, Janice and Lindsay Gibson killed their 12-year-old son in an exorcism ritual. Health workers and the police had visited the family just days before the death. Both were judged to be not guilty of murder on the grounds of their insanity at their trial in New Plymouth, New Zealand.[24]*

People with mental health problems were quickly being associated with danger in the minds of the New Zealand public. In 1995, another inquiry focused on high youth suicide rates. In 2018, the He Ara Oranga report resulted in the re-establishment of a Mental Health and Wellbeing Commission to provide system level oversight of mental health services in the country. The conclusions of the 2018 inquiry will be echoed in almost all developed countries: 'Many people in the system receive good care but the system is under pressure with escalating demand for specialist services, limited support for people in the community and difficulties in recruiting and retaining staff'.

Patient Suicides

Psychiatric hospitals have consistently had safety problems with patients who have found ways to commit suicide on their premises. In England, 224 patients died in mental health hospitals between 2010 and 2016. Of the 35,000 suicides a year in the US, around 6% are inpatient suicides. A psychiatric nurse working in the US can expect to experience a suicide every 36 months on average.[25] The majority of patients take their lives through hanging or strangulation, a situation that has led to determined efforts to remove all ligature points. In mental health institutions suicide is an ever-present danger. The policy of making checks every 15 minutes on at-risk patients has not proven to be very effective in mitigating this issue — over half of all patients who committed suicide in US hospitals were theoretically being checked. The times of greatest risk are in the first week of admission and shortly after discharge. Given these known risks, psychiatric hospitals really should do better. However, the persistence of the problem clearly indicates that there are no easy solutions. An important meta-analysis undertaken in 2018 concluded that suicide risk models did not provide an adequate basis for clinical decisions in inpatient settings. Doctors and nurses will instead have to rely on training and instinct.[26]

Psychosurgery

Psychosurgery, once popular in the post-war years, has now largely been phased out as long-term studies of post-operative patients have confirmed that the treatment had far greater adverse effects than any benefit patients may have received.

The Lobotomy

An ice pick or orbitoclast was inserted above the patients eyeball and through the bony orbital ridge to sever connections to and from the prefrontal cortex. A mallet was then used to drive the orbitoclast through the thin layer of bone and into the brain. The procedure was repeated from several directions. Dr. Walter Freeman, a leading exponent of the procedure, performed an assembly line of lobotomies at State mental hospitals in the US where resident psychiatrists would identify suitable patients and prep them before he arrived. On one occasion, he lobotomised 228 patients over a 12-day period in what has become known as the West Virginia Lobotomy project.[27] Freeman claimed success but others were doubtful and thought that the lobotomy was palliative, making uncontrollable patients docile to the point where although they could be released from hospital, they suffered from a blunting of volition, abstraction and personality. The project was terminated in 1955.[28]

In the UK, although psychosurgery has all but disappeared, eight were recorded in 1999 and four in 2015–2016. Australia and New Zealand had an average of two per year in the 1990s but the procedure was banned in 2011. It has been banned in Russia since the 1950s but still continues in very small numbers in some countries, including Spain, where 121 operations were performed between 1999 and 2003, mainly in private clinics. It also remains in limited use in China.

Deep Brain Stimulation is increasingly being used as an alternative to surgery. The implanted stimulator sends electrical impulses to the brain, interrupting the abnormal signals that are causing the symptoms. The wires used for this intervention remain in place for life. The electrical impulses are controlled and adjusted by the neurologist or nursing specialist using a handheld device.[29]

ECT has been in use for many years and is performed under anaesthetic, passing small electrical currents through the brain. It is, according to the Mayo Clinic, much safer than it used to be. In the UK it is only used to treat patients with severe symptoms and with their express consent.

The Links Between Mental Health and Crime

The link between mental health and crime is apparent in all countries, and the medical specialty of forensic psychiatry has emerged to assess and treat mentally disordered offenders. Until the 1970s, such patients were treated in criminal lunatic asylums that were closely linked to the prison system. In many US states they still are. England now has only three special hospitals that provide care in a high-security setting and are linked to a network of medium-secure units. The number of places for high-security patients has fallen sharply in recent years. Despite their high fences and strict internal security, they portray themselves as hospitals rather than prisons.

In 1997, Stephen Daggett, a patient at Ashworth High Security hospital in Liverpool, made a series of allegations about life in the hospital including the misuse of drugs and alcohol, financial irregularities, the availability of pornographic material and possible paedophile activity. A public inquiry followed which confirmed that most of his allegations were well founded.

Adult patients with a history of paedophilia were grooming young visitors to the hospital. The Inquiry had much to say about the definition and treatment of patients with a severe personality disorder. The diagnostic boundaries and treatability of patients with such a condition had been and still was a controversial issue in the medical community. Should offenders be treated in a hospital or punished in prison?

The Inquiry found the hospital's negative, defensive and blame-ridden culture was so deeply engrained they doubted that even the most talented managerial team could ever turn it around. They recommended closure.[30]

However, the UK government did not accept the recommendation that the hospital be closed, and it continues to operate in 2020 albeit in a much-diminished form, now caring for 228 patients. In recent years it has received good reports from the Care Quality Commission. Security has been improved and children can only visit when strictly supervised. In this case the hospital seems to have learned lessons from a bad experience.

In a number of countries, efforts are being made to divert defendants with mental illness from prisons into social security systems.

According to Judge Steve Leifman, there are ten times as many people with serious mental illness in Miami-Dade County Jail than in any State hospital. In 2000, he created a programme to steer people with a mental illness who had committed low-level offences away from incarceration and into community-based care. A person accepted onto the programme is provided with case management assistance to claim benefits and help find housing so as to reduce their likelihood of reoffending. Speed is of the essence as most recidivism occurs within 25 days of release from prison.

The next stage of the development is a Mental Health Diversion facility that will provide short-term housing, a crisis unit, rehabilitation areas and a court room.[31]

Racism and Mental Health

In the UK, the NHS has, on occasion, been accused of institutional racism in its provision of mental health services.

> *David 'Rocky' Bennett, a black Rastafarian with a long history of mental illness was being treated for schizophrenia at a modern medium secure unit in Norwich. In October 1998, following an altercation with another patient in which blows had been exchanged, Bennett was transferred from one ward to another. There he assaulted a female nurse, prompting an immediate response from the rest of the nursing team who applied restraint procedures in an attempt to prevent further harm. He was held on the floor in a prone position for at least 25 minutes. Towards the end of the restraining period, he collapsed and became unconscious. Attempts to resuscitate him failed. An inquiry into the incident, chaired by Sir John Blofield, a retired High Court Judge followed. His report made a number of important recommendations about restraint practices but also went on to accuse the NHS of institutional racism. He detailed excessive medication, restriction and control of many black and ethnic minority patients in the system as well as the lack of black staff and managers. The poor care offered to these patients was, he said: 'a festering abscess and a blot on the good name of the NHS'.*[32,33]

The problem identified was systemic rather than down to the conduct of individual members of staff. Politicians became involved and one Minister claimed that young black men were six times more likely to be sectioned under the Mental Health Act than their white counterparts.

A five-year plan to halt racial discrimination in the NHS followed. However, it has made little progress, and by 2017, Prime Minister Theresa May had commissioned another review that found that patients from a black or ethnic minority background were still four times more likely to be detained under the Mental Health Act. They were also 10 times more likely to be the subject of a community treatment order. It was, May claimed, a 'burning injustice that must be corrected'.[34]

Issues in Ireland

Ireland has also had its problems with mental health services. The Irish Inspector for Mental Health first reported in 1999 and then again in 2006 that services were under pressure and described inadequate accommodation, unnecessarily locked and dirty wards and concerns about fire safety. The transition to community care in Ireland has been slow. The North of Ireland has also had problems at Muckamore Abbey Hospital, one of its larger long-stay hospitals for patients with learning disabilities.

In the summer of 2017, whistleblowers reported to the police that patient abuse was rife at Muckamore Abbey Hospital. Police inquiries started into a number of individual cases but then extended to a systemic investigation into the hospital as a whole. Two years later the inquiry had extended to 400 incidents and over 1500 crimes. The police had access to 240,000 hours of CCTV footage all of which had to be viewed and evaluated. The relatives of patients complained about the delay and demanded a public inquiry. By January 2020, 40 staff had been placed on precautionary suspension and five had been arrested. Meanwhile, in December 2019, it was reported that 39 patients awaiting transfer to community care would have to remain in hospital as no suitable community placement was available.[35]

Treating Mental Illness in the US

Some years ago the state of Michigan had 16 psychiatric hospitals. Most of these have now closed but there are still patients with mental illnesses who need hospital care for at least a short time both for their own safety as well as the safety of others. For the most part there is now nowhere for them to go. The community health centres that had been promised to provide the backbone of a community-based service never materialised — at least on the scale that was required. Milton Mack, now Michigan's State Court Administrator explained: 'We are now using jails and prisons as our de facto mental health system'.[36]

In 1928, the transition from institutional to community care in the US was boosted by a Supreme Court Ruling, The Olmstead Case. This case gave institutionalised mental health patients more leverage in seeking community care. Two women with mental health problems who were confined for treatment in a psychiatric hospital in Atlanta argued that they could be treated better in a community setting. The court ruled in their favour, determining that institutionalisation limited a person's ability to interact with other people, to work and make a life for themselves.[37]

By 2018, New York had reduced its beds for long-stay patients to just over 500,[38] but policy experts claimed that three times that number of seriously ill individuals were now living on the city streets, with 20 times that number in the shelter system.

A Failure of Community Care in Canada

In September 2004, Sandra Pupatello, the Minister for Community and Social Services for the province of Ontario in Canada, announced that all of its long-term institutional facilities, including those for people with a learning disability would close in five years. At its peak, in 1974, the province had 8000 people living in 16 long-stay institutions. This mass closure approach was at the time very much in vogue with mainstream policy thinking about mental health. However, it proved to have unplanned and extremely disturbing side effects. As the long-term facilities closed, some patients ended up in detention centres, prisons and homeless shelters. A national scandal followed, but according to some experts, the answer was not a return to institutional care but the development of a community care system that worked and was properly funded. Other professionals, working on the frontlines of emergency care, disagreed. They argued that some patients could not survive in a community setting and their needs should not be forgotten.[39]

Patrick, a 24-year-old with cerebral palsy, was placed in a nursing home for seniors. Later, 'in a fit of frustration', Patrick broke the ankle of one of those seniors. His punishment was to have his wheelchair taken away. For four months Patrick crawled to get where he needed.

Layla was placed in 22 different group homes and shelters over a span of 34 days. Cindy waited seven years for a community placement. Guy drowned in a cistern while living with a 'host family' in Ancaster.[40]

An earlier Canadian case had centred on 20,000 children — the 'Duplessis children', as they came to be known[41] — who had been certified as being mentally ill in Quebec and confined to psychiatric institutions in the 1940s and 1950s. This had enabled the province (and the Roman Catholic Church) to claim additional subsidies from the Federal Government — far more than would have been provided for a more appropriate placement such as orphanages. The scandal was exposed in a report from a 1960s Commission that found many of the children involved had problems properly functioning either socially or emotionally in their adult lives. Over 50% had undergone physical, mental or sexual abuse. Those affected secured damages from the government in 2001, including a sum for being wrongfully institutionalised. As part of this settlement, the orphans agreed to drop any further legal action against the Roman Catholic Church.

Inappropriate financial incentives or payments can clearly and grotesquely distort health and social care policy. Referrals to Child Adolescent Services in England rose sharply when schools received a financial incentive to refer.

Dementia

Dementia in its various forms is a challenge for all societies. Symptoms include memory loss, confusion, mood changes and difficulty with daily living. Globally, the number of people suffering from dementia is expected to rise from 50 million in 2018 to 152 million in 2050.[42] In Australia, nearly half a million people were living with dementia and 1.6 million people were involved in caring for them in 2019.[43] Many people with dementia are cared for in family or community settings but others, with no family support or who are difficult to manage, end up in care homes or hospitals. Between 2015 and 2020, 25,000 dementia patients were sectioned under the Mental Health Act in England.[44] Age UK, an English charity, has argued that the large number of dementia patients being locked up is a symptom of a profoundly dysfunctional social care system: 'It is horrific that any older person suffering with dementia is being incarcerated in a mental health establishment that is woefully ill-equipped to meet their needs'.

Care homes are expensive, which explains in part why so many patients end up in free institutional care.

Recent advances in treatment have yielded a temporary improvement in memory and problems with thinking and reasoning. The treatments boost the performance of the chemicals that carry information from one brain cell to another. However, they do little to stop the underlying decline and death of brain cells; as more brain cells die, the disease continues to progress.[45] A better understanding of how the disease disrupts the brain has not yet led to a cure. Increasing international investment into the search for a better understanding of the disease continues. Pharmaceutical companies are also increasingly sharing data from their clinical trials in order to accelerate more effective treatments. This is a problem that will not go away and will place increasing strain on health and social welfare systems.

The issue does raise important questions: what level of institutional (hospital) support does a fully functioning community-care-based mental health system need; and whether there is a role for a limited number of caring asylums for those who cannot cope in normal society even with constant support. What is now clear is that the promise of better care at lower cost — central to the move towards deinstitutionalisation — will not be realised. Community care may be better for most patients, but it is not cheaper.

Deciding on the Pace of Change

The pace of change from hospital to community care has always needed careful judgement. South Africa provides an example of how not to do it with the closure of Life Esidimeni, a cluster of privately run mental healthcare facilities, with some 1700 vulnerable patients. Over eight months between 2015 and 2016, the Gauteng State Health Department moved patients to various unlicensed care homes — many of which were simply repurposed suburban residences. At least 91 patients died in the aftermath of the move from causes including starvation, dehydration and cold. Survivors described how they were transported, many with their hands tied, and bundled onto buses to head for their new homes. Many were transferred without their clinical records, medications or identity cards.

Families were largely left in the dark on where their family members had been sent. Why it happened remains unclear, but some speculate that cronyism, corruption and fraud played a part. It was not, as claimed, an experiment in a move to a different and better pattern of care, or a strategy to save money. The case was eventually investigated by Dikgang Moseneke, a prominent lawyer, who found that the officials 'had acted unconstitutionally and had behaved literally as though they could get away with murder. The death and torture of those who died in the Life Esidimeni tragedy stemmed from arrogant and irrational use of public power'.[46]

> *Andrew Pieterson was with his uncle, Victor Truter, on the day he left Life Esidimeni. Truter had been diagnosed with chronic schizophrenia and had lived at the hospital for 40 years. Clutching his small bag of belongings, he limped to the transfer bus. No one could tell him where he was going. When Pieterson tracked down his uncle two months later, he found him in a psychogeriatric facility — a different man. 'He was emaciated, he hadn't eaten and had not been given his tablets'.[47]*

Autism in France

The French system of mental health has come under considerable criticism for its treatment of autistic children. The United Nations became involved and reported that autistic children in France: 'continue to be subjected to widespread violations of their rights. They do not have access to mainstream education, and many are still offered inefficient psychoanalytical therapies, over medication and placement in psychiatric hospitals and institutions'. Parents who object to the institutionalisation of their children are 'intimidated and threatened and in some cases lose custody of their children'.[48] There are, said Vincent Dennery, who heads a collective of autism associations, 'thousands of autistic children in psychiatric hospital day units who have no reason to be there, but their parents cannot find any other solution'. Emmanuel Macron, the French President, has described the problem as a 'civilisational challenge'.

> *Catherine Chavy privately organised home schooling support for her son Adrien. The local authorities had told her: 'Why are you insisting on school? Put him in an institution'. Her high-functioning autistic seven-year-old is now doing well academically. According to Chavy: 'In France there is an autism of the poor and the autism of the rich. If I did not have the money and skill to fight, my son would have ended up in a psychiatric hospital'.*[49]

The French government's plan for reform was published in April 2018 and heralded a shift in aiming to keep autistic children within the education system and offering free nursery school places.

Meanwhile, pressure was growing in the UK for a speedier transition to better social, educational and medical support for autistic children and adults. Research continues into causes of autism though it seems unlikely that there will be a magic bullet. Progress in dealing with the problem will be made by improving early detection rates in children, followed by lifelong support.

Personality Disorders

One of the most challenging areas of psychiatry relates to personality disorders. There are many types of these, the most common of which are obsessive-compulsive, narcissistic and borderline personality disorders. Some of the cases discussed in later chapters involve individuals with one of these diagnostic categories. People with such disorders find it difficult to make or keep close personal relationships with work colleagues, friends or family. They often get into trouble, find it difficult to listen to others and struggle to control their feelings or behaviour. They are often unhappy, distressed, upset or harm others. There has been much discussion in professional circles about whether such disorders can be treated. Most psychiatrists believe they can provide help and support, though many such patients find themselves in secure treatment centres.

Dissociative identity disorder

A 55-year-old Caucasian woman with a history of substance abuse and a comorbid bipolar disorder presented to a local hospital with a history of the fragmentation of a single personality into different personalities when under emotional stress and under the influence of drugs. Her many personalities included a 7-year-old child, a teenager and a male person in addition to her normal 55-year-old self. While transitioning between these personalities she was found to be violent, both to herself and to those who were close to her. This vacillation from being suicidal to homicidal had resulted in her being arrested on two occasions and being referred to hospital. Cognitive behavioural therapy has been helpful but she remains under treatment and will probably need lifelong care and support.[50]

In 1998, the apparently motiveless murders of a mother and two of her children when they were travelling home from school in a rural area shocked the British public. Subsequently, a patient with a personality disorder, being monitored by psychiatric services, was convicted of their murders. The government responded by introducing a new concept: 'dangerous and severe personality disorder'.[51] *Programmes are being developed for this disorder but as yet, no clear successful treatment has emerged. This patient will remain in a high-security psychiatric hospital for an indeterminate sentence and will only be released on parole after a vigorous risk assessment to ensure public safety. He may never be released.*

Learning Disabilities

People with a learning disability are now largely cared for in the community or at their homes with specialist support. In many (but not all) cases, the outcomes are positive as the following case illustrates.

Thomas Johnson, from Worcestershire in England, has profound and multiple learning disabilities. He has Lennox Gastaut Syndrome that requires one-to-one support in all aspects of his life and also suffers from life-threatening epilepsy. For some time he lived in a specialist residential centre some 100 miles from his home. This did not work and so Thomas returned home and care was provided through specialist support funded by his local authority. When he was 18, the payment for this support was paid for through a personal health budget provided by the NHS. He now has ownership of his life and lives in an annex to his parental home. He chooses who looks after him and how he lives his life. According to his parents: 'Our son is safe, healthy and happy, thanks to choice and control'.[52]

Other children and young adults who suffer from learning disabilities and need hospital care are less fortunate.

Whorlton Hall was a privately run NHS-funded unit caring for patients with learning disabilities and autism. Many were detained under the Mental Health Act. Undercover filming by journalists showed staff intimidating, mocking and restraining patients. Whorlton Hall was one of scores of such units in England looking after a total of 2300 patients. What the reporters found was, one academic said, 'the absolute antithesis of good care' and amounted to psychological torture. The hospital had a very deviant culture. The CCQ quality inspectors did not pick up the abuse when they visited and later apologised.[53]

These were very difficult patients to manage who demanded staff with high skills and in sufficient numbers. The hospital had found recruitment difficult and had resorted to engaging a significant number of transitional locums. Clearly, this was a contributory factor.

Refugees and Migrants

The provision of mental health services for refugees and migrants is proving to be a particular problem for some countries and has highlighted the ineluctable intersection of mental health, human rights, ethics and social policy. The migration policies adopted by many Western governments have seen major resettlements of thousands of children from war zones such as Syria, Iraq and Afghanistan. These are further discussed in Chapter Ten of this book.

Parents and children in Australian immigration detention centres are often vulnerable to mental health problems before they reach the country. Experiences in prolonged detention add to their burden of trauma, which has an impact not only on the individual adults and children but also on the family process itself. Immigration detention profoundly undermines the parental role, renders the parent impotent and leaves the child without protection or comfort in already unpredictable surroundings where basic needs for safe play and education are unmet. This potentially exposes the child to physical and emotional neglect in a degrading and hostile environment and puts children at high risk of the developmental psychopathology that follows exposure to violence and on-going parental despair.[54]

Post-traumatic Stress Disorder

The absence of adequate mental healthcare services for armed forces and their families has now been recognised by many governments. Now that post-traumatic stress disorder (PTSD) is better understood, it can be treated. However, the scale of the problem is sizeable. Almost a third of active and reserve soldiers in the British army deployed to Iraq and Afghanistan returned from active duty with a mental illness that needed treatment. A similar percentage of US service men and women who served in Vietnam also suffered PTSD at some time in their life.

PTSD is not just a problem for soldiers affected by their experiences in warzones. It is also extremely prevalent in the survivors of genocides, ethnic cleansing events, racial or ethnic persecution and other forms of direct and indirect violence. A sexual assault, the impact of a natural disaster or a car accident can all prompt a harrowing reaction which individuals will continue to battle with for much of their lives. PTSD affects 3.5% of the total US adult population — some 8 million Americans — according to the National Alliance on Mental Illness.[55,56]

Jared was a 36-year-old married veteran who had returned from Afghanistan. He turned up at an outpatient mental health clinic complaining of 'a short fuse' that was easily triggered. He experienced out-of-control

> *rage when startled, constant thoughts of death-related events and vivid nightmares of combat that affected his sleep patterns. He was most worried about his extreme anger and concerned that he might accidentally hurt somebody. He was jittery and always on the lookout for danger. On leaving the Army he had gotten a college degree but elected to work as a plumber as this enabled him to protect his personal space.*[57]

Given what is now known about the disorder and its lifelong effects on some of those affected by it, investment levels in treating PTSD are far too low, a situation that is particularly true for armed forces veterans.

Lessons for the Future

Mental health is a major problem in all societies. The closure of long-stay asylums and move to care in the community has now been a central feature of mental health policy for 50 years or more. The asylums were actually not all as bad as we might now think, but too many had become professionally isolated and distanced from their local communities. Many patients were placed many miles away from their families in County or State institutions. Containment and the protection of the public has been the dominating ethos in managing patient with mental illnesses, and until relatively recently, few treatment options were available. Abuse and neglect occurred on too many occasions in many institutions. Public attitudes to these issues could best be summed up as 'out of sight, out of mind'.

The great promise of care in the community has worked for many patients but not for all. Some patients needed the safety of a caring institution, including some of those with a learning disability. Some psychiatrists are now calling for the return of a new type of asylum as a safe sanctuary for those with intractable mental health problems.[58] Such asylums would need to have a local or city focus and be fully integrated into their local communities. The greatest danger that they will face — as previously — is public and professional isolation. This suggests that they should be small in scale.

Mental illness often occurs as a comorbidity with other diseases and therefore needs to be identified at an early stage and treated in both specialist acute centres and in primary care.

Mental health still has an inadequate science base. The brain and the mind have been slow to give up their secrets. Clinical knowledge of mental illness is increasing, but very slowly, and the conversion of scientific understanding into really effective treatment is not on the short-term horizon for patients with severe mental illnesses. Coping, care and human rights will be the dominant drivers of public policy.

Mental hospitals experience many of the same problems as those in acute sector when staffing levels become too low and they are forced to employ too many short-term locums. Such situations must trigger alarms for managers and health authorities.

Investment in mental health needs to be increased almost everywhere. One key reform may be to ring-fence mental health investment so that it cannot be diverted to other areas of the health budget. In 2013, NHS England introduced a programme to promote 'parity of esteem'; an initiative to equally value mental and physical health. The aims are admirable, but delivery will not be easy.

It is clear that many countries have pushed care in the community too far, too quickly and have underinvested, leading to some catastrophic breakdowns. Italy, one of the leaders of the move to community care, is now experiencing difficulties in consolidating its reforms in a period of economic austerity. If the community care breaks down in Italy, there are few places for a patient to go even if they are categorised as dangerous.[59]

Most people will probably take the view that the move to community care was the right thing to do but this change of strategy is not without its critics. As P. D. James, an international author put it: 'Care in the community could be described as the absence of care in a community still largely resentful and frightened of mental illness'.

Some countries have also seen an interesting shift in the balance between public- and private-sector mental health provision, with frontline mental health services provided by public sector organisations and long-term specialist care provided by the private sector. In

2018, the independent sector in England provided 53% of inpatient beds.[60] In many countries there remain wide geographical disparities in the provision of services that result in patients being cared for a long way from their families and local communities, making future integration with community care more difficult.

The link between mental health and the prison service has never been satisfactorily settled. Prisons clearly need much more support in dealing with inmates suffering from mental health problems. The practice of dumping mentally ill people into prison systems in the US (and elsewhere) should stop. Specialist forensic mental health facilities for convicted and dangerous patients with a mental illness need to remain in place and are better located in health systems rather than prisons.

Drug misuse and its impact on mental health is approaching a crisis point in some countries. There is little consensus about the right way forward. Some countries, like Portugal, have completely decriminalised the possession of all drugs and as a consequence, levels of drug use are now below the European average, the prison population has reduced as have HIV rates.[61] However, other countries remain reluctant to follow suit. Opioid misuse is a growing problem, particularly in the US, and treatment services are usually located within the mental health domain.

Mental health services demand skilled personnel, so long-term investment requires increased and targeted funding for medical, nursing and other schools mixed with incentives for practitioners to practice in the field of mental health. The NHS in England had vacancy rates for mental health in both medicine and nursing of around 12% in 2018. There are few short cuts to solve this mismatch between the need for competency and the willingness to pay for it.

Quality assurance agencies have a mixed record of identifying abuse in residential settings and this has led to increasing pressure for the use of internal CCTV in shared areas. Whatever the counter-arguments about privacy, it seems certain that this is going to happen. Whether it will deter some of the deviant behaviour we have seen in the chapter is still an open question.

Mental health and cancer have one thing in common. Some patients need to be helped to live with their illness rather than constantly focusing on an elusive cure.

The dark side of the mental health story is that the alternative to asylum care has generally not been properly funded, leaving too many vulnerable people with nowhere safe to go except prisons, shelters for the homeless or living lonely lives in a community without any care at all. Image, branding and reputation have always been a problem for mental health services despite the undoubted progress that has been made in the last decade. For many patients, community care has worked. The case studies in this chapter should not devalue this progress but act as a stimulus for greater research and targeted investment for a better future.

Chapter Seven
Fraud and Corruption

There are few reliable estimates of the extent of corruption in health-care organisations. However, it certainly exists and it appears to be growing. Some estimates put the cost of fraud and corruption at 6% of annual global expenditure.[1] Perhaps surprisingly, one third of OECD citizens consider the healthcare sector to be corrupt.[2]

The US healthcare system is particularly vulnerable to corruption as it is insurance based and healthcare delivery is largely contracted out and delivered by private sector or independent not-for-profit entities. The Clinton Administration declared that healthcare fraud was the second most important problem in the US after violent crime.[3] Medical providers perpetuate a large amount of the fraud found in the American system. When physicians accept payment to give people unnecessary prescriptions, pressure patients into treatments they do not need or submit bills to public programmes for services they did not provide, most people see this as corruption. Automated payment systems do not help and are very attractive to fraudsters. New forms of fraud have emerged in recent years that are harder to detect and prosecute (because there is no false claim around which to build a case) and include the embezzlement of capitation funds provided by the state (a fee per registered patient), overstating patient numbers and the use of fraudulent subcontracting to benefit friends or family. Perhaps even more serious are improper enrolment or disenrollment practices such as driving out seriously ill patients or refusing them admission to a health plan.

Insurance Fraud

Individuals and institutions can both commit insurance fraud. Individuals could, for example, allow someone else to use their identity to obtain healthcare services. Institutions sometimes bill for services that were never provided. The following examples illustrate the range of offences.

> - *Chris was the only one in his family with health insurance but he let his brother and cousin use his card to receive healthcare benefits.*
> - *A nurse in Dr. Smith's office became addicted to painkillers and with access to patient records she called in forged prescriptions to a local pharmacy and posed as a family member of the patient when she picked up the drugs.*
> - *Dr. Talbot billed his patient's health insurer for both the services he actually provided and for services he did not provide. He falsified the patient's records to reflect office visits and treatments that never occurred.*
> - *Dr. Salazar was employed at a medical centre where low-income and indigent families were recruited to undergo unnecessary exams. Dr. Salazar saw few patients, but medical records falsified by an assistant were used to bill insurance programmes for procedures that were never performed.*[4]

Kickbacks

Kickbacks are normally described as a form of negotiated bribery and are not uncommon. A key example involved the Columbia/HCA hospital chain and its involvement in a Federal probe that became the longest and costliest investigation of healthcare fraud in US history.

> *In 1993, lawsuits were filed against Columbia/HCA by former employees who drew attention to the company's questionable billing practices to Medicare for hundreds of millions of dollars. The company was accused of paying kickbacks to physicians for referrals, keeping two sets of books, inflating the seriousness of diagnoses and giving doctors loans that were never intended to be repaid. The Federal investigation drew to a close in 2003 with the government receiving over US$2 billion in criminal fines*

and civil penalties from the company for systematically defrauding federal healthcare programmes.[5] In November 2015, the Attorney's Office in South Carolina announced that the company had settled allegations of billing for unnecessary lab tests and double billing for foetal testing for US$2 million.[6]

In February 2020, a Chicago woman, Angelita Newton, was found guilty by a federal jury of being involved in a scheme to defraud Medicare of approximately US$7 million by submitting claims for unnecessary home health services for unqualified patients or for visits that did not happen as billed.[7] This crime was detected by the Medicare Fraud Strike Force, an organisation founded in 2007 and, as of the end of 2019, responsible for charging 4200 defendants.

Starting in 2016, a New Jersey man, Zachary Ohebshalom, admitted violating the federal anti-kickback statute. Along with others, he got involved in prescribing and dispensing expensive, but medically unnecessary, pain creams which generated an improper benefit of US$1.5 and US$3.5 million.[8]

In 2019, Philip Esformes, a Miami Beach businessman who operated a network of nursing homes and assisted living facilities, was ordered to pay US$44 million after been found guilty of bribery, kickback and money laundering charges. He had submitted fraudulent claims for services not provided and not medically necessary. He had bribed doctors to admit patients into his facilities, where those residents often failed to receive appropriate medical services that were then billed to Medicare and Medicaid. He also bribed an employee of a state regulator to receive advance notice of surprise inspections of his facilities. He was jailed for 20 years.[9]

India

India has many of the same problems as the US. According to Dr. David Berger, who served as a volunteer physician at a small charity hospital in the Himalayas: 'The corruption strangles everything. It's like a cancer'. Referring doctors often receive kickbacks for unnecessary private sector diagnostic tests and examinations. One senior doctor was renowned for the use of ultrasonography as a profligate revenue earning procedure.[10] Endemic corruption has lowered both the national and international reputation of Indian doctors and until it is tackled, according to Berger, 'the doctor patient relationship will be in tatters'.

China

Information about healthcare service corruption in China is scarce but their healthcare professionals are clearly not immune from it as the following cases illustrate:

> *The anxious Chinese woman wanted to ensure that her mother would receive the best care during her upcoming gall bladder surgery. So, the woman cornered the surgeon at her local hospital and pressed an envelope into his hands. Inside the hongbao or 'red packet' was 1000 yuan. The doctor took the envelope without question. Everybody does it.*[11]

> *A number of senior managers at a Shaanxi hospital have been dismissed after one of their obstetricians sold a newborn baby after convincing his parents to give him up. Since the news broke other parents have made similar allegations.*[12]

Bribery and Privileged Access

In 2017, the European Commission[13] published a new study on corruption in the healthcare sector which focussed on privileged access to medical services, improper marketing and the potential risks of 'double practice' by doctors in public and private clinics. Some examples that were quoted in the study follow:

Heads of hospital departments in Greece typically have the right to reserve three to four beds for themselves, to allocate to patients as they wish. Other physicians typically have one to two beds. It is an unwritten law of the Greek system that patients can secure preferential treatment via a relative or for payment. In addition, there is an interconnection between staff, such as nurses and physicians, that exacerbates the problem. Patients may pay a nurse or have a nurse in their family who can then ask a physician to reserve a bed on their behalf, sometimes for payment.

In Lithuania, a Minister was forced to resign in 2016 after she admitted giving a bribe to physicians to operate on a relative. In 2018, senior staff were suspended following a report by the Lithuanian Special Investigation Unit that 'winning a public procurement contract could be as easy as making a hefty donation to the institution'.[14]

Waiting list mismanagement is causing major problems in Italy. As waiting times lengthen, patients bribe their way to the front of the queue. The Rome-based research institute, Censis, reported that in 2016, 13.5 million Italians were able to skip waiting lists by using friendships, recommendations or giving presents.[15]

In Bulgaria, it has been reported that young doctors are pressurised by older physicians to ask patients for 'informal payments', a practice that is widespread in the country. Politicians and their relatives are not subject to pressures for informal payments as they already have privileged access to publicly funded government hospitals with the best equipment.

As is the case in the US, the EU and its individual member states are now starting to take action against such practices and a European Health Care Fraud and Corruption Network has been created. In 2016, Germany introduced new anti-corruption in healthcare laws.

In the UK, the NHS has a number of counter-fraud organisations to combat a problem estimated to cost £1.3 billion a year in 2019.

Much of this fraud is low-level criminal activity by individuals, but the cumulative amounts are evidently very large. In a case in Scotland, a hospital worker stole surgical equipment worth £1.3 million. Another senior manager tricked her hospital into paying for animal sperm for a private stud farm business. One dentist stole more than £1 million by charging for work she had not conducted and making claims for people who were dead or did not exist. Another fraudster was the sole locksmith at a major hospital who fraudulently increased the price of locks he purchased for the hospital from a company he had once been a director of.

Building Projects

Corruption has often been associated with building and construction projects in all sectors, and healthcare is no different.

A former hospital manager who pocketed a CAN$10 million bribe in return for helping SNC-Lavalin win a Montreal building project worth over CAN$1 billion was sent to prison in 2018. He had given privileged information to the engineering firm to help with its tender for building the new McGill University Health Centre. Others were also prosecuted.[16]

In 1974, the architect, John Poulson, was jailed for five years after being found guilty at Leeds Crown Court of bribing public figures in order to win contracts. Poulson's talent was in offering an integrated design and build service that sharply reduced fees. He recruited people from the sectors he was interested in, including civil servants, and drew some of them into what turned out to be shady partnerships. George Braithwaite, a senior figure in the NHS, commissioned him to work on two major hospital projects in return for which Poulson helped him modernise his manor house and helped his wife set up a business. Braithwaite was jailed for three years. The Minister of Health took the unusual step of removing his NHS pension.[17]

Counterfeit Drugs

According to some physicians, counterfeit drugs have become a public health emergency, and there are now moves to reach an international agreement on drug quality and inspection. The scale of the problem is enormous. The European Union Intellectual Property office estimated that the pharmaceutical industry in Europe lost €16.5 billion between 2012 and 2016.[18] Other estimates claim that up to 10% of drugs in low- and middle-income countries are of poor quality or outright fakes. In 2011, the World Health Organization (WHO) estimated that 64% of Nigeria's imported malarial drugs were fake. Counterfeit drugs include those with less or none of the stated active ingredients, with added, sometimes hazardous adulterants, substituted ingredients, false brand names and drugs that have had their expiry dates removed. WHO issues product alerts such as the one below relating to a fake cancer drug.

World Health Organization
Medical Product Alert No. 2, 2019
This alert relates to confirmed falsified versions of ICLUSIG circulating in the WHO regions of Europe and the Americas. The drug is used to treat different forms of leukaemia. Instead of Ponatinib, the proper active ingredient, the product contains paracetamol.

The expansion of online pharmacies selling products directly to the public has added a further complication to efforts to stamp out this corruption. Some governments, such as several countries in the EU, have taken action, including a mandatory requirement for medicine to have a unique identifier and an anti-tamper device on the packaging.

Counterfeiting is also rife in recreational drugs. Some products are sold with no active ingredients at all, such as lactose powder passed off as heroin. Other drugs are sold with diluents that radically reduce their potency. Viagra is a very common target for counterfeiters.

Technological advances may provide solutions. Innovations such as the use of blockchain technology that can track drugs through the supply chain from the manufacturer to the end user will help to reduce fraud.[19]

Organised Crime

Organised crime has a big impact on the healthcare sectors of some countries. An Italian parliamentary report claimed that 126 deaths were linked to hospitals plagued by mafia corruption. The hospitals were offering substandard care as mobsters creamed off the money.[20] The police attached to Italy's Finance ministry concluded 'Ndrangheta hadn't simply infiltrated Vibo Valentia Hospital; rather they effectively ran it'.

San Raffaele Hospital in Milan has had a very troubled history with a string of scandals defrauding the Italian National Health Service. Double accounting, junior staff being substituted for senior surgeons and the 'San Raffaele system', whereby entrepreneurs working under contract for the hospital would intentionally overbill clients and divert the money to corrupt politician slush funds. The Vatican were drawn into the scandal when the hospital's administrator committed suicide after the level of debt was exposed. They offered a bail out sum, but the hospital was eventually sold to the San Donato group in 2012.[21]

Organ Trafficking

Organ trafficking and transplant tourism has become big business. The organs being traded include the kidney, liver, heart, lung and pancreas. The trade is estimated to be worth US$1.7 billion a year. WHO estimates that, in 2007, organ trafficking accounted for 5%–10% of all kidney transplants performed throughout the world and that 2000 Indians sell a kidney each year to pay off debts.[22]

> *Said Ahmed was held hostage for three months, with 24 others, by an organ trafficking gang in Rawalpindi, Pakistan, waiting for the removal of his kidney. He was told that he would be paid the equivalent of £2300 for the organ. The police intervened and he was saved. Zafar Shahab was not so lucky and had his kidney removed whilst undergoing surgery for another complaint.[23]*

> *In 2002, a London GP was struck off the Medical Register after he told an undercover journalist that he could obtain a kidney from a live donor in exchange for a fee: 'No problems, I can fix that. Do you want it done here, do you want it done in Germany or do you want it done in India?'[24]*

Behind these desperate stories of criminality and unprofessional conduct lies a deeper ethical issue. Thousands die each year waiting for an organ transplant that never becomes available. If market forces could save some lives, we should at least give it some consideration. Erin and Harris[25] have proposed an ethical market for organs with strict quality controls. The market would be operated by an agency licensed by national governments and the organs distributed according to some notion of clinical priority. Those who reject such ideas argue that this would reduce altruistic donations and exploit the poor. In any case, they argue, there are other ways forward. From 2020, all adults who die in England will be considered a potential donor unless they have specifically opted out. This new law is named after Max Johnson and Keira Ball (Max, a young boy, received a heart from Keira, who was killed in a road traffic accident). The government estimates that over 700 lives per year will be saved by this reform — still far short of the number of patients on waiting lists.

> *Simon Howell was born with a serious kidney condition called renal dysphasia. Despite this, he became a doctor specialising in the field of pathology. He had his first kidney transplant in 2005, thanks to his mother offering to be a living donor. In 2009, the kidney failed, and he was added to the*

> *transplant waiting list. Thereafter his life was dominated by his illness. He had dialysis four times a day, indescribable fatigue and constant anxiety about his future and that of his family as he waited for a suitable donor.*[26] *He had to wait eight years before one became available.*

There have been consistent reports that large numbers of the organs of condemned prisoners have been harvested in China, but allegations that this practice has been extended to include political dissidents have been strenuously denied by the Chinese government.[27]

International action to combat organ trafficking has been led by the Transplant Society and the International Society of Nephrology through their Istanbul Declaration. However, until fully functioning artificial organs become widely available, criminal activity is likely to continue unabated.

Criminal Negligence

> *In 2012, a crisis unfolded at the Punjab Institute of Cardiology in Pakistan causing harm to over 1000 patients and the death of at least 100. What was first thought to be an outbreak of dengue fever turned out to be an adverse reaction to a cardiac drug manufactured in Karachi. It was later established that a 25 kg drum of pyrimethamine had gone missing and been mixed into a batch of cardiac medicine. At 14 times its normal dosage levels, the pyrimethamine was causing folate deficiency, destroying the platelets in bone marrow and triggering heavy internal bleeding. WHO issued a global alert.*[28]

This was a case of criminal negligence, rather than fraud or corruption, although during the investigation, another company was found to be continuing to manufacture drugs when its licence to do so had long expired. In the light of this case, the Federal Government created a National Medicines Regulatory Body.

Examination and Inspection Fraud

Corruption of a different sort has been exposed in India. A criminal network had obtained a leaked copy of a pre-medical and pre-dental entrance test exam paper and sent the answers to candidates via WhatsApp during the examination. They also provided several candidates (who had each paid up to 2 million rupees to cheat) with tiny bluetooth devices, vests tagged with micro-SIM cards and wristwatches fitted with cameras so that answers could be relayed to them in real time from other medical students and doctors. The Indian Supreme Court demanded that more than 600,000 students retake the exam. However, some students still managed to gain admission to medical and dental schools without sitting the entrance exam at all. They paid criminals to get others to sit the exam for them.

Matter got even worse in Pakistan when the government closed down its main medical registration body in October 2019 and sent the police into its headquarters. Officials at the Pakistan Medical and Dental Council had, the government alleged, been taking kickbacks in return for providing good inspection reports to medical and dental schools in the private sector. A new body, The Pakistan Medical Commission, took over the registration process.[29]

Patient Data

Recent times have seen a growing problem in keeping patient data — that has a high commercial value — secure and safe. Anonymised data, sold to pharmaceutical or insurance companies under licence, is permissible in most countries provided that individual patients can never be identified. However, some companies are stretching the boundaries of legitimacy in the ways that they are now sharing data with third parties.

Health Engine, an online booking service for healthcare services, has been one of Australia's digital success stories and is used by thousands of healthcare professionals. However, it also asks about patient's symptoms when

> *appointments are booked and it transpired that this information was being shared with lawyers looking for personal injury cases. Health Engine has also been accused by the Australian Competition and Consumer Commission of not including negative reviews of patient experiences.*[30]

Identity theft has been detected through the use of hospital patient records. To a knowledgeable insider, security is usually light in healthcare systems.

> *Evelina Sophia Reid, a hospital unit secretary in Florida, was a prolific identity thief who passed large amount of personal patient information, including birth dates and social security numbers to an accomplice. Over a five-year period, she stole over 24,000 records.*[31]
>
> *Betty Cole, a respiratory therapist in Miami, pleaded guilty to aggravated identity theft by giving patient details to an accomplice who then used them to file fraudulent tax returns.*[32]

> *In 2003, NHS manager Debora Hancox was jailed along with her partner for a sophisticated IT fraud. The couple had pocketed £300,000 by supplying the NHS with goods at inflated prices. When the scam was discovered in 2008, they had fled to Northern Cyprus. The couple were arrested in 2014 and she was sentenced to two years in prison. After her release she went back to work for the NHS through an employment agency for almost a year before her past history was discovered.*

Public Sector Ethos

The public sector ethos is a defined set of principles or values that all public servants adhere to when performing their duties to the public. The Parliamentary Committee on Standards in Public Life describes seven principles: selflessness, integrity, objectivity, accountability, openness, honesty and leadership.[33]

As public sector organisations have been urged by governments of all political persuasions to become more business-like and competitive, the boundaries separating legitimate and illegitimate behaviour in public sector organisations have shifted and blurred, causing problems in UK health, education and local government organisations. The UK Parliament has not been immune from similar problems, notably the expenses claims scandal that emerged in 2009.

The public sector ethos is in part an instinctive set of attitudes and conducts which inevitably means that individuals do, on occasion, stray across the lines of probity. Some further examples are found in Chapter Nine of this book.

For private sector organisations, the law of the land draws the line of probity, but they too need moral and ethical guidelines built into their corporate cultures.

The Pharmaceutical Industry

The pharmaceutical industry has often found itself in trouble with regulators and the courts throughout the world. Poor manufacturing standards or badly designed testing programmes are sometimes to blame for faulty — or dangerous — products, but the principal criticisms of 'big pharma' are usually related to their marketing practices and the sometimes less-than-ethical incentives provided to doctors to prescribe or recommend their products. They have also been found guilty of promoting drugs for use by patients well beyond their licence.

In 2013, the generic drug manufacturer, Ranbaxy USA, pleaded guilty to charges relating to the manufacture and distribution of adulterated medicines made in its factories in India. Site inspections found incomplete testing records, an inadequate programme to assess the stability characteristics of medicines and significant Good Manufacturing Practice (GMP) deviations. The company also made false, fictitious and fraudulent statements to the FDA in its annual reports. The company paid a criminal fine of US$150 million and agreed to settle civil claims for US$350 million.[34]

Examples of a sales team promoting a drug for use beyond what it had been licensed for is below.

Between March 2002 and December 2003, Janssen Pharmaceuticals, a subsidiary of Johnson & Johnson, introduced 'Risperdal', an antipsychotic drug into the US market for unapproved use. Risperdal was for most of this time approved only to treat schizophrenia, yet sales teams also recommended its use on elderly dementia patients with symptoms such as anxiety, agitation and depression. It was also suggested that it had been promoted for the treatment of children with mental disabilities. The company paid speaker fees to doctors willing to promote the drug. The company played down the risks involved but eventually paid more than US$2.2 billion to resolve their criminal and civil liabilities.[35]

In 2012, GlaxoSmithKline pleaded guilty to the unlawful promotion of the prescription drug 'Paxil' by recommending its use by patients under the age of 18. The US government had claimed that GlaxoSmithKline had prepared, published and distributed a misleading journal article that misreported a clinical trial; instead of demonstrating the efficacy of Paxil in the treatment of people under the age of 18, the trial actually failed to show any benefit. At the same time the company did not make available data from two other studies in which Paxil failed to demonstrate efficacy for this group of patients. The company paid US$3 billion to resolve its criminal and civil liability.[36]

A whistleblower exposed AstraZeneca of promoting the drug 'Seroquel' for use beyond its licence. It had been approved for the short-term treatment of schizophrenia and later bipolar depression but sales teams promoted its use for other conditions including Alzheimer's disease, anger management and post-traumatic stress disorder. The company paid US$520 million to resolve civil settlements.[37]

In 2019, John Kapoor, the head of a leading pharmaceutical company, was found guilty of defrauding insurance companies in a push to sell 'Subsys', a spray made from fentanyl, a synthetic opioid many times stronger than morphine. The spray had been approved for use by terminal cancer patients but the company targeted sales to the much bigger and more profitable market of patients with non-life-threatening chronic pain. They hired doctors with high prescription records as seminar speakers for large fees. Kapoor was sentenced to 5.5 years in prison in 2020.[38]

In Croatia, the officers of a pharmaceutical company were indicted for the criminal offence of bribing a large number of physicians and pharmacists in order to achieve high sales figures. The bribes were provided in the form of value tickets, money, paid travel arrangements as well as other gifts to the value of five to ten percent of the value of the prescribed drugs.[39]

Two former UN consultants rigged contracts to supply drugs to the Democratic Republic of the Congo in return for bribes. Their company received contracts from a UN development programme to tackle HIV and malaria. They leaked details of the contract to Mission Pharma, a Danish pharmaceutical company, so that it could win the contract to supply the drugs. Their fee was US$1 million. A UN investigation team uncovered the corruption and the men were jailed in 2015.[40]

In 2012, Abbott Laboratories pleaded guilty and agreed to pay US$1.5 billion to resolve its criminal and civil liability arising from the company's unlawful promotion of the prescription drug 'Depakote' for uses not approved as safe and effective by the FDA. The drug had only been approved for three uses: epileptic seizures, bipolar mania and the prevention of migraines. The company also promoted the drug to control of behavioural disturbances in dementia patients and to treat schizophrenia despite the evidence from two studies it had funded that failed to show a statistically significant treatment difference between anti-psychotic drugs used in combination with Depakote and anti-psychotic drugs alone. As the Acting Associate Attorney General put it: 'As this criminal and civil resolution demonstrates, those who put profits ahead of patients will pay a hefty price'.[41]

Eli Lilly pleaded guilty in 2009 to actively promoting olanzapine (sold under the trade name Zyprexa among others) for off-label uses. including the treatment of dementia. The company began its promotion by encouraging doctors who treated patients at nursing homes to prescribe olanzapine because one of the drug's side effects was sedation. The company had also violated privacy rules by culling patient lists at doctor's offices at weekends in the hope of switching patients to Lilly products. The US$1.4 billion penalty included an US$800 million civil settlement. Robert Rudolf was one of nine whistleblowers who took allegations against Eli Lilly to the Federal Authorities and shared a US$78 million reward.[42]

Retail pharmacies

Retail pharmacies have also been accused of fraud. In a highly disputed report, PFK Littlejohn estimated that the cost to the NHS was £83 million a year. The stated losses included claims for services not provided and failures to declare prescription charges that had been collected from patients.[43]

In the US, 4% of community pharmacies submitted suspicious or excessive bills to Medicare amounting to about US$5.6 billion, according to the Inspector General of the Department of Health and Human Services.[44] A report by the Australian Corruption and Crime Commission investigated the theft and misuse of dangerous drugs by pharmacy employees. They had discovered repeated thefts by a senior pharmacist at a hospital in Murdock, Western Australia. Their advice was better recording, immediate investigation of discrepancies and better staff training.

The ethics of big pharma

For the most part, international pharmaceutical companies operate within their own ethical guidelines, which include a description of proper relationships with healthcare professionals. However, some companies actively circumvent their own industry rules. A number of UK pharma companies have been named and shamed by their own arm's length Prescription Medicines Code of Practice Authority for breaches. In 2017, there were a total of 72 complaints, 56% of which were upheld and with one company having its membership suspended.[45] Naming and shaming is a weak sanction. There needs to be a greater effort by pharmaceutical companies to walk the talk with regard to ethics.

Competition regulators

Competition regulators in a number of countries have been scrutinising the pharmaceutical industry for some years, imposing heavy fines when they have found infringements. Most cases centre on mergers and takeovers, but others relate to improper conduct and lead in some cases to the disqualification of company directors.

> *In 2020, The Competition and Markets Authority in the UK issued two separate infringement decisions. They found that two companies had shared the supply of nortriptyline tablets to a large pharmaceutical wholesaler. One would supply only 10 mg tablets and the other 25 mg tablets. They also agreed between them, the volumes and prices of the drugs to be sold. Both companies admitted the infringement and had their fines reduced as a consequence. The fines still amounted to over £2 million.*
>
> *In a separate decision, the Authority found that three other companies had shared commercially sensitive information about prices for nortriptyline tablets, the volumes they were supplying and one of the company's plans to enter the market. More fines followed and one director was disqualified for seven years.[46]*

Self-regulation

Whether these numerous and continual breaches of good practice and ethical conduct across the whole of the pharmaceutical sector are sufficiently serious to justify the further strengthening of oversight is a matter for government. The fines that have been imposed, particularly by the FDA in the US, are substantial, but some speculate that they are being regarded as a business expense — such is the scale of the profits that the companies generate. The companies may, sometimes with justification, blame rogue employees, but they remain vicariously liable. A strong and ethical corporate culture, married with authentic leadership, should theoretically block such inappropriate behaviour. The industry is already highly regulated and further tightening of the rules under which they operate may persuade such companies to relocate to countries with weaker rules and laws. On balance, asking the industry for bolder self-regulation is probably the most sensible path forward unless the serious breaches and infringements we have seen above continue. If they do, then governments should act; imposing fines that really hurt the companies and holding directors to personal account.

Conflicts of Interest

Conflicts of interest can be defined as a situation where a person is in a position to derive personal benefit from actions or decisions made in their official capacity. If declared, such situations may be acceptable but leaders need to be exceptionally careful not to get embroiled in controversy. Memorial Sloan Kettering Cancer Center in New York lost its medical director after he failed to disclose a financial relationship with Roche, the Swiss drug company. The same hospital's Chief Executive resigned from the boards of the pharmaceutical companies Merck and Charles River Laboratories after *The New York Times* reported 'undisclosed industry relationships'.[47]

Paula Vasco-Knight was a high-flying Chief Executive of an NHS Trust in Devon and also served as the head of equality and diversity in the NHS. She commissioned her husband to produce a newsletter and a document on leadership for a fee of £20,000, but failed to declare an interest. She later claimed that her husband was the MD of a design business when in reality he was a one-man business working from home. Both admitted fraud and received suspended sentences in March 2017.

Her troubles had begun earlier in January 2014 when a nurse at Torbay hospital, Clara Sardari, claimed that her boss, Vasco-Knight, had shown nepotism and favouritism in the workplace by promoting a member of her own family to a senior post. With another nurse she took her concerns to a senior colleague who told them that they would lose their jobs if they continued to question Vasco-Knight. Sardari left her job and claimed at an Employment Tribunal that she had been effectively forced out after she had blown the whistle on her Chief Executive. She won her case and was awarded £230,000 in damages. The Tribunal found that Vasco-Knight had breached the code of conduct for NHS managers and the South Devon Healthcare Trust's recruitment and selection policy. She had also tried to prevent the release of documents showing evidence of her wrongdoing. Vasco-Knight said the charges amounted to a personal slander and mused, as a BAME[48] person, whether a middle class white male would have been treated with such disrespect. Vasco-Knight resigned in May 2014.

Two years later she was appointed interim Chief Executive at St. Georges Hospital, London, but was suspended once the criminal proceedings involving her former employer began. There was an unusual twist to this case. In 2015, a third party referred the Vasco-Knight case to the Care Quality Commission (CQC) asking that her conduct be reviewed against the 'Fit and Proper Persons Requirement' test which is an essential prerequisite for a senior post in the NHS. The CQC decided that Vasco-Knight had not breached the test. The Parliamentary Ombudsman found that this judgement had not been transparent, fair or proportional. If they had dealt with the case properly Vasco-Knight would not have been able to secure another senior post in the NHS.[49]

A case in England, 'The Read Codes', led to a major parliamentary inquiry into public sector probity rules. The Read Codes were a clinical coding system developed by Dr. James Read, an English general practitioner. The system consisted of a coded thesaurus of medical terms used to record data on clinical computer systems.[50] The NHS bought the copyright to the system in 1990 and a company, part owned by Dr. Read, was given the exclusive rights to distribute the codes within the NHS and provide support for their further development. Dr. Read was appointed Head of the Centre for Coding and Classification. This Centre had a catalogue of failings, including serious weaknesses in its personnel management arrangements, failing to seek competitive tenders for external consultancy services, shortcomings in financial controls and arbitrariness in setting pay levels. The parliamentary committee judged that Dr. Read had been placed in a position where he had a clear conflict of interest and that this should never have happened.[51]

Sharp Practice and Corruption

The difference between sharp practice and corruption came out into the open when NHS England reported that the NHS could be losing as much as £88 million a year as a result of fraud within general practice. The causes for these losses included list inflation, claiming for services not provided, quality payments manipulation, conflicts of interest and self-prescribing. The British Medical Association objected strongly to the report on the grounds that it was wrong to extrapolate a conclusion from a few detected cases. They may have been right but some level of fraud and corruption does undoubtedly exist in primary care in the UK.

In talking about leadership, the Director of Audit New Zealand said: 'Ethics are at the heart of good leadership. Professional connections are grounded in shared skills, knowledge and experience but also in our ethics. Managers need to know the difference between what we have a right to do and what is right to do'. Professor Karin Lasthuizen,[52] also from New Zealand, said: 'This whole idea of ethical leadership is not just about being an ethical person yourself but about cultivating that behaviour amongst employees and within the organisation. Achieving this is no mean feat'.

Government

What about the role of governments? Do they always act with the highest ethical values, or is corruption an issue? Certainly, corruption is endemic in some countries but if we were to define it more widely and in historical terms we might include the health ministers who, in the 1950s and 1960s, denied the known causal links between smoking and cancer because of the problems a ban would have produced for their treasuries.

> *In the 1950s, five reports were published in the UK on the link between smoking and lung cancer. None offered conclusive proof, but the evidence was quite strong. The tax take from tobacco sales was extremely high and the tobacco lobby had a strong relationship with government. When, in 1956, Minister Robin Turton admitted the possibility of a link, he was quickly corrected by his officials. He made an oral 'slip', they explained. Behind the scenes, the issue was managed by John Hawton, the permanent secretary under pressure from the Treasury not to rock the boat. He stymied new research, made sure any briefings did not attack the industry and always included a note about their contribution to on-going research.[53]*

This was a dark corner in the history of the NHS. The defence used by the Ministry of Health of waiting for the evidence 'before I can act' did not work for individuals (see Chapter One) and nor should it apply to ministers. Despite the pressure being applied by the Treasury, health ministers should have made the public health argument about the dangers of smoking much more forcibly and much earlier than they actually did. It could certainly be argued that there is an uncomfortable parallel here with the COVID-19 pandemic.

Politics and corruption have all too often been close bedfellows, as the next case study illustrates.

> *An A&E department in England had struggled for some years to recruit acceptable doctors and, at weekends was often reliant on poorly qualified locums. The hospital never closed its A&E department because that was 'unthinkable' and would weaken its future as a general hospital. Instead, a regional manager proposed an operational link with a major hospital nearby. They would cope with complicated cases whilst nurses provided a local minor injuries service. Local politicians were up in arms and protested to Ministers. The regional manager received a call at home from a minister who accepted the arguments for change but was concerned about the timing. The sitting local politician was about to retire, and an election would follow. Could the transfer of service be delayed? Was this just run of the mill politics or was it corruption?*

Payroll Fraud

Corruption at a much lower level is often picked up by corruption detection organisations that now operate in many jurisdictions. It often involves payroll fraud of one sort or another.

> *The Australian Corruption and Crime Commission in reporting to a State Parliament in 2019 referred to the case of an employee, Judith Innes-Rowe, a clinical trials manager, who made unsubstantiated overtime claims amounting to half a million dollars, and took unauthorised absences from work resulting in a false final leave payment.*[54]

In the above case, the Commission reported: 'Strong internal controls, detection strategies and effective oversight are the best defence against serious misconduct and corruption'.

Academic Fraud

Academic fraud, amounting to scientific misconduct, has been widely reported, but some of these cases are so serious they can be properly categorised as being corrupt.

> *Piero Anversa was Director of the Cardiovascular Research Institute at Brigham and Women's Hospital in Boston (BWH). His specialist field was the regenerative properties of stem cells. He claimed that his research had shown that injecting bone marrow cells into the heart muscle could treat coronary heart disease. However, others in this field failed to replicate Anversa's experimental work and raised an alarm.*
>
> *In 2017, the US Attorney's Office accepted a payment of US$10 million from BWH to resolve allegations that Anversa's laboratory had, as a result of falsified or fabricated data, fraudulently obtained grant funding from the National Institute for Health. A total of 31 publications were judged to have been based on such data and were withdrawn by the scientific journals concerned.*[55] *Despite the fine, BWH were commended for self-disclosing to Federal Authorities the problems they had uncovered in one of their laboratories.*

Lessons for the Future

We need to examine the role of organisational culture as the principal defence against fraud and corruption in the healthcare sector. How do organisations build a culture where fraud is neither ignored nor tolerated? There is no single answer to this question but sensible and well-organised detection measures must be part of the solution. The rights of whistleblowers must also be protected. There should be no disincentive for exposing wrongdoing by medical practitioners, pharmaceutical companies or governments. In some societies, payments for services that should be free, or bribes paid to gain faster access to services are commonplace but difficult to deal with without major cultural change involving both patients and healthcare professionals. It is as much a political challenge as it is a problem of criminality.

As far the relationship between healthcare professionals and the pharmaceutical and medical device industries is concerned, some practical steps might include prohibiting healthcare professionals from accepting anything at all from pharma companies, directing all research funding to institutions instead of individuals and creating ethics committees to advise individuals when difficult choices emerge. Public hospitality registers are less effective but would be better than nothing. A requirement that individuals should make professional declarations of interest when appropriate is also essential in avoiding unethical behaviour. Strong, honest and authentic leadership is vital in setting an example for others to follow.

Insurance fraud is a problem in many jurisdictions. It will only reduce when such fraud becomes more difficult and detection rates increase. Clearly, the US healthcare system is more prone to such abuses than single payer systems.

Corruption has often been found in hospital building projects either during the contract letting process or in the way that the construction project is organised. Auditors should always be alert to this risk.

National or regional anti-corruption agencies appear to be good at picking up major fraud and corruption and increasingly operate across national boundaries. Stopping the manufacture and sale of counterfeit drugs, for example, needs international action as their supply expands through the Internet. This is particularly important as many lives are at risk.

The problems of the digital age, such as how to protect data, apply to all industry sectors, but healthcare systems must step up and take more seriously the issue of patient privacy. Robust systems to protect patient data must become a higher priority.

Sadly, fraud and corruption are present in all walks of life and healthcare is no different. To minimise the risks that we have seen in this chapter, there should be greater emphasis throughout the sector to prevent and detect abuses.

Chapter Eight
The Sexual Exploitation of Children: The Health Response

The sexual exploitation of children has usually been regarded as a problem to be dealt with by law enforcement agencies and has been recognised as a major health issue only in recent years. In England, the tipping point was reached with the scandal in Rotherham, exposed in 2014, and which led to harsh criticism of the social and healthcare services.

The impact on health of such abuse is devastating and detrimental to a child's physical, psychological and emotional well-being, with a lasting impact on both the child and other family members. One Australian study found clear evidence of a link between child sexual abuse and depression, suicide, post-traumatic stress disorder and adult sexual promiscuity.[1]

The signals of sexual exploitation taking place are varied and include children going missing from their homes and schools, mental health problems, the detection of sexually transmitted diseases, unplanned pregnancies, unexplained injuries, misuse of drugs or alcohol and committing petty crimes. Many abused children were in health or social care institutions when the offences happened. Children's homes have historically proved to be an easy target for predators.

Children are, by nature, vulnerable to those more powerful than they are and often ashamed and afraid to report incidents of abuse. Indeed, in many cases they do not understand what is happening to them or that this is abuse. The Internet has made it far easier for abusers to groom children and produce and distribute child pornography. In a conference at the National Press Club in 2020, the Australian Federal Police Commissioner said:

> *Today I want to lift the lid on society's dark secret. I want to shine a light on the ever increasing online exploitation of our children, by those who seek to do them harm. Deviant and perverted offenders, with global reach, who are using the dark web to evade law enforcement detection and commit heinous crimes against our most vulnerable. We all think we can use the clear web, or surface web safely as long as we follow some basic precautions. Yet this is where the predators hunt for our children. And the dark web is a more sinister place, where these predators lurk and hide in complete anonymity. Over a decade ago, the Australian Police received about 300 referrals for online child exploitation material a year; in 2019 there were almost 17,000. In the USA it's in the millions. We are seeing more videos, younger children and more violence. We are seeing the rape and torture of our children all for sexual gratification. This is organised crime but the commodity is our children.*[2]

In the UK, another senior police officer, Simon Bailey, the Chief Constable of Norfolk said: 'We are seeing exponential increases in the reporting of abuse year on year ... do I think there are more people with a sexual interest in children in the population? Probably not. What there is though, is a greater opportunity for them to fulfil these desires. Technology has opened up new opportunities for people to do that'. A colleague, Peter Wanless, added: 'Child sex abuse is about abuse of power. Victims are cowed into silence'.[3]

In the UK, a number of major scandals have exposed the problem to the public and, as a consequence, forced health and social care services to develop plans to better protect children in their care, support the child victims and provide services that support the affected families. However, this is an international problem. In the US, it is estimated that between 100,000 and 3 million children a year suffer the horrors of sexual exploitation.[4]

> *On the day she met Thompson, the girl later told the FBI, she was only 15, alone on the streets and contemplating suicide. He promised to make her a model. But it was a lie and in the summer of 2015 Thompson and his wife forced the girl on a six-week trek across the southern US. Photographed in suggestive poses and marketed online, she was sold for sex out of hotel rooms and truck stops. She was beaten if she refused. She was eventually recognised as sex-trafficking victim at a hospital in St. Louis. Thompson and his wife were arrested and he was eventually sentenced to 20 years in prison.[5]*

A European task force estimated that between 10% and 20% of children are sexually assaulted during their childhood.[6] Another report showed that thousands of people, including children, are being sexually trafficked in Europe every year. Organised criminals are making considerable profits from the suffering and abuse of children.

Cleveland

One of the earliest examinations of child sexual abuse took place in Cleveland in the northeast of England. A total of 125 children were diagnosed by a consultant paediatrician as having been sexually abused, as shown by evidence of anal dilation. The children were subsequently removed from their families or foster homes. However, the families, supported by other clinicians disputed the evidence. The Butler Sloss Inquiry[7] was established to investigate and criticised the original medical reliance on a single test to separate children from their families. The use of anal dilation as a signifier of abuse was not new and although it was unusual in children it was not in itself evidence of anal abuse. A diagnosis of abuse should not be made simply on the basis of a medical examination but on the rounded opinions of medical, nursing, social work and police professionals. Children should not, the Inquiry said, 'be the subject of repeated examinations or confrontational disclosure interviews for evidential purposes'.

The US State Department publishes an annual report[8] on human sexual trafficking and ranks countries on their efforts to combat it.

Most developed countries are found in tier one but there are some exceptions, including Ireland, that are rated in tier two. Ireland did not have specialised accommodation and adequate services for victims and had chronic deficiencies in victim identification, referral and assistance. They had also not secured any trafficking convictions.

An Optimus Study of South Africa showed that the sexual abuse of children was widespread with one in three adolescents questioned reporting at least one incident in their lives.[9] A Royal Commission in Australia reported 361 cases of abuse in out-of-home care to the police and interviewed 160 survivors of sexual abuse in healthcare settings.[10]

From about 2012, journalists in England began reporting that organised groups of men were able to groom, pimp and traffic girls across the country with virtual impunity. Offenders were identified to police but not prosecuted. In part this was because the girls declined to give evidence.

Rotherham, England

The Jay report into child sexual exploitation in Rotherham, an English town in South Yorkshire in 2014, raised major alarm bells.

No one knows the true scale of child sexual exploitation in Rotherham over the years but a conservative estimate suggests that 1,400 children were sexually exploited between 1997 and 2013. Just over a third of these cases were children previously known to social services because of interventions made for reasons of child protection and neglect. Children were raped by multiple perpetrators, trafficked to other towns and cities in the North of England, abducted, beaten and intimidated. There were examples of children being doused in petrol and threatened with being set alight, threatened with guns, made to witness brutally violent rapes and threatened that they would be next if they told anybody.

All of this happened in plain sight. Damaged children were presented to many services, but officials judged the reports to be exaggerated and little effective action was taken.

One of the common threads running through child sexual exploitation across England has been the prominent role of taxi drivers in being directly

> *linked to the children who were abused. This was the case in Rotherham from a very early stage in the 1990s when the heads of residential care homes met to share intelligence about taxis and other cars that collected girls from outside their units. In the early 2000s some secondary school teachers were reporting girls being picked up at lunchtime at their school gates and being taken away to provide oral sex to men in the school lunch break. The majority of victims were white British children and the majority of perpetrators were from minority ethnic communities. At least 1400 children were thought to have been abused.*[11]

The government blamed everybody. According to the Prime Minister at the time, Theresa May: 'The Jay report is a terrible account of the appalling failures by Rotherham Council, the police and other agencies to protect vulnerable children'.

Other UK cities began to look at what was happening in their areas and found similar evidence of widespread abuse. Large-scale police inquiries followed and these led to numerous convictions over the next few years and urgent action to upgrade the capacity of health and social care organisations to cope. Before the Rotherham report, few had the necessary skills or insight into how to deal with children damaged by sexual abuse.

The Savile Case

In 2012, another huge story broke in the English press. Sir Jimmy Savile, a famous and popular star of TV and radio, who had died in October 2011, was accused of sexual abuse against hundreds of individuals, many of them children. He had worked for many years in family and children's TV, undertaken a huge amount of charity work and volunteered to work at many hospitals in the NHS. The accusations were staggering in their scope and number; the police had 400 lines of inquiry. To many in the general public, Savile was not only a talented entertainer but also something of a hero, associated with film of the many patients that he pushed down hospital corridors as a volunteer porter. Hospital managers picked up few signals about the dark side of his character but rumours had begun to circulate while he was alive, and at one hospital some ward sisters had banned him from their wards. The evidence began to emerge after his death, first in a trickle and later in a deluge. An investigation into Savile's time with the BBC found that he had abused 72 people and raped eight, including an eight-year-old.[12] Inquiries into the conduct of other radio and television stars of that period followed. After the Savile scandal, many more victims came forward and a national police inquiry named 'Hydrant' was established, leading to over 4000 convictions.

Other inquiries into Savile reported that some healthcare staff members were aware of complaints against Savile but did not pass on the information to senior management, fearing retribution against reporting a national 'hero'. Clearly, the amount of money Savile raised for particular hospitals led to a culture of him being 'untouchable'.[13]

The Savile case and other such high-profile cases led to a national investigation into child sexual abuse led by Professor Alexis Jay[14] that, from March 2018, began to publish a series of reports. One of the earliest reports focussed on the UK government's role in allowing children to be removed from their families, care homes and foster care homes in England and Wales and sent to institutions or families abroad, without their parents. We will discuss this policy further in Chapter Ten.

International Peacekeepers and Charities

Multilateral organisations, such as the United Nations (UN), have been extremely active in highlighting and responding to the sexual trafficking of children, but their impact has been blunted by the behaviour of some of their peacekeepers. International charities have also been caught up in scandals involving the abuse of children.

In 2017, an investigation by the *Associated Press* revealed that more than 100 peacekeepers had run a child sex ring in Haiti over a 10-year period and none were ever jailed. The report further found that over the previous 12 years there had been almost 2000 allegations of sexual abuse and exploitation by UN personnel around the world. Many of the abused women and children ended up contracting HIV/AIDS and other diseases that were not prevalent amongst the local population. The UN leaders were, of course, appalled, but peacekeepers are formed from the military ranks of multiple nations — many of which have been guilty of such crimes in war and conflict zones. As Gita Sahgal of Amnesty International put it: '*Quis custodiet ipsos custodies*' (even the guardians have to be guarded).[15]

> *In 2018 it was reported that Oxfam had allowed three men to resign and sacked four others for gross misconduct after an inquiry in Chad and Haiti concerning the sexual exploitation of minors. The most senior of the perpetrators was allowed to resign in a phased and dignified exit because sacking him risked 'potentially serious implications for the charities work and reputation'. According to Penny Mordaunt, International Development Secretary, 'Oxfam had failed in its moral leadership over the scandal'.[16]*

Yet again, the protection of an organisation's reputation had been prioritised over doing the right thing. The actions of these men were neither a secret in the organisation nor were they condoned. Other leaders were just too busy with other concerns to act against one of the most senior members of their team. Resignations did follow, as did new measures for the tougher vetting of staff and mandatory safeguarding training for new recruits.

Children need rescuing from abusive settings and some also need long-term support from mental health and social services. Many governments have established inquiries and later published their plans for improvement.

Australia has established a Centre to Counter Child Exploitation built on four pillars: prevent, prepare, pursue and protect. It works closely with a similar team recently created in the Philippines. New Zealand also has a task force. The US has a Crime against Children research centre. Canada has a Centre for Child Protection and published a report focussed on the abuse of children by teachers that included some painful victim stories. Some of these follow:

> '*My mind will be forever scarred*', a Canadian student said in a victim impact statement about abuse by her teacher. '*You took my childhood and my hope for happiness. I went from a child to an adult in a matter of moments and there is no way back*'.[17]

> *Another student explained: 'keeping my mouth shut for three years was one of the most horrific and destructive experiences of my life so far'. The student contracted an incurable sexual infection from a teacher whilst being abused.*

Following these cases, Canadian licensing bodies started making public their disciplinary decisions against teachers.

Clearly, many agencies must be involved in combatting and dealing with the consequences of child sexual abuse. From a healthcare perspective, the NHS in England has developed a plan:

> *Our vision is in two parts. Firstly, for those who have recently experienced sexual assault and abuse and who are in the immediate aftermath, we must provide highly responsive, personal services delivered by trained doctors, nurses and support workers in settings that respect privacy and are easy to access. These services should include specialist medical and forensic examinations, practical and emotional support and support through any judicial process. Secondly, for those who have suffered historic sexual assault and abuse, we must provide therapeutic care that recognises the devastating and lifelong consequences on mental health and emotional wellbeing. Underpinning both parts is the need for all commissioners and providers of services that support victims and survivors to work together to create a seamless approach that recognises personal needs and reduced fragmentation and gaps in service.*[18]

One obvious omission from this plan is mental health support in prison for the men and women who have abused and need treatment programmes that will minimise the likelihood of them committing a reoffence. Such plans do now exist.[19] One unforeseen consequence has been the need to provide support to the families of perpetrators who often live and work in the same communities as the victims and families of the abuse.

Child Sexual Abuse in Religious Institutions

There are many reports of child abuse involving clergy from many denominations. The Catholic Church enforces a vow of celibacy on its clergy, but has been hit particularly hard by a flood of scandals. These were worsened by the practice of either quietly moving on offenders to other parishes or allowing them to finish their ministries without reporting their alleged offences to the police. Some offenders also moved into other jobs with a close link to children, including nursing.[20] In the US, dozens of Catholic priests who had been credibly accused of abuse found work abroad with the blessing of the church.[21] This pattern of avoiding organisational responsibility and sweeping malfeasance under the carpet has been seen in many settings throughout this book and again, the result was untold suffering for extremely vulnerable people. The Anglican and Methodist Churches have also had to come to terms with the existence of abusive clergy, as have the Muslim communities. We shall hear more in Chapter Ten about other forms of abuse in residential homes and orphanages operated by religious organisations.

> *At the age of nine or ten when delivering the priest's breakfast, I was made to stand beside him whilst he rubbed his hand up and down my leg. Later he put his hand inside my pants. I had to stand whilst he did this waiting for him to tell me to take the covers off the food dishes and dismiss me. I would cry afterwards and a nun asked me why. I said I did not like the priest and was not going into the parlour again and if made to do so would run away. The nun gave me tea and toast in the kitchen. I never saw the priest again.*[22]

In Spain, bishops created a commission to investigate child sex abuse allegations in response to a number of scandals involving Catholic clergy. In 2015, 10 Spanish priests were convicted of child sexual abuse; an outcome that led to the extraordinary consequence of the Pope speaking directly to the victims to apologise. The Spanish government extended the statute of limitations so that victims could bring more cases to court. The Pope declared zero tolerance for abusers in 2019 and changed the canon law to require offences to be reported to the police. Other denominations offered apologies and took action to ensure that future offenders were referred to the police. However, they left ill-prepared healthcare services to offer long-term treatment and support to victims.

The Lucy Faithfull Foundation believes that child sexual abuse can be stopped through preventative programmes, counselling and support. It argues that one of the best ways of protecting children is to work with the offenders, including former members of the clergy. In 2019, it received a major grant from the UK Home Office in England to help fund its helpline 'Stop it Now!'[23]

A Scottish Child Abuse Inquiry reported that in some care homes children had lived in harsh rigid regimes where scant regard was paid to their dignity and they suffered physical, emotional and sexual abuse. At one orphanage, children were sexually abused and beaten with leather straps, hairbrushes and crucifixes. At another, it concluded that some children were subject to sexual abuse of the utmost depravity. 'Many children did not find the warmth, care and compassionate comfort they needed', Lady Smith who chaired the inquiry said.[24]

Margaret Oliver, a former detective with the Greater Manchester Police says that senior officers dismissed her as 'unreasonable' and 'too emotional' when she voiced concerns about the conduct of two investigations into child sex exploitation.[25] She contacted her Chief Constable who replied with a bland email. Getting nowhere, she resigned in 2012 and went public with her allegations, prompting the Mayor to order an independent review. The review agreed that the first police operation had been closed down prematurely and children at risk of sexual exploitation put at risk. She later launched the Maggie Oliver Foundation to help support abuse survivors and whistleblowers.[26]

Reverend Keith Osmund-Smith, who served as a chaplain with West Mercia Police, was suspended in November 2016 for passing reports to the media about hundreds of young British girls being groomed by British Pakistani gangs in the Telford child sex abuse ring. The reports stated that the local Council, as well as the police, knew about the abuse but did nothing to protect the victims. He was reinstated two months later.[27]

Lessons for the Future

We find many echoes from other chapters in this book in the issues and cases discussed here: senior managers who put the reputation of their organisations first; organisations that are either blind to misconduct or hide it when it emerges by quietly moving perpetrators to other areas; agencies that find it difficult to work together; staff who look the other way; and the importance of good organisational culture and institutions that can be openly challenged so that staff and others can safely raise questions and concerns without the fear of reprisals.

One of the key lessons we can learn from these case studies is the importance of local agencies working together and sharing intelligence. Each agency has their own rules about operational or client confidentiality and this can make the sharing of sensitive information and effective collaboration problematic. Formal agreements between organisations can help but sensible professionals who trust each other should be able to find a way of working together without breaching important principles of patient and client confidentiality. Professionals from different disciplines need to be able to share suspicions of abuse with each other without a fear of retribution. As this has generally not been the case, many of the cases of abuse we have seen were exposed by whistleblowers who were unable to find support and protection.

Five years after the Rotherham scandal, actors from different support services have significantly more knowledge and evidence of the needs of victims in order to help them to become survivors. Statutory and voluntary partnerships have matured in their approach and there has been progress in working together towards common aims. An integrated system has been created that provides people with an alternative narrative, helps them build protective factors to increase their resilience and, above all, gives them the skills to navigate a new path forward in life.

Children need to feel safe when talking to health and social work professionals and know that they are supported when they make 'good' decisions. Working with communities and exploring their values and expectations is a fruitful way forward for all of the agencies concerned.

High standards of professional training is also clearly important, particularly in relation to maintaining professional boundaries when dealing with children in trouble. Training staff in primary and community care to identify abused children, understanding how to react once suspicions are aroused and, if appropriate, being able to refer them on to specialist teams is essential. Of course, such specialist teams and services need to be available. Hospital staff in departments such as Accident and Emergency also need specialist training. The whole system would be far more joined-up and effective if multi-agency training programmes could be developed. Treatment services such as specialist cognitive behavioural therapy units are woefully scarce and need to be funded and developed so that they can be made available at short notice and continued for as long as are clinically necessary. A waiting list for such services amounts, in effect, to no service at all for these children.

Some abused children will need lifelong support and this needs to be available when they need it. This support cannot be dependent on one-off grants provided at the start of a specific crisis. Haphazard funding streams are dangerous. A reliable and consistent way of financing such support should be a priority.

Organisations that hide perpetrators by quietly moving them on should be publicly shamed and made to compensate both victims and the state or organisation responsible for the long-term support of the victims. Some, but by no means all of these cases of sexual abuse involve unacceptable behaviour by members of communities that knew what was going on but kept quiet. The voices of concerned parents and professionals should not be stilled by fears of being threatened with defamation or accused of racial discrimination.

Chapter Nine
Managerial Scandals and Problems

Managing healthcare services is not an easy job. The science of medicine is constantly evolving, stimulating changes in clinical practice and working methods. Finance is always a problem as demand always exceeds supply even in the richest countries. Infinite demand is a truism in the case of healthcare. Rationing, or if you prefer it, informed choice, is part of day-to-day life both at the frontline of medicine and in the management boardroom. The sheer complexity of modern medicine demands a high level of coordination and finely tuned process management. Healthcare is a labour-intensive activity and this brings with it the challenges of recruiting, training and retaining the right people as well as maintaining morale within organisational settings — a factor closely linked to providing excellent care.

Contemporary healthcare systems require that complicated teams function effectively with each other and that speedy interventions are made when this breaks down. Specialisation in medicine and nursing has been on the rise for many years but now disciplines such as information technology, biomedical engineering, management and finance are increasingly important. These new healthcare professions are just as committed as their clinical colleagues to excellent patient care and have become established as part of the extended team in modern medicine.

Clinical Freedom

Doctors have always valued their clinical freedom in treating patients in their best interests. This freedom has been increasingly constrained in recent years on both economic and quality grounds. The economic argument centres on issues such as tackling the wide variations in length of hospital stay for the same treatment. Is it acceptable that some surgeons can perform cataract operations on a day-case basis while others insist on an expensive and lengthy stays in hospital? Questions like these persuaded politicians such as Margaret Thatcher to introduce internal competition into the NHS. Many countries have now developed organisations such as the UK's National Institute for Health and Care Excellence (NICE) to advise on the economic value of treatments, including the effectiveness of drugs, and doctors are now required to follow this advice. In Germany, the law dictates that health procedures that are not approved cannot be reimbursed. Many quality initiatives have led to the increased recording of clinical activity and the creation of recommended patient pathways for specific diseases.

Some clinicians welcome these developments as a sensible way to improve good practice, but others resent managers insisting that they follow recommended patient pathways written by professional or specialist societies as an intrusion into their clinical freedom. Some physicians believe that such decision-making should be left to them.

The occasional diversion from an approved pathway can be justified to match the unique clinical situation of an individual patient but the complete rejection of an agreed pathway is rarely tolerated. This unresolved tension in healthcare delivery has continued to emerge from time to time and, when it does, generates a great deal of organisational stress.

Left to our own devices, most of us physicians try our best to provide high-quality care to our patients. But almost none of us provide perfect care to all of our patients, all of the time. In fact, most of us get so caught up in our busy clinics we occasionally forget to, say, order a mammography for women overdue for such tests, or we don't get around to weaning our aged

> *patients off unnecessary or potentially harmful medications. Because the quality of medical care is so uneven, third-party payer insurance companies and government programmes such as Medicare increasingly measure clinician performance and reward or punish physicians who provide particularly high- or low- quality care. The result of all this quality measurement is gazillions of hours of clinician time spent documenting care rather than providing it. Physicians spend almost three hours a week documenting the care they provide.*[1]

Some managers have been accused of demanding that doctors adjust their clinical practices in order to boost a hospital's income.

> *Every day the scorecards went up, so that they could be seen by all of the hospital's emergency room doctors. Physicians who hit the target of admitting at least half of the patients seen over 65 years old were colour coded green. The names of doctors who came close to the target were coded yellow. Physicians who failed to get close to the target were coded red. The scorecards were just one way in which Health Management Associates, the managing company, increased hospital admission rates regardless of a patient's needs. The Chief Executive resigned when this practice became public.*[2]

Health insurance fraud is almost endemic in the US and federal regulators have multiple investigations underway into questionable hospital admissions. Is this smart accounting, or fraud? 'Gaming the rules' became commonplace in England with the introduction of the internal healthcare market and required tough action to curtail.

Bureaucracy

The association between management and bureaucracy is firmly rooted in the minds of most physicians. Recording, measuring and pricing what doctors do has become standard practice for quality assurance in modern medicine. However, the use of competition to spur efficiency has brought with it a flood of bureaucracy, although the greater use of information technology is now mitigating some of this burden.

Many governments want to reduce the cost of managing their healthcare systems and regular purges are made to cut spending. In England, the King's Fund has estimated that the cost of managing the NHS is 8% of the total healthcare budget.[3] This analysis actually suggests that the NHS in England is under- rather than over-managed — in per capita terms England is 30th in the world with regard to its health management spending. The administrative costs in the US, with a system based on medical insurance, had risen to a huge 34.2% in 2017. In Canada, the cost was 16.7%.[4]

Managers do, of course, make mistakes. However well-motivated they and their boards may be, misjudgements are not uncommon and should be the source from which new learning flows. Managerial misjudgements have been centrally involved in a number of the case studies we have seen in earlier chapters. In the case of the Mid Staffordshire hospital scandal discussed in Chapter One, an inflammatory mix of managerial incompetence, a single narrow objective with little clinical relevance and professional infighting created a toxic culture. Managers launched a radical restructuring of the hospital wards with insufficient clinical support, made unreasonable cuts to the number of frontline staff and were in denial about a high level of avoidable deaths. They also cast patient campaigners in the role of the enemy. The basic elements of the Stafford story are certainly not unique and can be found in other examples in this book.

The Professional Background of Managers

Managers routinely operate throughout healthcare systems, with some going on to key leadership roles such as becoming a Chief Executive. In public sector organisations, an increasing number will have a clinical background. In the private sector, lawyers, accountants and business people predominate.

The professional background of managerial leaders in healthcare has changed in many countries over the past decade. The role of medical director is now standard practice in most hospitals. Nurses have always supplied professional leaders and it is now commonplace for them to serve on governing boards. In some countries, doctors have been reluctant to move into Chief Executive roles because of the high degree of employment risk and problems with returning to frontline medicine after an extended break. Nurses are less inhibited and many have moved into Chief Executive positions, particularly in mental health and community services. General managers from non-clinical backgrounds still provide valued support to clinical teams.

The question of what is the most appropriate background for managerial leaders in healthcare systems is widely debated. Some argue that doctors make the best leaders, while others argue that they are too pre-occupied with individual patient outcomes, irrespective of the consequences for other patients and are reluctant to challenge colleagues outside their specialty (as was the case in the Bristol Inquiry outlined in Chapter Three). The skill sets needed for clinical practice and managerial leadership are, of course, very different. Physicians, some argue, focus on outcomes rather than the overall patient experience. Nurses have strong clinical backgrounds but sometimes have difficulty building a managerial relationship with senior doctors. Some believe that managers from a non-clinical background have a wider organisational focus, understand how the whole system works and manage upwards better. They are also, it is argued, more able to focus on government priorities such as the financial bottom line and targets. The truth is that any discipline can produce excellent leaders, but whoever takes on such a role should aim to build an interdisciplinary team around them. In healthcare, teamwork is essential in both clinical and managerial settings.[5]

Alert managers might have spotted some of the serial killers discussed in Chapter Two or the sexual predators of Chapter Eight rather earlier had they developed more open organisations where talking about adverse and unusual events was actively encouraged.

Managers are, as part of their role, the custodians of an organisation's rules on probity. They need to enforce them sensibly. However, in some cases, it is clear that managers can lose their moral compass and stray from the boundaries of probity themselves.

The most serious problem faced by managers is when they lose the confidence of their clinical staff. A vote of no confidence is often terminal unless they can demonstrate that the action that caused such offence was in the interests of patients and consistent with the values of the organisation. Tensions are most acute when political targets jar against professional ethics. The political priority to reduce patient waiting lists is one such example. Politicians want patients at the bottom of waiting lists to be treated within set time limits; professional ethics dictates that the patients most in need should be given priority.

Politics

Healthcare service managers are always influenced by the political systems in which they operate. Politicians get involved because of their responsibility for ensuring that communities have a healthcare system that is fit for purpose and can be easily accessed. Of course, they are also responsible (in most countries, at least) for largely funding it. Most developed countries invest around 10% of their total GDP on healthcare and so it plays a major role in national economies.

Healthcare systems can come in many forms, but the two principal models are those based on health insurance and those provided directly by governments and paid for out of general taxation (single-payer systems). In almost all countries, the state, even in an insurance-based system, provides a safety net for its poor or disabled citizens, licenses healthcare professionals and makes the fundamental decisions about the type of healthcare system in operation. Governments on the left of the political spectrum usually aim to provide universal care to all their citizens and keep healthcare systems predominantly within the public sector, whilst those to the right tend to prefer private health insurance and private or not-for-profit providers of care. The value of competition had become commonly accepted in UK politics as a means of stimulating how the healthcare economy worked, although thinking is now gradually shifting towards integrated systems where there is minimal competition. Constructive collaboration is becoming the new objective.

There is plenty of evidence that policies aimed at reducing social inequalities often have a positive impact on health indicators such as infant mortality and life expectancy at birth.[6] The US, with by far the highest level of investment in healthcare — 17% of GDP in 2018 — has world-class standards of technical excellence but also the most citizens with little or no access to good healthcare. This equality gap is a growing problem which is now stimulating a major political debate in the US about a move towards a more universal system of care. An end to the ubiqitious health insurance system seems unlikely but the Federal government and some States may become more directly involved in first controlling the price of premiums and then paying them for large sections of their population, thus replacing the Medicaid programme for the poor. Making health insurance premiums fully tax deductable is an alternative policy being discussed. An even more radical option would be for a mandatory State or Federal health insurance scheme with defined benefits and employer contributions. Politicians may also want to get involved in reshaping the US provider networks in order to reduce the domination of the hospital sector. Whichever direction US health policy moves in will be highly controversial.

Most healthcare systems have a strong orientation on care and treatment and whilst prevention is much discussed, it usually lags behind in terms of investment because it needs long-term sustained funding to yield results. Some public health policies, such as reducing smoking, cutting sugar content in fizzy drinks or providing better public information about preventing HIV, are political rather than managerial.

Local or National Priorities?

The political debate between national, regional, state, county or even more local decision-making has always been a tension point in healthcare. In many countries, reponsibility for the bulk of healthcare service provision is located at a state or provincial level. In the UK, healthcare is a devolved competency for each of the four countries of England, Scotland, Wales and Northern Ireland. The inevitable variations that local priority-setting creates is an easy target for critics and pressure groups who argue against a post code lottery where the location of a patient affects their entitlement to care and the level of service that they should expect.

In most jurisdictions, the heads of healthcare systems are appointed by politicians and can be sacked for missing their targets. In some countries, like China, the heads of hospitals can only be appointed with political approval.

Most ministers of health find themselves, at some point, in conflict with healthcare professionals who constantly seek higher levels of investment to enable them to use their skills to save or improve lives. Rationing, or 'policy priority choices', as the politicians prefer to call the process, is a mixture of rationality and politics. In large public sector systems, pay and the terms and conditions of service for staff are always contentious and whilst industrial action is unusual in healthcare systems, when it does happen, managers are usually forced to the forefront of any conflict in trying to protect emergency services. In these events their loyalty to governments or to their staff is severely tested.

Ministers come from all sorts of backgrounds and often have little direct knowledge or experience of healthcare policy and even less understanding of the complexities of healthcare management. In some countries, a clinical background is regarded as appropriate, or even required, for a health minister role, but in others (including England) this is almost never the case. Some politicians regard health and social care as the toughest job in government.[7] All too often they use constant initiatives for organisational change to create the illusion of progress or create ever-moving targets for managers to achieve. These often include reducing waiting times for non-emergency surgery, lowering infection rates, decreasing inpatient suicides and achieving efficiency targets. They have, on occasion, also stretched further into clinical practice including setting targets that demand faster thrombolysis and speedier diagnosis of cancer. A small number of strategically important targets may work but when healthcare systems are swamped by multiple and diverse targets, they become ineffective.

Attempts to reduce political involvement in the day-to-day management of healthcare systems have had mixed success. Even when statutory independence is created, politicians still find ways to intrude. They launch independent inquiries, demand resignations and withdraw funding. While keeping healthcare at a distance from politics is possible, achieving complete separation is not. In 2021 ministers in England announced that they planned to regain control of the NHS after their experience during the COVID-19 pandemic.

The civil servants that support and advise ministers of health may be experts in healthcare policy but few have any real experience of managing healthcare services. Ministers value them for their unemotional objectivity, sharp intelligence and their inate loyalty. They offer their advice in private and put into action whatever their minister decides, provided that it is within the rules of probity. Healthcare managers, on the other hand, operate largely in public, even if their organisation falls within the private sector and have a wide span of personal operational responsibility and accountability. They are much more exposed to public and political challenge and criticism. Attempts to integrate managers and civil servants in ministries of health have a mixed history.[8] Ministers in England closed down a semi-independent NHS Executive in 2002. Politicians prefer control and they have been instrumental in encouraging the growth of public-private partnerships that have caused considerable distress for the hospitals who took this option to modernise their estates.

Organisational Change

Health ministers appear to be addicted to organisational change. All too often such efforts create only the illusion of progress. Reorganisations are disruptive, very expensive, rarely achieve their objectives and, of particular relevance to this work, can result in a loss of corporate memory and hard-won quality gains. They also create major cultural problems as organisations downsize, merge and refocus or rebuild, often under new leadership. The difficulty of persuading local politicians that local hospitals produce poorer results than major specialist centres has already been illustrated in the case studies in Chapter Three of this book.

Andrew Lansley took office as the British Secretary of State for Health in 2010 with his own plans to reform the NHS in England. In order to create distance between his Ministry of Health and the day-to-day operations of the NHS he firstly created a new quango, NHS England, to organise and oversee the commissioning process, and then also developed independent Foundation Trusts to manage hospital and community services. The Chief Executive of the NHS moved to lead NHS England and his old post in the Department of Health was abolished. The commissioning of NHS services was transferred from Primary Care Trusts to a consortia of General Practitioners. This was, said his critics, wholly unnecessary, expensive and very disruptive. The same effect could have been achieved by increasing the GP membership of the Primary Care Trusts. It would not be the first time that a politician had felt the need to strip out an old organisational structure to ensure that his or her policies would be delivered. He wanted his structural changes locked in by law. Lansley also strengthened the role of local government in the field of public health and, some claimed, expanded the role of the private health sector. Parliament demanded that he remained ultimately accountable to them for the performance of the NHS, a point he was eventually forced to concede.[9]

His ideas were, in fact, not paticularly radical but they were poorly presented and attracted enormous opposition from almost every quarter. Though he stated that he wanted doctors to be far more involved in managing the system he received little support from medical organisations and there were calls for him to resign. His focus on forcing change through an Act of Parliament was misplaced — he could have achieved much of his reform programme without major changes to the law. Eventually, the opposition became so intense that in 2012 the Prime Minister transferred him to another governmental post. His reforms remained in place but were gradually remodelled over the following years without another statutory reorganisation. Some of his promised cost savings were achieved but became swallowed up in the financial crisis that began to hit the healthcare sector in 2010 through the imposition of austerity policies. Creating wholly independent foundation trusts (made up of individual hospitals or individual community groups) ran against the grain of medical progress which was moving towards much greater service integration.

The central idea of Thatcher, and echoed by Lansley — that independence and self-reliance would generate financial prudence in hospital trusts — was only partially successful. In 2021 the English NHS began to move towards Integrated Care Systems. Partnership working was now valued more than competition.

Professional Politics

Professional rivalries and competition can be destructive. The leadership role of physicians in clinical decision-making is widely accepted by other healthcare professionals. The principal exception to this is maternity care, as has sadly been demonstrated in a number of news stories. Personality clashes between senior professionals generate major problems.

> *The National Women's Hospital in Auckland had been dogged with controversy since an unfortunate experiment that went terribly wrong in the 1990s and the Cartwright Inquiry that followed.[10] Streams of managers failed to secure long-term stability. It closed in 2004 and was replaced by a new unit at Auckland City Hospital. Bryder's history of the hospital[11] attributes its problems to: 'a change not in medical practice but in the social relations of medicine, specifically a distrust of the medical profession as guardians of health. Such misgivings were fuelled by the feminist movement and by territorial disputes between doctors and midwives as well as a media receptive to scandal'.*

Another example from New Zealand highlights the tension between political ambition and managerial reality.

> *Wellington Hospital in the capital of New Zealand has had a turbulent history and a high turnover of managers. One Chief Executive resigned in 2007 when a report was released detailing a list of serious and fatal accidents at the hospital. One patient had died when doctors realised halfway through surgery that equipment was not available in the right size. Another patient died after surgery was postponed three times. In another*

case, a baby died after being discharged early after a long and difficult labour. Some argued that the problems were systemic while others claimed 'clinicians, nurses, management and the board are all engaged in what appears to be a civil war'.[12]

In the middle of 2018, nurses threatened to go on strike to protest about pay and poor staffing. A staff survey had reported that more than half of all nurses and midwives felt under pressure, were emotionally drained, and had witnessed bullying behaviour by their managers. Some highly qualified staff began to search for jobs elsewhere. The Health Board did not have the resources to respond to the pay claim but took what action it could to improve morale. A new Chief Executive arrived in 2019 and came through an audit reasonably well. She was still in post as of the end of December 2019 but high levels of concern about unsafe staffing levels were still rife and being reported to the board. In March 2020[13] the hospital was forecasting a financial deficit of NZ$16.9 million for the year and its waiting lists were continuing to grow. Some were of the view that politicians had built a hospital they could not afford to run.

Value-based Healthcare

The idea of value-based healthcare, central to the Swedish Karolinska case study discussed in Chapter One, is to focus on reducing variations in clinical care. International interest in the concept continues to grow with managers in England, Australia and the US all exploring its potential.[14–16] Value-based healthcare requires hospitals or healthcare systems to redefine the business that they are in by concentrating on their clinical specialties and then organising and managing their services into medically integrated practice areas. As the Karolinska study demonstrated, this is not an easy process. Radical hospital reorganisations, particularly when led by external organisations, rarely succeed. The most sustainable change programmes have strong internal commitment, are flexible in their implementation, are well led and do not offer promises of unrealistic financial savings. Striving for improved clinical quality is a better motivator than cost reductions. Better and safer care often provides improved economic results as a by-product. However, sometimes, a crisis like the COVID-19 pandemic can create the perfect storm for real radical change to take place. For example, we may see a further concentration of hospital specialities, the nationalisation of the increasingly broken social care sector or accelerated dilution of the NHS internal market.

New Hospitals

Building and then opening a new hospital is both an exciting and a dangerous time for healthcare managers. Capital costs often prove difficult to hold within budget. New hospitals usually herald the beginning of an era of expansion of clinical staff with an inevitable impact on the budget.

If a new building has been funded by a public-private partnership, then the on-going costs act as a financial drag for years to come. Public-private partnerships take the pressure off governments to directly fund expensive public infrastructure. In return for building new facilities, private sector companies in effect charge a rent for a serviced building for an agreed number of years. In some countries it has become the only source of capital funding for major hospital building projects.

Some NHS Trusts in England end up spending a significant percentage of their income on such service charges. One of the most expensive deals was struck in Mansfield, near Nottingham in England, which had a partially new hospital built for £326 million that now costs £56.3 million a year in service fees, eating up 16.5% of its revenue budget. The total mortgage costs over the period of the 38-year contract are likely to exceed £2.6 billion,[17] although £234 million of accumulated debt was written off by the government in 2020.

The Royal Liverpool Hospital has a long history but efforts to rebuild it have proven to be difficult. The first attempt, in the 1970s, had 'an intrinsic flaw' in its design. The second, started 2012, agreed in a private finance deal with the company Carillion, a British multinational construction and facilities management services company. There were major problems during the construction process when cracks appeared in three of the concrete floors and asbestos was discovered on the building site. The company filed for bankruptcy in January 2018 — in the largest trading liquidation ever in the UK — with about 20% of the work still to be completed. The government agreed to buy out the private finance deal and restart building from public finances. The completed hospital was due to open in 2020 but the date has now moved forward to 2022.[18] According to a local member of parliament, the whole process was 'a creaking monument to greed'.

In 2006, a large teaching hospital in England moved into its brand-new building funded by a private finance initiative (PFI). The revenue costs of the finance agreement were crippling; representing 12% of their revenue budget, and debt quickly began to accumulate. The management team chose to hide these problems for as long as possible in the hope that a change in government policy might rescue them and buy out the PFI contract. This never happened and senior management faced an impossible decision. Should they strip out highly specialised services, which were not properly funded, but upon which their clinical reputation depended, or sustain basic medical services for their local community? They chose not to make this choice public for fear that it would damage their reputation as a major regional hospital. Instead, they produced an overly ambitious cost improvement programme that bought some time but was never properly delivered. They staggered on, with morale plummeting and the debt increasing until they were finally rescued through a government debt write-off in 2020. However, the underlying problems remain and debt will no doubt accumulate again.

New PFI schemes have now been banned in England and there are calls for the Treasury to buy out all existing schemes. Public-private partnerships are, however, still being used to build hospitals in Australia and other countries, causing much of the same problems. These schemes can only realistically work if future revenue costs are accurately profiled in advance and built into the commissioning prices. New hospitals rarely produce cost savings, though they can evidently enhance quality.

> *The Chief Executive of Sydney's newest hospital, Northern Beaches, a partnership between the Government of New South Wales (NSW) and Healthscope, resigned only two days after the opening in 2018. Deborah Latta had led the Healthscope bid through a competitive tender process to design, build and operate the hospital. The total capital costs had ended up at around AUS$1 billion. The private sector partners would be paid AUS$ 2.1 billion over the life of the contract until 2038. The hospital had been dogged with quite serious teething problems, such as staff, medicine and supply shortages that undermined the support of senior medical staff for the leadership. The Chief Executive had to operate in a very difficult political climate with opposition politicians describing the new hospital as 'part of the Americanisation of Australian health care'.*[19]

This was not the first public-private partnership in NSW that had found itself in difficulty.

> *In 1994 the NSW government entered into a 20-year agreement with a private company to build, own, and operate the Port Macquarie Base Hospital. Under the terms of the agreement, the government paid the hospital to treat public patients. However, the hospital quickly ran into problems and ended up with lengthy waiting lists. In February 2005 it was taken back into public ownership. It was, said the NSW Auditor General, an example of the public sector being left to shoulder the burden and the risk, adding, 'the government is, in effect, paying for the hospital twice'.*[20]

Organisational Culture

Poor organisational culture comes up as a common cause of problems in many inquiry reports. It was the root cause of the problems at the Mid Staffordshire Hospital discussed in Chapter One. Culture is an elusive thing; often referred to as 'the way we do things here' or 'what our values are'. Culture is never static but evolves over time and can be disrupted by changes in professional and managerial leadership. Organisational culture is usually written down in some form (a mission statement or credo), but to become really valuable it should be understood, and the behaviours that it demands have to become second nature to everyone working within an institution.

An independent review of an NHS Trust providing community services in Liverpool reported that the root cause of the Trust's problems was an inexperienced and bullying management and leadership obsessed with obtaining Foundation Trust status and the freedoms that this would bring, irrespective of its impact on patients. They had expanded the organisation well beyond their competence to manage it, including running complex services at Liverpool Prison. In pursuit of Trust status, the managers imposed drastic and immediate cost cuts in order to pass crucial financial tests. Managers set a target for cuts of 15% in a single year. The Trust had arbitrary disciplinary processes and prolonged suspensions without reason. It was not uncommon to see staff crying in the car park. A toxic managerial culture seeped into every part of the organisation breaking the morale of front-line staff and inflicting serious clinical harm'. There was a climate of fear, intolerance, disbelief and insecurity.[21]

If staff are not able to speak out about the concerns that they may have, something was rotten at an organisation's core, said media reports.[22] Perhaps more alarming than all of this was the decision by the national body to whom the organisation was accountable to arrange for the transfer of the Chief Executive without telling his new employer about his history at Liverpool.[23] An unforgivable mistake by an organisation charged with oversight.

An example of a more positive organisational culture comes from Airedale Hospital, in Yorkshire, which has a code of conduct for staff:

Our Right Care Behaviours: Let's make them part of our DNA.
How do we live our right values?
What we love to see:

- *You take the time and effort to understand people and their situations;*
- *You stand up for our values and challenge others who do not;*
- *You are genuine and authentic in everything you do;*
- *You value and acknowledge the experiences and feeling of others;*
- *You go out of your way to help others learn and develop;*

- *You always see things from the patient's perspective;*
- *You are positive and enthusiastic about delivering right care;*
- *You treat patients as you would wish to be treated yourself.*[24]

The Cleveland Clinic in the US has a similar code with a message aimed at patients.

- *We will keep you safe*
- *We will partner you*
- *We will care for you as a person*
- *We will make it easier*

Safety Culture

Building a safety culture is central to success in many industries and is particularly important for healthcare. It requires constant vigilance to protect the safety of patients and staff and demands that all adverse events and near misses are reported so that learning and change can follow. Investigations into any incidents should search for explanations and learn from mistakes, but all too often they degenerate into apportioning blame.

An insistence on the highest safety standards is not an easy option. It brings with it consequences, costs and ethical dilemmas. For example, there is plenty of evidence that hospitals that have a bed occupancy rate higher than 85% over an extended period time are potentially dangerous for patients, yet they still exist and in some jurisdictions have become the norm. Should non-emergency admissions be stopped if bed occupancy rates exceed the safe limit of 85% even though this may result in a disastrous loss of income? A hospital in England that cancelled all surgery until it fully understood a report that concluded their avoidable death rate was higher than expected took major risks with their financial viability and public reputation.[25] Nevertheless, this was the right thing to do and enhanced rather than tainted their reputation in the long term. We have seen many examples in this book of leaders doing the absolute opposite: covering up shortcomings to protect their organisation's reputation.

A probity issue that is currently hotly debated is whether to allow the public access to internal reports on adverse events. One view is that transparency is essential in building public trust. Others argue that any commitment to make sensitive information public will reduce the willingness of staff to report such events and result in a flood of legal claims. One consequence of publically reporting adverse events at Wellington hospital, in New Zealand, was political and public pressure to sack the Chief Executive and the hospital board. Public summaries of anonymised events that include details about corrective actions that have been taken may be a sensible compromise going forward.[26]

Staff Safety

Managers have a legal as well as a moral responsibility for staff safety. Health settings — particularly hospitals — can be dangerous places to work.

Every year, thousands of staff working in healthcare are injured or die whilst caring for patients. The COVID-19 pandemic has brought these numbers to worldwide media attention. The World Health Organization (WHO) estimate that in some countries 1 in 10 of all staff were infected[27] and a yet unknown number died, although the international death total is likely to run into thousands. Some of these deaths will almost certainly be shown to have been avoidable. A similar situation is evident in care homes for the elderly.

There were over 100 COVID-19 linked healthcare sector staff deaths in England during the early weeks of the pandemic and a still unexplained high proportion of these came from the black and ethnic minority community. At highest risk were those of Bangladeshi ethnicity.[28,29] Most of the staff that died were employed in the public hospital sector.[30] It certainly appears that hospitals may have been one of the principal loci for the spread of the disease. The discharge of elderly hospital patients to care homes also resulted in an untold number of infections and fatalities — including those charged with caring for patients.

Italy has reported the death of over 100 physicians.[31] The US was reporting 735 deaths of frontline healthcare workers in early July 2020 and many more are expected.[32] An inadequate supply of personal protection equipment for frontline staff has been a major issue in many countries.

Healthcare workers in a small hospital in Brooklyn took to the streets in protest at the number of colleagues who were dying of the coronavirus. The New York City Council acknowledged the death of 26 employees at public hospitals but details were not available for private hospitals or nursing homes.[33]

Tributes were forthcoming for Jean-Jacques Razafindranazy, the first doctor to die from the coronavirus in France. He had retired as a doctor in A&E and returned to work on an emergency ward at Compiegne to support his colleagues. France's health minister acknowledged the very heavy price healthcare professionals had to pay in the struggle against the virus.[34]

Concerns about the safety of staff working in healthcare services have been around for some years and go far beyond the risks associated with infection.

The US Congress and Work-related Injuries

In 1996, the US Congress asked the Institute of Medicine to determine whether there was a need to increase the number of nursing personnel in hospitals in order to reduce the prevalence of work-related injuries and stress amongst such healthcare workers. At that time, the US healthcare services sector employed almost 9 million people who had between them suffered 6.7 million injuries and illnesses, at a rate of 8.5 cases for every 100 full-time workers — and the rate was worsening. Back injuries were the most commonly reported problems, with older staff in nursing homes particularly at risk. Needle stick injuries were also common with over 800,000 cases a year, often resulting in the transmission of Hepatitis B and, in rare cases, HIV infections.[35] Although the Institute made a number of recommendations for improved safety, with the exception of back injuries, they were unable to substantiate conclusively a linkage between staffing numbers, the skill mix and work-related problems.[36]

Between 2003 and 2011, there were 263 work-related deaths in US hospitals. The highest numbers involved motor vehicles and violence. A total of 33 deaths involved exposure to harmful substances and environments. Injury and illness rates in hospitals were nearly double the rate in the private sector and higher than the rates in the construction and manufacturing — two industries thought to be particularly hazardous.[37]

In England, the health and social care sector reports higher rates of total illness than any other sector but marginally lower workplace injuries than any other part of the economy. There were more than 8000 serious injuries to nurses, midwives and healthcare assistants in the three years ending in 2011.[38] These included 2057 strained backs, 300 broken arms or legs, five amputated fingers and one loss of sight. Later figures, released in 2015, showed that injuries reported to the UK Health and Safety Executive included musculoskeletal injuries, slips, trips and falls, needle stick injuries, workplace violence and stress.[39] There were few deaths other than those caused by infections.

Some hospital departments present special dangers that, although are known about, require clear safety procedures. One example is radiation safety. Clinicians and radiographers need to be very careful about overexposure, follow strict safety protocols and wear dosimeters at all times and, when appropriate, personal protection equipment.

A more common example of preventable healthcare injury follows.

Amelia Anne Covey, who worked as a physiotherapist at Charters Tower Hospital in Queensland, tripped while climbing some stairs. Two engineers said that the gaps between the steps in the staircase were inconsistent and outside the tolerances allowed under the building code. Two other people had also previously suffered injuries. According to the judge, there was no evidence that the employer, through its servants and agents, turned its mind to the safety of the stairway or sought advice. Ms. Covey was awarded AUS$1.6 million in damages.[40]

Physical Assaults on Staff

Hospitals in England reported a 9.7% increase in physical assaults on NHS staff in the year between 2015–2016 and 2016–2017, with over 200 reported attacks each day.[41] Such numbers were clearly unacceptable. More recently, Matt Hancock, the Secretary of State for Health and Social Care said: 'I have made it my personal mission to ensure that NHS staff feel safe and secure at work'.[42] In order to improve matters, the recording of violent incidents was improved and the police and Crown Prosecution Services instructed to act quickly and decisively to prosecute alleged offenders. The maximum prison sentence for assaulting an emergency worker was doubled from six months to a year.[43]

When Miranda Roland (not her real name), a doctor working in the A&E department at a London Hospital, was held hostage by a patient brandishing a pair of steel scissors in a cubicle, she did not panic. Moments earlier she had gone in to check on the young patient, who was having a mental health episode after taking drugs and had closed the door behind her. Although she was alone she thought she was safe — all sharp and dangerous objects had been removed. Unfortunately, the patient had managed to hide a pair of scissors that she pulled out before backing the doctor into a corner. Roland stayed calm and talked the patient out of stabbing her. The police were then called and restrained the patient. Roland then returned to work.[44]

Paramedics in the UK face their greatest danger from young men and women encountered after the pubs close on Saturday and Sunday nights. Paramedics have also often been caught up in public disorder events whilst trying to rescue and treat injured people. In 2018, it was announced that paramedics would be provided with body cameras.[45] In mental health settings, the majority of assaults on staff occur in a morning. In the acute sector, patients over 75 years old are most likely to be responsible for assaults.[46] Long waits in A&E departments are part of the problem as tempers become frayed. Staffs in nursing homes are subject to regular verbal abuse by residents, often linked to their dementia or other medical conditions.

Violence against health and social care staff is also a growing problem in the US; healthcare is regarded as America's most dangerous profession due to workplace violence.[47]

> *'I've been bitten, kicked, punched, pushed, pinched, shoved, scratched, and spat upon', says Lisa Tenney, RN, of the Maryland Emergency Nurses Association. 'I have been bullied and called very ugly names. I've had my life, the life of my unborn child and of my other family members threatened, requiring security escort to my car'.*[48]

According to the US Government Accountability Office, workers in healthcare service facilities experience substantially higher estimated rates of non-fatal injury due to workplace violence compared to workers overall.[49] A research study in 2017 confirmed a continued rise in violence and reported that nursing assistants and nurses faced the greatest risks.[50]

Reports from Australia also state very high industrial injury rates for health and social care staff of 5.5 per 100 employees, with an accident profile consistent with that reported in other countries.[51] There were 521 violent incidents in hospitals in New South Wales recorded by the police in 2018.[52] Hospital-recorded violent incidents and threats over the same period are much higher.[53] In Australia, 16% of all worker compensation claims come from the healthcare sector, with 5514 cases recorded in 2017–2018.

> *Former nurse Graham Levy has a 15-cm hole in his stomach wall, limited movement in his neck, hearing loss and psychological injuries after being assaulted by a patient. He no longer works and has been assessed as having '32 per cent total body impairment'. Sitting across the road from Macquarie Hospital, a mental health facility in Sydney's north, Mr. Levy recalls the day he was attacked. 'This is the first time that I've been here since I was assaulted in February of 2016 … I'm very, very uncomfortable about being here.'*
>
> *On that day, his life was changed in an instant. 'I went to work, as I usually did. I was given a patient to look after who was critically unwell.*

> *I said, "Hi, my name is Graham, I'm a nurse, would you like some hot water for a cup of coffee?" He's turned around to me, started screaming at me, swearing ... and he hit me. I was stunned. (He) hit me again. I went to the ground. He then kicked me twice in the head, abdomen'.*[54]

Policies that take a zero tolerance approach to violence against healthcare workers do appear to reassure staff. Placing police or security staff in high-risk areas such as emergency departments at times of peak risk is also an effective strategy. Training employees on how to spot the early signs of someone becoming potentially violent and to handle attacks can also be helpful. Workers in mental health services are better and more regularly trained to handle aggression. The training emphasis, of course, has to be defence without causing injury to a patient.

Occupational Health and Stress

Dealing with life and death generates its own levels of stress, even for the most experienced staff, and healthcare services need to get better at spotting the early signs and taking corrective action. The way that the airline industry monitors the physical and mental health of its pilots represents the benchmark required. The US, UK and most other countries now insist that pilots undergo rigorous medical examinations each year as part of their licence to fly. In some jurisdictions, this also extends to other flight crew and staff working in air traffic control centres.

Strong occupational health standards and services for healthcare sector employees should be an example for employers in other parts of the economy but this is not always the case. Many health organisations do not invest enough despite extremely high levels of sickness in their workforce. The UK government's Black review[55] of the working-age population reported that 175 million working days were lost annually in the wider economy in England and that the cost of ill health was over £1 billion a year. The healthcare sector is likely to have made up a significant component of this total.

The services needed for healthcare workers must go far beyond health screening prior to appointment and responding to illness and accidents at work. Active steps should be taken to identify health hazards and monitor much more closely the health of staff in critical areas. Requiring physicians and nurses to have renewable medical certificates, or at least to undertake an annual health check, should be considered for those working in surgery and key wards. The lack of investment in such measures is frankly surprising given the clear economic case.

Another area of stress, as noted in Chapter Four, is that of professional staff under investigation by their regulatory bodies or suspended by their employers whilst their conduct or performance is under review. Employers still owe these staff a duty of care and regulatory bodies also need to protect, as far as they can, the health and welfare of registered practitioners whilst they are under investigation.

Security

Security staffs are now a constant presence in most hospitals — particularly those with A&E departments. In many US hospitals, these security guards are armed.

Cleveland Clinic is dedicated to providing a safe and secure environment, enabling the delivery of world-class care. Our force, consisting of Cleveland Clinic Police Officers, Security, Traffic Control and Communication Officers, operates 24 hours a day, 7 days a week to assist all who visit our facilities. Our Officers, in coordination with other Protective Services departments, provide many services, including:

24/7 Safety Escorts;
Active Patrols to Prevent Crime;
Alarm and Code Response;
Community Policing;
Crime Investigation Emergency Alerts (Cleveland Clinic Alert Service);

Emergency Response;
Non-emergency Support;
Responding to Calls for Assistance;
Safety Awareness Education;
Vehicle Assistance;
Victim Advocacy.

The medical centres at the University of California have large security teams, some armed with taser stun guns. This is not just a US development. St. Georges Hospital in London has a team of 22 security staff, as do many Australian city centre hospitals. Security is now a significant component of hospital costs.

Health and Safety Laws

Most countries have laws designed to protect people whilst they are at work and breaches can lead to prosecutions with penalties, including prison sentences and substantial fines. Managers and their boards are particularly at risk. In 2018, five NHS Trusts were fined a total of over £3 million.[56]

Dundee City Council in Scotland was served with a legal improvement notice in 2006 because of the lack of an in-house occupational health service.

Dorset General Hospital in England was served an improvement notice after an employee complained about the high stress levels at work.[57]

The duty of care for NHS Trusts covers not only employees but also visitors and patients. Prosecutions for harm to patients are now beginning to take place in England. In 2019, a private healthcare company in the UK, in what was claimed to be the first prosecution of its kind, was charged with breaching the health and safety legislation after the death of a young patient in its care.

In 2012, 14-year-old Amy El-Keria was admitted to a private psychiatric hospital as an urgent referral from an NHS hospital. She had complicated healthcare needs and a history of attempts at self-strangulation. On admission, she was assessed as high risk and placed under observation every 15 minutes. Four months later she strangled herself with a football scarf. An inquest found that staff levels were inadequate, risk assessments were not properly carried out, staff missed chances to remove the scarf and there had been a delay in the scheduled check.

The hospital pleaded guilty to a charge under the 1974 Health and Safety at Work Act in respect of failing to perform its duty as an employer to ensure people other than employees were not exposed to risk and was fined £300,000.[58]

In 2018, the Southern Health NHS Trust (a public sector provider) was fined £2 million for two offences under the Health and Safety at Work Act. The Trust had pleaded guilty and admitted systematic failures that had led to the deaths of two patients. Connor Sparrowhawk had drowned in a bath after an epileptic seizure and Teresa Colvin died after she was found unconscious in an adult mental health unit. An aggravating feature in these cases was the failure to properly investigate and learn from previous incidents and concerns raised by staff, service users and their families.[59]

The Families of Healthcare Workers

Looking after the families of healthcare staff who are injured or die in service is routine in some, but not all, jurisdictions. As part of its response to the COVID-19 pandemic, the NHS in England made a £60,000 lump sum available to all of the families of staff who had lost their lives.[60] This time-limited scheme applies to the families of all front-line staff who die with COVID-19 including locums, general practitioners, retired staff who returned to work in the crisis and final-year medical students who took up paid frontline roles during the pandemic.

Information Technology

Poorly performing information technology systems have caused problems for many managers around the world.

In 1984, JH, a well-respected English NHS manager, launched his invest-ment plan for computing systems in the Wessex region of England. It was a bold and forward-looking initiative that blended together five key systems of accountancy, manpower, hospitals, estates and community. Every part of the NHS in the region would be involved and contribute to the cost, then estimated to be £26 million with annual running costs of £17.5 mil-lion. Matters began to go wrong during the tendering process, as Anderson Consulting, an advisor on the development of the plan from its early days, became a bidder. They were awarded the contract in partnership with IBM after a reopened round of tendering had moved them from fourth place to that of prime contractor. Accusations made about undue influence and conflicts of interest and at least one of the other bidders complained to the ministers involved.[61]

In Wessex itself, support for the project began to fade as IBM systems were imposed on the health authorities, delays became commonplace and costs began to escalate. In 1990, a new regional manager cancelled the project. A flurry of legal action was then initiated and the police briefly became involved. Wessex Regional Health Authority was heavily criticised by the parliamentary watchdog, the Public Accounts Committee. The Brit-ish Medical Journal was even more critical: 'The Regional Health Author-ity Board had lost control over its managers who were left to go their own way without challenge'.[62]

The managerial vision in Wessex may have been right, but the implementation was extremely poor and delivering the project suc-cessfully may have been beyond anyone's skill base at that time. Adopting leading edge technologies always comes with risks and pub-lic sector organisations do not normally have the capacity to cope with upheaval involved.

In 2003, the Queensland State government decided to introduce a stan-dard payroll system across all of its services, including Queensland Health. IBM won the tender and became the prime contractor. In late 2008, the scheme was scrapped at considerable cost but a decision was made to continue the development for Queensland Health. The system went live, without adequate testing, in March 2010. It cost Queensland in excess of AUS$400 million to run the system that made 35,000 payroll mistakes.

> *A Commission of Inquiry was highly critical of the procurement process.*[63]
> *The State premier described the project as: 'Arguably the worst failure of public administration in Australian history'. If the payment system had been simplified, the software properly tested and a realistic timetable applied, the scandal might have been avoided.*

Similar comments were made about an NHS IT system dubbed by critics as 'the biggest IT failure ever seen'. Its development was abandoned in 2011 at a cost approaching £10 billion. An in-house developed track-and-trace system for the coronavirus was abandoned in June 2020 and the NHS moved to a commercially developed system. 'Stick to the knitting' is managerial shorthand for concentrating on core skills.

The future of leading edge, modern healthcare lies in IT support and the increasing use of artificial intelligence but is unlikely to come from large national systems. Locally developed projects that are proven to work and then disseminated more widely will be a more productive way forward. National IT policy could sensibly concentrate on ensuring excellent connectivity and maintaining quality standards. International systems sometimes have problems in adapting to local cultures. IT specialists with expansive visions but no experience of complex implementation should be treated with caution. Knowledge transfer from other sectors is another poorly exploited opportunity. Companies like Google, Amazon and Apple, with their sophisticated software, are already looking for opportunities in the healthcare sector and may disrupt traditional thinking. They have international systems that work but are very focussed on marketing, ordering, sales and delivery, although the volumes involved are huge. Remote consulting in primary care, adopted so readily in the 2020 pandemic crisis, may be an early target for the further expansion of IT into healthcare.

Delayed Maintenance

During periods of austerity, all budgets come under pressure and routine maintenance is often postponed or cancelled with potentially serious implications for safety.

> *The decrepit and decaying state of many of the buildings at Middlemore Hospital in Auckland came out into public view in 2018. There was rot, sewage leaking into walls and power supply problems. Maintenance budgets were grossly underfunded. Things were so bad that there was talk of the need to rebuild the hospital from scratch. The national backlog maintenance shortfall was estimated to be over NZ$10 billion.*[64]

Managers are blamed for such issues but in juggling reduced budgets they are often left with the unenviable choice of spending on struggling clinical services or on backlogged maintenance. Underfunded maintenance budgets are a common problem in hospitals in all jurisdictions. The shortfall in the NHS in 2017 was put at £6 billion.[65]

Fiddling the Figures

Managers have, on occasion, been tempted to manipulate the data, to disguise growing financial problems, hide clinical errors from patients or obscure a lack of progress in achieving government targets such as reductions in waiting times. The NHS Chief Executive threatened managers in England with instant dismissal if they were caught 'fiddling the figures'. A few cases were detected, resulting in resignations. The boundaries between deliberately misreporting information and fraud are quite small.

> *In May 2002, health managers at The Royal United Hospital in Bath, England, found themselves being investigated for an alleged manipulation of waiting lists and a serious deterioration in their finances. Barbara Harris, the Chief Executive during much of the period under investigation, had been seconded to run the NHS Leadership Centre. She was sacked by the NHS Trust but later won substantial damages for unfair dismissal at an industrial tribunal. The Trust had not followed its own disciplinary procedures nor taken account of her disability (depression) at the time. She denied falsifying waiting lists but admitted that others in her organisation had done so.*[66]

There was a similar case in Scotland.

In 2012 there was a major public row at NHS Lothian after 1000 patients were offered unrealistic outpatient appointments in England and, when they declined, their names were removed from the Scottish lists. Patients who were close to the 18-week waiting limit were managed away in the last few days of each month to prevent a breach. Nicola Sturgeon, then the Minister for Health and Wellbeing, established a full inquiry which reported in May 2012. The Inquiry blamed the culture of NHS Lothian with its focus on 'just do it' and 'no bad news'. Internal reports always had a positive spin. Some in the managerial community knew things were not right but it was easier to keep quiet and get on with their job. The Chief Executive took an early retirement package.[67]

This case and others that followed raised the question of when does a forceful management style cross over into bullying. Forceful managers give their organisation a clear sense of direction and set challenging targets. They listen to and support those that are set the task of achieving targets and help remove obstacles in their way. Bullies, on the other hand, use phrases like 'just do it — or else' and then use penalties or threaten the removal of incentives as a way of ensuring that their wishes are followed. They intimidate rather than explain and inspire.

In 1996, a TV programme alleged that the North Yorkshire Ambulance Service had wasted money on a control and command centre, failed to invest in heart defibrillators and was behind schedule in its paramedic certification process. The programme also criticised the management style of the Chief Executive. A subsequent inquiry rejected much of the criticism but did confirm that the Chief Executive had a harsh, arbitrary and inflexible management style that impacted badly on the operational efficiency of the service. He had a manipulative approach to staff management. Nevertheless, he had a clear and single-minded vision for the Service and gained some national recognition by offering paramedics to cover weekend shifts alongside doctors at the local hospital. He eventually retired on ill health grounds. When the Inquiry report was debated in parliament[68] the local member said: 'there are some essential national lessons to be learned from

> *this sorry tale. The management structure and style failed to deliver an honest team-working spirit and failed to establish a no-blame culture'. The Chairman, a former army general, knew nothing of many of the issues discussed in the report but nevertheless resigned because he judged that this was the right thing to do in the service of the public.*

There are many examples of Finance Directors massaging data to produce a more favourable picture than the facts would justify. In this respect, healthcare organisations are no different from other sectors of the economy. The accountancy professions need to embrace openness and transparency whilst at the same time protecting commercial confidentiality.

> *In 2017–2018, Tayside NHS Trust in Scotland was heavily criticised for covering up overspending in its day-to-day expenditure from endowment funds accumulated from charitable donations. The Trust, said one of the professional accounting bodies, had been window dressing its accounts for some years.*

Wilful Blindness and Denial

How managers deal with external criticism is an important measure of their competence and style. In the Mid Staffordshire scandal discussed in Chapter One, managers chose to challenge the veracity of the alleged number of avoidable deaths at the hospital rather than search for the causes. This might be termed wilful blindness or denial.

Leaders at a famous children's hospital decided to remove criticism that it did not accept from a report submitted to its own board and its external regulator.

> *In 2015, world-famous Great Ormond Street Hospital in London received a series of highly critical reports from a team of external experts about the treatment of children with inflammation of the gut. The gastroenterological team had, they said, overinvestigated and overdiagnosed their patients*

> *resulting in invasive procedures and treatments that could compromise their physical or psychological well-being. This was not the first critical report on this area of clinical practice at the hospital. The hospital later admitted: 'that some approaches had been at the aggressive end of the spectrum' and 'some patients were exposed to the risks of unnecessary invasive investigations, difficult food exclusion diets and drugs with potentially serious side effects'. A follow-up report in 2017 indicated that some improvements had been made but also that some of the gastroenterologists had not accepted the need to change their practices.*
>
> *When the report was sent to the hospital's board and external regulators, a crucial appendix containing complaints from patients had been removed. The Medical Director at the time defended the exclusions, stating that: 'some anecdotal information had been included which is unsubstantiated and not adequately triangulated'. It was, he said, 'important that the progress the department had made over the last two years is not undermined by unverified information'. This highly defensive approach was later criticised by the regulator. Great Ormond Street got it wrong.*[69]

The Leapfrog Group, a national non-profit organisation based in in Washington D.C., produces the Leapfrog Hospital Safety Grade that assigns letter grades to hospitals from A (excellent) to F (very poor). Their latest report, published in 2019, found that the risk of patient death nearly doubled for those using hospitals in grades D–F (6% of all hospitals). Managing a hospital with poor grades presents exceptional problems for the managers and staff but should provide some impetus for action.[70]

Whistleblowers

Whistleblowers initially exposed much of the wrongdoing discussed in this book. Such individuals can sometimes be difficult as their motives may not always be altruistic. For example, some may have a grudge against colleagues or management. However, the information that they provide should always be evaluated with care and never ignored. In many countries, whistleblowers are protected from repercussions by the law and the process for them to come forward has been made easier with online reporting. Senator Grassley, a long-standing US champion of whistleblowers said, 'whistleblowers stand on the front lines of defence to root out misconduct'. They have been increasingly visible in recent years, exposing fraud and corruption, money laundering, tax evasion, the abuse of vulnerable patients, incompetent managers and other poorly performing professionals.

In 2002, an inquiry into the Campbelltown and Camden Hospitals in NSW, Australia, was initiated after nurses complained that their efforts to improve patient care had been frustrated by managers. Their credibility had been consistently challenged and their comments ignored. The inquiry found that the nurses had paid a heavy personal price for their decisions to come forward. Some were no longer working as nurses. Those that were still working at the hospitals reported vilification and isolation by some colleagues because of the public criticism generated by the inquiry.[71]

Dr. Hayley Dare, a Consultant Clinical Psychologist at the West London Mental Health Trust, expressed her concerns about patient safety and staff welfare to her Chief Executive in 2013. She also complained about bullying and harassment. After speaking out, she fell sick with anxiety and depression. Dare discussed a gradual return to duties after an approved period of annual leave, but was told that after an assessment she had been sacked. She appealed to an Industrial Tribunal but lost on a legal technicality after which the Trust claimed legal costs against her, claiming that she had acted 'vexatiously, abusively, disruptively or otherwise unreasonably'. The Trust CEO, in discussions with colleagues, referred to her as a very disturbed woman. Dr. Dare, a single mother of two, was left paralysed by the affair: 'If this does not terrify anyone from speaking out in hospitals ever again, I don't know what will'. Two years later the Trust acknowledged that her claims were made in good faith and in the interests of the public. Her legal costs were reimbursed. The CEO, who had a good national reputation, clearly mishandled an admittedly difficult case. He moved on.[72]

In 2000, a rehabilitation physician at Canberra Hospital in Australia, frustrated by his unsuccessful attempts to get managers to address patient safety concerns, convinced a Minister to order an inquiry into the neurosurgical services at the hospital. The inquiry, which reported two years later, confirmed his concerns about the standard of care but reported that some surgeons had claimed that they were unable to comment on the patients of their colleagues, thus hampering the ability of the inquiry to come to firm conclusions. In these circumstances, peer review was impracticable. The report was never published and when the whistleblower tried to present anonymised case histories from the suppressed report at a hospital grand round, he was threatened with defamation proceedings. The inquiry did, however, prompt the establishment of a 'hot line' for concerned patients.[73]

Two nurses working at a small hospital in Winkler County, Texas, sent an anonymous complaint to the Texas Medical Board (TMB) detailing their concerns about the clinical practice of Dr. Rolando Arafiles, who had trained in the Philippines before obtaining a licence to practise in Texas. He was an advocate of alternative medicine and performed surgery for which he was not credentialed. Arafiles became aware of the complaint and talked to his friend, the local sheriff, about harassment. The TMB sent the sheriff a copy of the nurses' complaint that he shared with Dr. Arafiles, identifying the whistleblowers. As a result, the nurses were sacked and a few days later arrested and charged with the misuse of official information, a felony that carried a maximum sentence of 10 years' imprisonment. The sheriff argued that the nurses had filed the complaint as a personal vendetta rather than as a good faith reporting of facts. National nursing organisations vehemently protested the charges and as a consequence, they were dropped for one of the accused. The second went to trial but was found not guilty. Ultimately, both nurses received a large financial settlement and Arafiles was forced to surrender his medical licence. New legislation prevented the TMB investigating other anonymous complaints concerning physicians. The sheriff was also jailed for the misuse of official information, retaliation and official oppression.[74]

Non-executive directors of health boards sometimes find themselves in difficulty when they disagree with other directors.

Kay Sheldon, a non-executive director of the Care Quality Commission (CQC) complained that the organisation was not doing its job properly and gave evidence to this effect to a legally-led public inquiry. The Chair of CQC asked the Secretary of State to remove her from the board alleging that she was mentally unstable. The Chair then commissioned an independent psychiatric report on Sheldon. This report, by an occupational health doctor, (not a psychiatrist) thought it possible that she was suffering from paranoid schizophrenia and should be assessed or removed from her post. The Secretary of State asked for an independent review of the situation that confirmed a 'fundamental breakdown of trusting relationships'.[75] Sheldon went to court where her lawyers argued that the independent report was unlawful as it breached the legislation protecting whistleblowers. The matter was finally settled and Sheldon returned to the board. The Chair resigned.[76]

Managers who attempt to expose a whistleblower almost always find themselves in trouble.

An unidentified whistleblower in England wrote to the husband of a deceased patient, highlighting errors in her surgery. The husband was 'knocked sideways' and the letter was passed to the police and the Coroner. The Coroner asked the Health Trust to investigate. The Trust launched a major effort to identify the whistleblower led by a non-executive who was a former senior police officer. They employed both handwriting and fingerprint experts to identify the writer of the letter. Senior staff were asked for fingerprint samples and were told that non-compliance would be regarded as an admission of guilt. Medical staff objected strongly to this action claiming that it was bullying and intimidatory behaviour.[77]

Protecting the confidentiality of patient data is an important principle but instead of a witch hunt to expose the whistleblower, the energies of this Trust would have been better invested in investigating the truth of the allegations about the quality of surgery and remedying the faults identified at an inspection by the Care Quality Commission.

Managers can themselves sometimes become whistleblowers.

Throughout the 1990s, medical and nursing staff at King Edward Memorial Hospital in Western Australia repeatedly raised concerns with managers about high error rates and a culture amongst the consultant medical staff that minimised accountability and supervision of junior medical staff. No action was ever taken. In 1999, a new Chief Executive exposed these quality and safety problems to the Metropolitan Health Service Board. An inquiry followed but when the Chief Executive attempted to implement its recommendations, he was blocked by senior clinicians who questioned his competence and refused to cooperate. One sought unsuccessfully to obtain a permanent injunction against the release of the inquiry report. As a result, the Chief Executive was forced to resign. Another formal Inquiry followed.[78]

Gary Walker was brought in as Chief Executive to the troubled United Lincolnshire NHS Trust in 2006. Within two years, hospital-acquired infection rates and waiting lists had both been reduced and its financial problems were starting to be resolved. Things began to unravel when Walker refused to keep meeting government targets for reducing waiting lists on the grounds that his hospitals were dangerously full of emergency patients who should have had priority. He was then accused of bullying and harassment and sacked for swearing during staff meetings. He appealed and at his Industrial Tribunal an out-of-court settlement was reached that gave him a six-figure severance payment but included a gagging clause which prevented him making any further comment. Despite this he gave evidence to a parliamentary committee about his experiences. Dame Barbara Hakin, the regional head, had insisted that he continue to meet the waiting list targets, but was later cleared of misconduct by the General Medical Council. As a result, the practice of using gagging clauses to silence whistleblowers was later banned in the UK.[79]

In 2019, NHS England rolled out a whistleblower support scheme for staff that raised alarms about unsafe practices. Similar schemes exist in other jurisdictions.

Loss of Financial Control and Rationing Care

The most common reason for the removal of healthcare managers is a loss of financial control and the failure of financial recovery plans. A simple but not always acknowledged question is: 'what is your underlying deficit and is it getting worse?' To put it another way, how much of your recurrent spend is covered by non-recurrent grants or one-off capital transfers. Healthy organisations do not have long-term recurrent deficits.

However, what is the ethical position for managers when patient demand outruns resources? In the short term the right response is to take action in the interests of patients but what if this becomes the new normal? Some, particularly those in the public sector, might take the view that the patient's needs must always take priority regardless of the financial consequences. Others argue that financial balance is essential to the integrity of the whole system and without it systems will collapse — an outcome even more dangerous for patients and their families. Politicians have, at different times, adopted both stances, making life difficult for management decision-makers. In the private sector, the choice is starker but clearer; loss-making will lead to closure.

Managers who lose financial control and have no agreed recovery plan find themselves descending into a black hole from which escape becomes increasingly difficult. The worst thing that they can do is cover up the problem as it will not go away.

Fixed Budgets and Rationing

What happens when care has to be rationed? Some medical treatments are extremely expensive. One key ethical dilemma for a manager is when patients and their relatives demand treatment that clinical teams do not think will work.

Child B was 11 years old with leukaemia and had initially been treated successfully. However, three years later the cancer returned in a more virulent form. A bone marrow transplant brought some immediate relief, but the effects did not last. The child became very ill. The specialists in Cambridge who were treating her thought she had only a few weeks to live and judged the chance of a second bone marrow transplant being successful at 2% at best. A second opinion from specialists in London confirmed this view. The child's distraught father did not accept this judgement and found yet another specialist who was willing to try a new and experimental technique. Cambridge Health Authority refused to authorise payment for further treatment on the grounds that they had been advised that another attempt was not in the best interest of the patient and they had many more claims on their limited resources. A large private donation ensured that the child received the transplant, but she died some months later.[80] The Chief Executive of the Health Authority was described as being 'not uncaring but actuarial'.

The legal position appears to be that as long as the decision-making on such procedures is evidence-based and carefully considered, a challenge made in court will usually be rejected. One international commentator put the bar rather higher: 'one clear message from international experience is that rationing can never be separated from values'.[81]

The Times added a further level of complexity to the subject and put it thus: 'The danger of orderly rationing is that no gambles will be taken, no hunches pursued. Every medical procedure that we now take for granted, from hip replacements to bypass surgery was experimental at one stage. Nobody expects health service managers to spend money on moonshine. Equally they must leave space for uncertainty and risk taking'.[82]

Managers must navigate a middle ground between such ethical dilemmas by attempting to shape or redirect demand, seek economies where available and present realistic choices to their boards, payers and politicians. Most clinicians understand the value of financial prudence and stability. The moral dilemma for government is whether to rescue the profligate organisations at the expense of the prudent. In

2020, the UK government did exactly that in writing off accumulated hospital debt in England as part of its response to the pandemic. However, if the underlying issues and pressures that created the problems in the first place are not resolved, the deficit will accumulate once again.

The 2007–2008 financial crisis affected healthcare systems across the world. Many governments made deep cuts to public services, including healthcare, as austerity became the favoured strategy to deal with the economic repercussions. Some countries, like the UK, were able to protect their healthcare systems from dramatic cuts but still experienced nearly a decade of minimal growth (2.1%) and pay freezes for staff over much of that period. Public spending on adult social care fell by 2.1% over the same decade. It was not until 2018 that the UK government announced a five-year NHS plan with an average growth rate of 3.3% and began to ease the downward pressure on social welfare spending. Throughout this period of austerity, most governments demanded ever larger and often wholly unrealistic cost improvement programmes in both health and social welfare that made the growth numbers look better than they actually were. Capital spending programmes were slashed. However, the demand on healthcare services continued unabated and so financial deficits began to gradually accumulate, some of them hidden by Trusts. By 2015–2016, two-thirds of NHS Trusts were in financial deficit. At the start of the financial year 2017–2018, the NHS in England was judged to have an underlying deficit of £5.9 billion.[83] The Royal Society of Medicine claimed that the impact of austerity on health and social welfare in the UK was likely to result in 30,000 extra deaths in 2015.[84] It was the same story in most of Europe as the EU insisted that countries paid down their debt until the financial markets recovered.

One of the first things to happen in a financial crisis, as demonstrated by many of the case studies in this book, is a strain on quality and safety standards. Managers should never knowingly provide dangerous services. Sometimes a higher theoretical risk can be justified but a known danger cannot. The argument that any service is better than no service is simply a slippery slope to disaster, as the Australian examples in Chapter One demonstrate.

> *Health services in Birmingham, England's second largest city, had been under financial strain for some years and were getting worse. A huge overspend was accumulating. Drastic cuts were required but were judged to be impossible in the local political climate. The alternative, a request for more money from government, fell on deaf ears. Plans to resolve the situation had been rejected by the City Council and were strongly opposed by the local press. The Regional Health Authority, whose remit included Birmingham, had not only failed to find a solution, they had also run into serious trouble with outsourcing commercial services. National audit teams swarmed all over the authority. The Chairman and Chief Executive both retired. Their replacements first clarified that the problems existed and were getting worse month by month and then built a new more open relationship with the City Council and local media, sat down with local hospital managers and talked about possible ways out of the crisis. What emerged was a frank and public disclosure of the challenges and the development of a shared vision on the way forward. Local managers and their clinicians were given time to reduce staffing numbers safely through a number of grants and loans. In a normal case this plan would have needed to go to ministers for approval as usually there were community council objections, but on this occasion no such referral was made. Birmingham emerged from its crisis and began to plan for its future, including building a major new hospital.*[85]

Ethics

Ethical problems are not limited to rationing. Most hospitals have, or have access to, ethical committees who anticipate problems and offer advice. There are numerous ethical decisions that need to be taken related to healthcare. None are easy. Should a surgeon undertake a transplant if he is suspicious about the provenance of the donor organ even though it is shown to be compatible for his patient? Should a transplant surgeon proceed if he is told that the death of the planned donor should be reported to the coroner and he should not go ahead without the coroner's consent even if it means his patient will die? Can age ever be criteria for access to essential services? In what circumstances can the spouse of a patient with HIV ever be told? When, if ever, is it ethical to prescribe powerful drugs to a dying patient in pain when it is certain that the consequence will be an early death? Can a psychiatrist or any other healthcare professional maintain confidentiality when a patient admits committing or planning a criminal or terrorist act? Individual cases are a matter for clinicians but managers are sometimes drawn in for advice and support.

Some of these problems are encapsulated in the following case study, often used in the training of healthcare managers.

Stunned, Carolyn Aubrey, the CEO of the Metropolitan Hospital, sank into her chair and stared out of the window for a very long time. She realised that something was a foot when Dr. Midmore's wife had angrily insisted on meeting her and then telling her that she was suing her husband, a popular orthopaedic surgeon, for divorce because he had given her AIDS. Was this just the ranting of an angry vindictive wife or could it be true? Dr. Midmore was still operating. Aubrey recalled he had played a major part in discussions about patient and surgeon safety when the surgical division had demanded to know the HIV status of all patients prior to surgery. The special risks to surgeons of torn gloves and cuts during orthopaedic surgery had been discussed at length. Aubrey asked her secretary to call the hospital's attorney and medical director and fix an urgent meeting. Mrs. Midmore had been right that something must be done. But what?[86] It was agreed that in the interests of patient safety, Dr. Midmore must be challenged and even if he denied having HIV be required to undergo an independent test to verify this. His operating schedule would be stopped until he was declared clear. He would also be encouraged to take a short spell of sick leave whilst the tests were being done. It would be for him to decide what to say to his colleagues. If the test proved positive a decision would have to be made about informing all his patients and inviting them in for review. If the test proved negative he should return to his duties immediately with thanks for his cooperation. Mrs. Midmore would be told that her information had been taken seriously but not informed about the agreed action or the outcome of the tests. She would be asked if she needed medical help herself.

Research ethics are well-established in most universities and teaching centres but practice must to be monitored for adherence.

Management Fads

Managers in healthcare are just as susceptible to managerial fads as any other manager in any other sector of the economy. Work study and bonus schemes became fashionable in the 1970s and were followed by consensus management, efficiency targets, process re-engineering, self-governing teams, total quality management, performance excellence and consumer delight with a friction-free client experience. Most had a short life.

Shapiro put it as follows:

'The practice of riding the crest of the latest management panacea and then paddling out again to ride the next one; always absorbing for managers and lucrative for consultants, is frequently a disaster for organisations.'[87]

Quality improvement has emerged as a managerial imperative in healthcare in recent years. However, many improvement gains are short-lived.

Sigma was a local quality improvement programme introduced into two English NHS regions in the late 1980s with the objective of improving the performance of their systems and making them more sensitive to individual patients. It set unthinkable standards using examples from other industries. A Sigma outpatient clinic was one where all patients and physicians arrived at the clinic at the appointed time. All case notes and ordered diagnostic test results were available to the physician together with interpreters if required. Every General Practitioner received a summary of the outcome of the consultation within 48 hours.

In order to achieve these targets (a 100% success rate was required), hospital systems had to be remodelled, some double banked and clinic preparation had to begin days earlier then had previously been the case. The philosophy was to get it right first time. Sigma clinics were very economic.[88] However, the leaders who had been inspired by this programme moved on and it lost momentum as hospital systems defaulted to their previous practices. The changes had not been locked in so that default was impossible. Five years later, it was another quality initiative lost in the past. This is the fate of many quality improvement programmes.

Courage

Bravery is not something normally associated with the day-to-day activities of a manager but speaking honestly to politicians, appearing before a hostile press or local community group, or confronting senior colleagues with personal conduct issues does sometimes require managerial fortitude. Healthcare managers can also face exceptional challenges in periods of war or conflict.

A manager in Northern Ireland let it be known to a terrorist organisation that doctors at his hospital had determined that members of the group would not be treated after some of their members had entered the hospital searching for their enemies. The terrorist organisation asked for a secret meeting with the manager. They vouched for his safety, but should he go or inform the security services? He decided to proceed, told only his deputy and waited outside the hospital to be picked up. At the meeting, the terrorist leaders explained that the hospital incursion had not been authorised and would not happen again. The manager accepted their explanation and said he would report back to the medical staff. The ban was quietly lifted.[89]

Managerial Codes of Conduct

As we saw in Chapter Four, managers are not regulated like other healthcare professions, although in some jurisdictions, like England, those working in the public sector are required to operate within a national code of conduct. Similar codes exist in Australia and other countries. HCA Healthcare, a large UK private provider, has a company code of conduct. This stresses the unique and intrinsic value of each individual, the need to treat other with compassion and kindness, to act fairly with absolute honesty and integrity, and trust colleagues and treat them with respect, loyalty and dignity.

Managerial ethics are rarely codified or enforced.[90] As a result, there are too many examples of managers being prepared to live with unacceptable levels of patient risk just to keep their services open.

Heads Must Roll

Managers and Chief Executives sometimes have to resign or are dismissed when bad things happen in their organisations in order to satisfy public demands for 'justice' or a public clamour for heads to roll. Some managers simply walk away so as not to create further damage to the organisation; others decide to fight but usually lose. The NHS, like many other organisations, has often failed to distinguish between those managers who have just not been good enough and may need help and coaching and those who have lost their moral compass and should never be employed again in a healthcare setting. A 'fit and proper person test', introduced in England for the directors on health boards, effectively bars individuals who have been convicted of crimes or previously struck off professional registers. Having a history of bankruptcy or being listed on a sex offender's register would also exclude an individual.

There is a relatively high turnover of Chief Executives in healthcare. This is problematic because one feature of an excellent hospital is managerial stability and strong leadership. Of course, Chief Executives are never free agents wielding unfettered power but serve at the behest of their boards. A widening gulf in thinking between the Chief Executive and the board (or the chair of the board) is an immediate sign of stress.

Hubris, excessive pride or overconfidence, has led some managers into trouble. They typically refer to 'my' organisation being the best and therefore attempt to place themselves beyond challenge or criticism. Such individuals often forget the boundaries of probity. They see only success and are obsessed with self-image and the protection of the reputation of their organisations. They are impulsive and inclined to make decisions based on instinct rather than fact. Some view hubris as a clinical syndrome — an acquired personality disorder.[91] Most studies of hubris have focussed on political leaders, but the trait applies to everyone who holds a substantial degree of power. It falls to management boards to spot such hubris in their managerial leaders and take steps to curb the worst excesses, as the individual is unlikely to have any personal insight into the problem. Actions that can be taken include closer oversight of decision-making, exit interviews for staff who leave in unusual circumstances, insuring that whistleblowing policies are working properly, close checks on how personal expenses are being managed and a focus on investigating erratic, impulsive and manipulative behaviour. The differences between an inspired, visionary leader and a hubristic one can be small.

Managing Pandemics

As we first discussed in Chapter One, pandemics have also created serious problems for both healthcare managers and politicians. There will be many inquiries into how the COVID-19 pandemic has been managed around the world, and this will be painful and challenging for everybody involved.

> *Angela Hernandez Puente, a surgeon and general secretary of Madrid's AMTYS medical association said: 'political rhetoric could not be used to hide missteps and mistakes in Spain's response to the virus. The excuse that "we are doing everything that we can", or "we're on a war footing", can't be allowed to cover up the managerial deficits we are seeing at both a regional and a national level'.*[92]

It is for governments to decide what action to take, if any, to protect their citizens, but this is usually decided on the basis of medical and scientific advice. The WHO eventually declared the epidemic a pandemic on March 11, 2020, based on the degree of international spread. Some have argued that this was too late and that they misjudged the timing of the declaration under political pressure from some members.

In many countries, public health is a state or provincial responsibility. However, the response demanded by the pandemic required action well beyond public health encompassing economics, education, immigration, travel and even the deployment of armed forces, some of which were the responsibilities of national or federal governments. This tension was noticeable in the responses from some countries to crucial decisions on how to manage hospitals, provide PPE and commence or end lockdowns.

Few countries were properly prepared to manage the pandemic despite multiple warnings of many years that such an event could and should be reasonably expected. COVID-19 was not, after all, the first pandemic of the 21st century.

In 2017, the plague reappeared in Madagascar and led to 2417 confirmed, probable and suspected cases and 209 deaths. Severe Acute Respiratory Syndrome (SARS) was unheard of until 2003 but infected more than 8,000 people in many countries, killing one in 10 of them. In 2009, a novel influenza, H1N1, spread widely across the world but the effect was not as severe as had been expected. In 2012–2013, a new virus, Middle East Respiratory Syndrome (MERS) surfaced in the Middle East and spread widely into other regions. The Ebola virus, which emerged in Africa in 2014, produced a viral haemorrhagic fever and spread across three continents. In 2015, the Zika virus, spread by mosquitos caused dreadful damage to the brains of unborn children. Since 1970, more than 1500 new pathogens have been discovered.[93]

> *In 2015 it took just one traveller to bring MERS to South Korea after spending time in the Middle East. The consequence was a Korean outbreak with 186 cases and 36 deaths. The outbreak had related costs of US$8 billion all in the space of two months.*[94]

The WHO traced a clear pattern for such events, including diseases that had thought to be eliminated like cholera, the plague and yellow fever, as they often return, as well as emerging new strains and types of viruses. The epidemics of the 21st century are spreading faster and further than ever before. Our globalised world is ideal for rapid transmission.

There will be much to learn from the different government responses to the COVID-19 pandemic and particularly when and how actions were taken, although the learning is likely to be blurred by those seeking to avoid or attribute blame. Some governments may have moved too early to close down their economies, schools and universities and some too late. Some will have relied too heavily on epidemiological models of disease spread that proved to be less than perfect. There will be many lessons to be learned about how the extended supply chains for personal protective equipment were organised and the most appropriate levels of strategic reserve stocks. We now know from the evidence in both China and the UK that it is possible to radically and rapidly expand hospital capacity with temporary new hospitals. Impeccable hygiene practice in hospital settings has been essential during the pandemic and good organisations will find ways of embedding this best practice into their future daily routines. Track and trace procedures have rarely been tested on the scale required in 2020 and will benefit from being reviewed so that they can be placed on permanent standby ready for the second wave of COVID-19 or the next infectious disease outbreak.[95] The safety of healthcare workers was seriously compromised in this pandemic. Doctors and nurses were, in many cases, inadequately protected and those most at risk of infection were left exposed instead of being deployed to safer areas. Care homes for the elderly proved to be at a particularly high risk, and support mechanisms for workers in these settings were slow to be put in place and wholly inadequate. The science makes a clear argument that health and social welfare systems should be integrated, but the politicians remain more focused on cost and ownership.

Visiting patients in hospitals by friends and relatives was severely constrained during the COVID-19 pandemic and may continue to be heavily circumscribed in the future as a means of reducing infections to a minimum. Electronic communication seems likely to become the main mode of contact between patients and their friends and family. Good hospitals will change their procedures in response to this new normal.

Lessons for the Future

The case studies in this chapter tell us quite a lot about what successful healthcare sector managers look like. They operate most effectively when they manage within a clear and well-defined and understood set of values and ethics and have the respect and support of their clinical community.

These managers secure the best results when they see themselves as part of a wider team providing support to those on the frontline of healthcare. Although it may be counterintuitive, it is not always the right answer for them to share the pain of difficult decisions. In some cases, it is better to explain the circumstances, make the decision and accept the accountability that this entails. If the decision is consistent with the organisation's values, it will be accepted. They will have built a positive and a safe culture and been in post long enough to see it firmly embedded.

Successful managers understand the stresses and strains of clinical practice and retain their respect for medicine in all its forms. They limit their intrusion into personal professional practice to issues or cases that really matter and even then deal sensitively with the professionals concerned. The best interest of the patient should always be central to their actions.

Major reorganisations of clinical services such as ward reconfigurations in hospitals need to be managed and handled with great care. Major system change is expensive and potentially hazardous and should only be embarked upon after the most serious consideration of the risks. Good managers know this.

In times of austerity and cuts to funding, managers need to be able to deal with difficult decisions and minimise risk for both the organisation and its patients. Any temptation to reduce safety standards must be resisted. When financial pressures weigh heavily, becoming wilfully blind to reality is a constant danger.

The health and safety of staff is just as important as the safety of patients and visitors. Building a robust safety culture is not easy but is essential — if staff are safe, so, usually, are patients. The physical and mental health of staff with close personal contact to patients should be closely monitored in everyone's interest.

Large hospitals and other healthcare organisations employing thousands of staff should consider appointing a Director of Staff Health with a seat on the managing board. People are the most valuable asset in any healthcare system. Reducing the extremely high rates of absence through sickness (both physical and mental) would almost certainly cover such an investment. Employees that are judged to be at the highest risk because of their health background or ethnicity should not, in situations such as the COVID-19 pandemic, be deployed in dangerous areas. Staff should never be placed in a position where they have to risk their personal safety for their patients. We can expect more prosecutions under Health and Safety Laws, particularly where employers have failed to provide staff with adequate personal protection equipment. The impact of the COVID-19 pandemic on healthcare staff across the globe may well come to be seen as 'never' or sentinel events, that require radical changes in how healthcare systems operate in the future. National and local emergency planning certainly needs far better preparation for future pandemics.

The safety of whistleblowers must also be ensured, with measures taken to protect their identities, remove gagging orders on staff and managers and crack down on any attempt to retaliate against them. Of course, ideally an open and inclusive organisational culture, essential for a healthy working environment, will mean that they are needed less in the future.

Zero tolerance policies to control violence against staff need to be backed up with practical measures, such as posting security staff or police in high-risk areas at peak times. Personal body cameras for staff may also be useful and employees should be trained to quickly identify potentially violent threats. All of these measures will add to costs, but are necessary.

The adoption of new technologies — whether in the operating theatre or through the use of new IT systems — provides enormous benefits for modern healthcare practice, but it needs to be introduced and managed carefully and properly tested, with staff buy-in. No technology is infallible and some can be dangerous.

Chief Executives of healthcare organisations change far too frequently to provide continuity to the organisations they manage. Supervising authorities need to distinguish between those managers who, for whatever reason, are judged to have failed but can learn from the experience, and those who have lost their moral compass, are hubristic or weak and should never be employed again. All managers, if there is no national scheme to regulate them, should adhere to and operate within the boundaries of accepted professional codes of conduct.

Managers who lose their respect for medicine and its practitioners never succeed. Poor or incompetent management impacts directly on the quality of care offered to patients, as is demonstrated by many of the case studies this book has provided from the dark side of healthcare.

Chapter Ten
Social Care

There is a wide international variation in the way social care is both defined and delivered. In some countries, it is integrated with, and in others, separate (though adjacent) to healthcare services. At an operational level, the two sectors are inextricably linked. A crisis in one generates problems for the other.

Social care is extremely expensive, and the average OECD cost for only long-term care was 1.7% of GDP in 2017.[1] Some country examples are provided below before we look at service failures and the lessons that can be learned.

Some social welfare systems, such as in Australia, are focussed on the poor with the option of a personal budget to access care. France has a mandatory social care insurance system to which every citizen contributes, which includes a subsidy for the poor. The US system also operates an insurance system but most citizens enter social care as a payer until Medicare kicks in for those without assets. The Scandinavian countries have generous social welfare systems but still have an element of cost sharing with the citizenship. In England, care is funded through general taxation once the assets of a citizen have reduced to a set (and quite low) level. In most countries the responsibility for providing social care lies with provinces, states or local governments. Their responsibilities usually encompass children and disabled people as well as the elderly. All are now trying to develop home-based rather than residential care. In all countries, social care systems are now under financial strain as the numbers of elderly people increase and required standards of care rise.

Australia

The Australian social care system is not universal as government assistance is focussed on those with low incomes. The services provided are based on an assessment of an individual's needs and charges are determined by a means test. National and State governments offer residential care and a range of community care packages. In residential care, individuals make a means tested contribution to their care costs but must pay accommodation and daily living expenses themselves. Regulations set out the maximum amount that each person can be charged. Since 2012 there has also been an option of a personal budget in order that an individual can tailor services to their own needs. Community and residential services are rationed by limiting entitlement approvals and waiting lists. Non-profit organisations provide the majority of residential care but there is also a private sector market. Attempts to expand private insurance have had mixed success as the system has a number of perverse incentives that drive individuals and their families to select the most economic rather than the most appropriate solution.[2]

France

France has had a universal and mandatory long-term care insurance scheme called Allocation Personalise Autonomie (APA) since 2002. It provides assistance to all citizens over the age of 60 who have care needs above a government-determined threshold. The needs assessed are 'carer blind' so do not take into account the availability of family support. In residential care, individuals pay for their own accommodation costs and personal expenses although those with low incomes are granted a subsidy. Nursing care is provided by the state health insurance system, while individuals pay other personal care costs through their APA insurance. There is a reasonably large, private, long-term care insurance market covering 15% of the population. Residential care is provided at three levels: collective housing with little if any dedicated medical support; retirement home care with minimal medical support; and long-term care units. Over half of all residential care homes are provided by public sector organisations with the remainder by for-profit or not-for-profit companies.

France spent 1.8% of its GDP on long-term care in 2019 according to the OECD.[3]

US

Most US citizens enter residential care as private payers, spending the assets that they have until they qualify for coverage by the Medicaid programme, which provides a means tested safety net for those with low incomes (but which does not include the family home as an asset). Medicaid does not cover residential assisted living, but many States provide waivers. A small number of individuals have private long-term insurance although this increasingly covers only catastrophic costs. A Commission of Inquiry set up by Congress in 2013 failed to find a consensus on the future of US social care, leaving States to find their own solutions. There are therefore great differences in how social care is funded and what is offered depending on where in the US an individual requires it. Washington has an old-fashioned compulsory insurance system operated via a payroll tax. A Maine proposal that would have raised taxes on higher income households to fund long-term care was defeated at the ballot box. Essentially, US families have to look after themselves, with Medicaid as a last ditch safety net. The OECD estimated that public spending on long-term care was 0.6% of US GDP in 2019.[4]

Netherlands

The Netherlands has a universal social insurance scheme called AWBZ that pays for the care of elders and disabled people. It covers both home care and care provided in residential settings including accommodation costs. It is closely linked to the health insurance system. The extent of care is determined by a needs assessment and a complex system of cost sharing. Individuals can opt for a personal budget, calculated on the basis of the number of hours of care needed. Theoretically, the individual must top up their budget with income-related contributions to meet the cost of the level of care they are assessed to need, but few do. People simply spend whatever is allocated to them. The budget can also be used to pay relatives. The Dutch scheme ran out of funds in 2010, which led politicians to restrict eligibility to reduce demand. The Netherlands' expenditure on long-term care was the highest in the OECD in 2019, at 3.9% of GDP.[5]

England

In England, local government authorities provide social care with funds allocated from the central government, topped up by a small amount of local taxation. In 2019, there were 410,000 people resident in 1300 care homes. Needs are assessed locally using national criteria. 25% of the population aged over 85 are in residential care of one sort or another. If an individual's assets are worth more than £23,250, they have to pay the accommodation and personal costs themselves. Their house is not included in the assessment of eligibility for funding for home-based care or if a partner remains living in the property. The rules are very complex and often disputed on appeal. Healthcare provided by the NHS is free, which has caused some tension when individuals transfer from free hospital care to paid residential care. About 41% of social care residents are self-funders. Residential care is provided by both the non-profit and for-profit sectors with little direct provision by the public sector. The main policy thrust is for more care at home. The whole system has been under financial strain for some years but by 2020, no political consensus about how to reform it had been possible. A reform plan for England has now been promised for the end of 2021.

The system also varies in the four countries that make up the UK. Personal social care is free in Scotland. Health and social care services in Northern Ireland are fully integrated and Wales and Scotland are moving in same direction. The OECD assessed that overall long-term social care spending in the UK amounted to 1.4% of GDP in 2019.[6]

Sweden

Sweden provides universal and comprehensive coverage for social care to all citizens with minimal cost sharing. The system is mainly funded through local taxation (85%). Need assessments are made at a local level where any co-contribution to residential care is determined through the income of an individual. One consequence of this decentralisation is variation in entitlements between municipalities. Private companies are commissioned by local government to run residential care facilities. Home help services are offered by a mix of public and private providers based on a policy of using competition to increase patient choice and quality. Sweden spent 3.2% of its GDP on long-term care in 2019.[7]

Who Should Pay?

All social care systems came under extreme strain during the COVID-19 pandemic but there were deep-seated problems clearly visible before this crisis. At a political level, the key issue is: who should be responsible for the care of the elderly and the disabled — family or state? In most countries individuals and families have the prime responsibility, with the state providing only a safety net for those with limited resources. Insurance systems, many mandatory, that provide at least catastrophic cover are common, as are efforts to focus the resources that are available on the most vulnerable and needy. It has proved difficult to find a political consensus on the best balance between individual, family and state responsibility in many countries.

The link between health and social care is very close. Many people in social care have complex healthcare needs. If social care breaks down, or is inadequate, vulnerable people remain in hospital occupying urgently needed beds. In England, there were a total of 5370 delayed transfers of care cases in February 2020[8] although this number will have reduced as the hospital sector prepared for the COVID-19 pandemic. If social care capacity is reduced, as a consequence of the pandemic, the pressure on the hospital sector will return. Many experts in the field of healthcare have argued that if new healthcare-related investments are to be made by governments, social care should be the priority.

For the most part, staff who work in the social care sector are poorly paid, and the operating costs of residential facilities are constrained by those who commission care because of increasing demand. A more effective integration of health and social care services will be difficult without major structural reorganisation. What may be easier is to merge the commissioning of health and social care rather than its provision. Social care is now provided predominantly outside of the public sector in most countries.

Welfare systems are full of complications and disincentives, particularly when hospital care is free and families have to pay or contribute to the cost of social care.

Ireland is an interesting case as its demographics means that it has more time than others to adjust to an ageing population.

Ireland is predicting large increases in the number of elderly people needing support in the next decade or two. The number of people over the age of 65 will treble by 2051 when there are predicted to be more old people in society than young. The demand for long-term care will increase substantially as will that for home care. The Nursing Home Support Scheme, more commonly known as Fair Deal, is already under strain and in need of supplementary funding from the government. Waiting times to access government-funded nursing home places are increasing, putting pressure on the hospital sector that is finding it difficult to transfer patients from hospitals into community care.

Private sector nursing homes (75% of those available) are under particular financial strain.

'If you do what you always did, you will get what you always got', said Jim Daley, the Minister of State at the Department of Health. Ireland plans to expand home care, with a financial contribution from recipients and reduce its reliance on long-term residential care. Elderly people will age in their own communities with support. They also plan to upgrade the regulation and oversight of an expanded home care sector.[9]

Finland

Finland has a history of generous state-funded health and social welfare but has recently run into serious political problems. In March 2020, the government resigned when their planned health and welfare reforms were defeated in Parliament. Their reforms would have included creating regional organisations to run the health and social care system, rather than local municipalities, as well as creating more choice for citizens by increasing the number of private sector companies sanctioned to provide services for the elderly. With one of the most rapidly ageing populations in the world, the government had judged that something had to change. There had been clear signs that the system was under stress.

Authorities found that a care home in Forssa, operated by Attendo, a large private sector provider with a good reputation, had left elderly patients in soaked diapers all night. Some private sector homes have now been shut down after investigations into fatalities and negligence. Shortages of staff and difficult funding issues were at the heart of these problems.[10]

Social Workers

Social workers have become registered professionals in modern times and are involved in dealing with the full range of social problems — particularly the care and protection of children. The profession's core values include social justice, the dignity and worth of their clients, the importance of human relationships, integrity and competence. There are nearly 700,000 registered social workers in the US and over 100,000 in the UK. Many operate in sensitive and at times controversial settings. A few fail to live up to the profession's standards and are either struck off or have their licence to practise restricted. Many were criticised in the reports on sexual abuse in Rotherham and in cases such as that of Victoria Climbie, discussed in an earlier chapter.

Roanna Althia John was employed as an agency senior social worker within the children's management team at Dudley in the West Midlands of England. Between July 2015 and April 2017 she was found to have failed to keep adequate case notes of numerous child protection visits. The disciplinary panel agreed that this amounted to misconduct and her fitness to practise was therefore impaired. She was suspended and when no evidence of learning from the experience emerged she was suspended again.[11] John was removed from the register in January 2021.

A social worker registered in Ontario, Canada, was assigned to a client in a correctional institution who had been imprisoned after being convicted of aggravated sexual assault. The social worker provided her client with counselling and psychotherapy to assist his anger management, depression and feelings of guilt for the crime that he had committed. The social worker then engaged in a sexual/intimate relationship with the client and allowed him access to the records of other patients. Once their relationship had been uncovered she agreed with her client how to 'get their stories together'. She was suspended for a year, required to complete a boundaries and ethics course, and on her return, to practise while being supervised for two years.[12]

Linda Elaine Fraser, a social worker from Bristol, England, was found to have fabricated evidence to bolster her case for removing a child from a mother's care and then lied to a court about what she had done. The judge in the case was highly critical of her conduct and she was referred to the Health and Social Care Professions Council. She received a written caution that would remain on her record for five years.[13]

Asylum Seekers and Refugees

Asylum seekers and refugees have added significantly to the caseloads of social workers in recent years. The United Nations High Commissioner for Refugees (UNHCR) estimated that the global number of forcibly displaced people could be as high as 65 million in 2016. The US, Pakistan and Turkey have many asylum seekers, as do European countries. In the fourth quarter of 2019, the highest number of first-time asylum applicants was registered in Spain (with 35,400 first-time applicants, or 21% of all first-time applicants in the EU Member States), followed by France (32,800 or 19%), Germany (31,600 or 18%) and Greece (28,000 or 16%). These four Members States account for 74% of all first-time applicants in the EU-27.[14] These are not easy clients to deal with. Many have hugely traumatic personal histories.

Long-term Care

Residential long-term care has produced some of the most serious examples of underfunding, understaffing and patient neglect and abuse, many of which are very similar to those we have seen in Chapter Six.

Bupa, one of Australia's largest providers of care homes, admitted in 2019 that 18 of its 72 homes fell short of required standards with problems including understaffing, a lack of staff training and assaults taking place on patients in care. One home failed to meet 26 of the 44 standards. Medication errors were common, as were dementia patients being allowed to leave unaccompanied. Dying patients were left in hunger and pain and there were multiple reports of patients assaulting one another. A male resident with dementia was found undressing a female patient who was crying. The Bupa Chief Executive apologised and promised to put things right: 'We lost our focus on what we were doing', he said.[15]

German police notified their Spanish counterparts that a 101-year-old German woman named Maria Babes had been reported missing. She was later found in a care home in Chiclana de la Frontera near Cadiz in a very poor condition. A Cuban-German couple had befriended her in Tenerife and persuaded her to move to Chiclana. They had then sold her house and emptied her bank accounts. When she arrived in Chiclana she was locked up in a rented flat with her hands tied for some months. Other care home residents reported that they too had been locked up, drugged and unnecessarily fed through stomach tubes. The day before the police arrested the couple, they had persuaded Babes to leave the care home with them. She was dead in a matter of hours and cremated the following day. The police continue their investigation.[16]

The owners of a care home in Nottingham, England, was found guilty of corporate manslaughter after a patient died after been found dehydrated, malnourished and suffering from a significant pressure sore. The evidence suggested that the care home records had been fabricated and that staff had taken short cuts in the care regime. The owners were fined £300,000.[17]

In a case with very familiar echoes from the world of medicine, New York state officials were found to have failed to process criminal background checks on an employee, leading to a damaging outcome.

> *Zymere Perkins, a six-year-old, was assaulted by a convicted murderer employed by New York Children's Services (ACS). A law enacted in 2013 required ACS to check the criminal history of any job applicant who would have contact with children. Whilst ACS finally started background checks in 2017, the issue was never dealt with retrospectively according to the State Office of Children and Family Services. They rather belatedly assured the public that 'a convicted killer would never get employed again'.*[18]

Transitioning from Residential Care

A current trend in social care in many countries is to move away from residential care and put more resources into home care. This is not as easy as it sounds. Coordinating visits by nurses and care staff two or three times a day is challenging and the system often breaks down, leaving clients in difficulty. Double banking staff to ensure this can never happen is expensive. New information systems that directly involve patients or their relatives in the process might secure improvements.

Children's Homes and Orphanages

Children's homes and orphanages have of course existed for many years. Many were initially established by charities or religious organisations. In more modern times, the state has become a major provider and commissioner of children's homes.[19] Although many homes have provided excellent services for the children in their care and successfully guided them into adulthood, there have been a number of high-profile cases of abuse (some of which have already been discussed in Chapter Eight).

A long inquiry about the abuse of children in the Channel Islands that finally reported in 2008 uncovered more than 500 alleged offences.

> *In 2008, Haut de la Garenne, a former children's home on the island of Jersey became the focus of international attention when bone fragments were uncovered that were thought to be human. It was a false alarm, but*

> *stories began to emerge that, when in use as a children's home, shackles, restraints and punishment rooms were commonly in use. An Inquiry covering all children's home and orphanages on the Island found evidence of similar abuse at other homes. Children had their mouths washed out with carbolic soap or were stripped and stung with nettles. Senior boys used an electric generator to administer shocks to younger children. A girl was punished by having to spend a night with a dead nun. It was, said one witness to the Inquiry, the place where all the abandoned children were dumped. At another orphanage a witness said: 'if a child wet the bed they would be put on a chair with their pants on their head whilst other children formed a circle and danced around them'. Children fathered by German troops were also placed in the homes. Criminal charges followed the Inquiry. Jimmy Saville, a serial abuser, was alleged to have been a regular visitor.[20]*

Senior people within the Jersey government were thought to be involved with or had at least known about the abuse. Witnesses were reluctant to give evidence because they were living so closely with those they were accusing and did not trust that any evidence they gave would be treated confidentially. In 2010, Jersey's Chief Minister offered an unreserved apology to those that had been abused. Local healthcare services have been providing support to victims ever since.

However, the stories of abuse did not go away and in 2013 another independent inquiry was launched, led by Frances Oldham QC, to examine what had gone wrong in Jersey's childcare system over many years.[21] The Haut de la Garenne case was revisited along with five others. All were judged to be ill-equipped to deal with the behavioural and emotional needs of children.

There was little if any oversight or inspection at the homes. Children were effectively abandoned in the care system. Foster care lagged decades behind accepted good practice. The inquiry was also damning in its criticism of family group homes and approved schools. It concluded that the State of Jersey failed to understand its role as a 'corporate parent'. The inquiry recommendations included the creation of a Commissioner for Children, a Children's Rights Officer, substantial investment and routine external oversight. All recommendations were implemented.

More Inquiries into Children's Homes

Given the prevalence of children's homes in accusations of abuse it is not surprising that many governments have begun to look at whether they should have a future at all. A Royal Commission in Australia heard evidence in 2017 that 2200 people had reported abuse in orphanages or children's homes. They also took evidence from 160 survivors of abuse in healthcare settings, including those being cared for by disability service providers. The inquiry recommended, amongst other things, a national redress scheme.[22]

In England, the government commissioned a review led by Sir Martin Narey, a former head of the Prison Services and Chief Executive of Barnardo's, the children's charity. He reported that whilst many believe that a family environment is the best placement for an orphaned child to grow up, for some children the best answer may be residential care. However, these homes could and should be better.[23]

Not everyone was convinced by Narey's conclusions as reports continued to emerge of children being treated like cattle and moved around sometimes unregulated care homes in England and Wales. Local authorities with a statutory duty to look after children in need were routinely including the personal details of children in online adverts, including details of previous sexual abuse and gang involvement, while inviting private companies to compete for contracts to provide care. It was, said the Under-Secretary for Business, Energy and Industrial Strategy, Nadhim Zahawi, unacceptable for local authorities to 'to promote or be seen to seemingly auction children in care'.[24,25]

There is clearly a role for some children's homes in the future, but perhaps substantially fewer than at present, once viable alternatives are developed. However, when children's homes become detached from their local community and children stop mixing outside, problems with such homes become inevitable. Children develop better if encouraged to join local youth clubs, football teams and events set up at local schools. In the developing world, charities and religious organisations remain in place as the major providers of such care.

Child Migration

The transfer of orphan children from the UK to other Commonwealth countries (principally Canada and Australia) in first half of the 20th century has resulted in many inquiries.[26] Children were transferred under the child migrant programme for adoption or care in state-run residential homes or those provided by charities and religious institutions. Between 1920 and 1970, about 130,000 children aged between four and 14 years — all from underprivileged backgrounds — made such journeys. The intention was to give them a chance of a better life in a new country, but it later emerged that some of the children had been the victims of abuse. For many years, the British government referred these allegations of mistreatment to the Australian and Canadian governments. They had been reluctant to close the scheme down earlier to avoid jeopardising relations with colonial governments and creating embarrassment and reputational risk for some of the major charities involved. Recently, the Jay Inquiry concluded that the scheme was eventually closed down not on policy grounds but because the supply of suitable children had dried up.[27] The last children sailed for Australia in 1967. In 2010, the government made a public apology and Prime Minister Gordon Brown offered financial compensation to those involved via the Family Restoration Fund, administered by the Child Migrants Trust. The migration programme was initially well-intentioned but the poor oversight and years of concerted efforts to promote a historical mistake as a success story is today correctly viewed as misguided.

> *John Hennessy was sent from an orphanage in England to the Bindoon Boys Town in Western Australia in 1946 at the age of 10. He later described life at Bindoon, which was run by the Catholic Church's Christian Brothers, as a catalogue of cruelty, where beatings and sexual assaults were daily occurrences. The boys worked as labourers on the grand buildings in the grounds and were flogged if they slowed down carrying loads of bricks up the scaffolding, and lime burns lacerated their legs. It was like slave labour, Hennessy said, and claimed that Bindoon was nothing more than a paedophile ring.*

Much later in life Hennessy traced his birth mother who told him that 'he had been stolen out of his cradle when only 2 months old and taken to be cared for by the Sisters of Nazareth. In those days being born out of wedlock was a mortal sin and we were classed as children of the devil'. The nuns had told her: 'Mary, you are not a fit and decent woman to have this child. John is ours and he belongs to God'.[28]

A former child migrant told the inquiry that his experiences at school were better described as torture than abuse. He described how he had been locked up in a place called 'the dungeon' without food or water for days. Others talked about backbreaking work and the sadistic killing of a pet horse as a punishment for alleged wrongdoing.[29]

Child Refugees

There are many lessons to be learned from the historical accounts of the child migrants to inform the management of the thousands of children orphaned as a result of recent conflicts in the Middle East. In 2019, over 10,000 children were being considered for resettlement in the EU; including 3000 planned for the UK. Many of these children were unaccompanied. The EU governments concerned hoped to provide these children with a new start in life. In doing so, they must accept the long-term responsibility to protect their futures and not simply pass the buck to other organisations no matter how outwardly reputable these may appear. Looking after young people with no family in an unfamiliar country is a substantial challenge that should not be accepted lightly. The role of the 'corporate parent' is an onerous one.

In 2018, the Trump Administration attracted global condemnation when it emerged that there was a policy of family separation being employed at the US–Mexico border for asylum seekers and refugees from Central America. Adults were being placed in detention centres (essentially prisons) while their children were being placed perhaps into care, many hundreds or even thousands of miles away.[30] The policy was eventually changed.

Difficult Inquiries

The difficulty of conducting inquiries in closely knit communities is highlighted by the following case in North Wales.[31]

In the mid-1980s, a residential worker, Alison Taylor, reported to her superiors at the local council that children were being abused in residential care. No action was taken so she took her concerns to the North Wales police, making a series of allegations against senior social work professionals working for the Council. As a result she was sacked for a breakdown in relationships with colleagues but later awarded an out-of-court settlement for wrongful dismissal.

In 1990, a police investigation found insufficient evidence to undertake a successful prosecution. The investigation had been hampered by a lack of cooperation by social services.

Taylor continued to pressure authorities and this eventually led in 1994 to an Inquiry led by John Jillings, a retired Director of Social Services from England. The Chief Constable of the North Wales police declined to assist the Inquiry. The publication of the Jillings Inquiry was blocked for some considerable time because of concerns about libel actions and warnings from the Council's insurers that should the report be published it would encourage multiple court cases and compensation claims.

Whilst the arguments about publication continued, another Inquiry was launched in 1996 chaired by Sir Ronald Waterhouse, a retired High Court Judge. He interviewed 250 witnesses and in 2000 published the report 'Lost in Care'. It concluded that 'the evidence before us has disclosed that for many children who were consigned to Bryn Estyn in the ten or so years of its existence as a community home, it was a form of purgatory or worse from which children emerged more damaged than when they had entered and for whom the future had become even more bleak'.

However, he found no evidence that there was a wide-ranging conspiracy involving prominent persons and others with the objective of sexual activity with children in care.

The Waterhouse report[32] led to a significant number of criminal charges and substantial changes in the way that children in care were dealt with by local councils. A total of 140 compensation claims were settled.

When the Jillings report eventually surfaced in 2013, it stated that: 'Our investigations have led us to conclude that the abuse of children and young people in Clwyd residential units had been extensive and had taken place over a substantial number of years'. The leader of the Council, who had been threatened with the sack if he spoke out, commented: 'Because it was suppressed the lessons from the Jillings report were not learned. It was the exchange of financial safety for the safety of real people'.

That was not the end of the tragic saga as allegations of a paedophile ring involving prominent people persisted. The head of the Serious Crimes Unit in London was sent to investigate. The first phase of what became known as Operation Pallial reported in 2013 that 140 allegations of abuse between 1963 and 1992 had been investigated. One outcome was the conviction, in 2014, of one of the men who ran some of the homes to a term of life imprisonment. Two years later, a former police superintendent was sentenced to 12 years in prison for the abuse of boys at the same home.

Whilst the multiple inquires in North Wales unfolded, other inquiries were underway in the rest of the UK. In all there were 10 public inquiries into children in residential care between 1990 and 1996. When the Utting Report was presented to Parliament in 1997, Frank Dobson, the Secretary of State for Health said: 'it presented a woeful tale of failure at all levels to provide a secure and decent childhood for some of the most vulnerable children'. The earlier Warner report had made recommendations that that led to the screening of staff being employed to work in children's homes.

Lessons for the Future

Social care is a significant political issue in many countries, including the UK. Some of the key questions include: whether the government or individuals should pay for social care, or the costs be shared in some way; Should the providers of care be in the public, private or not-for-profit sectors; and how should they be regulated? These issues have all stimulated polarised political arguments and, as a result, there has so far been limited progress in reforming any national system.

Perverse incentives that mean many families prefer elders to remain in free hospital rather than paid-for social care clearly need to be removed.

The COVID-19 pandemic has clearly demonstrated that the interdependence between health and social care is real and can have terrible consequences if not managed thoughtfully. The early discharge of elderly patients to care homes in order to free up hospital beds for an expected surge in COVID-19 patients looks to have been a huge strategic mistake. Many patients with the virus were transferred from hospitals, resulting in major outbreaks in almost 50% of all care homes in the UK and thousands of unnecessary deaths. A similar situation was apparent in New York.

However, fully integrating health and social care through structural reorganisation is an expensive option that needs very careful thought before implementation. Even where services are currently fully integrated, such as in Northern Ireland, operational and cultural boundaries still exist.

Social care needs a higher professional profile if it is to attract better-qualified staff. This means that the current debate in countries such as the UK about the terrible pay on offer to care workers is urgently reassessed. Low pay also means a less able workforce resulting in the fact that long-term residential care has many of the same problems as those found in mental health. Inadequate, poorly paid staffing levels leads to unprofessional behaviour. Risks increase if they become closed institutions.

As we have seen, children's homes have proved difficult to manage and some have failed to keep children safe from sexual exploitation and other forms of abuse. They need to be fully integrated into local communities so that children can access the same services as their peers living in normal family environments. Alternative forms of long-term care for children also need to be developed. Child migrants, refugees and asylum seekers also need exceptional long-term health and social care support from their corporate parents. This is clearly a work very much in progress at the moment.

Social workers play a challenging and difficult role in all societies. In many countries they are regulated and required to practise within defined standards of conduct. A few fail to meet these standards and either lose their licence to practise or have conditions imposed on them. Poor and fraudulent record keeping has been a common problem. Weak oversight by senior professionals is clearly a problem that needs to be addressed. However, social workers are often under great pressure with large caseloads of difficult clients. Their work is stressful. Better support systems for the profession are needed.

In conclusion, the complex healthcare needs of citizens in need of social care have rarely been fully met and services around the world need to be improved. However social care systems are paid for, demographic trends mean that for most developed countries the cost is only going to increase in coming years. Governments need to step up to the challenge. The problem is not going to go away.

Chapter Eleven
From Darkness into the Light

This final chapter pulls together the themes that have been covered and looks for what we can usefully learn from the case studies in the book. The aim is to identify some of the practical steps that can be taken to reduce harm to patients and staff and support healthcare services and systems that are in trouble.

Organisational Culture

The best healthcare organisations build an open organisational culture based on a foundation of ethical conduct and where learning from adverse and 'never' events is second nature to all employees. External opinions about clinical or managerial performance are treated with respect and while they may be challenged, this should only be undertaken after a thorough examination of their validity. They can never be ignored. Healthy organisations are financially robust and responsible.

Leaders will know if they have the right culture if:

(1) Information systems are in place that will alert them when danger signals are being triggered. Such alarm systems will go off in the case of adverse and never events, lapses in effective infection control measures, overstretched intensive care capacity, excessive and prolonged bed occupancy, low staff morale, high sickness absence rates, significantly compromised staffing levels, high

levels of locum staff, a growing backlog of routine maintenance and delayed equipment replacement. A package of clinical alert indicators, agreed with the clinical staff, will be in place and include avoidable death and readmission rates, slow diagnostic processes, high medication errors, the occurrence of pressure sores, inappropriate antibiotic prescribing and comparative clinical outcomes. The comparative data will be interpreted with care but never hidden. Staff will have been trained in adverse event reporting, investigations and recovery processes.

(2) The learning process in the organisation is active and deeply rooted in clinical practice. The organisation recognises that it owes a duty of care to patients who may have been harmed whilst in its care. Clinical audit data is open to hospital management and made public in an anonymised form so as to protect patient and staff confidentiality. When published, it includes details of the corrective action that has been taken. This will enhance rather than damage an organisation's reputation. Clinical audit investigations are separated from disciplinary processes.

(3) The suspicion of a problem is always enough to justify an investigation without attributing blame. Waiting for the evidence is never an excuse for inaction.

(4) Any illegal or aberrant behaviour (such as the surgeons who carved their initials on patient's organs or staff who abuse vulnerable patients) is simply not tolerated. Any breaches in the code of ethical conduct are dealt with firmly but fairly. When staff 'look away' or are afraid of reporting incidents, the organisation has problems. Whistleblowers who come forward in such situations must be respected and protected.

(5) The organisation does not tolerate no-go areas or opt-outs from its processes. Participation in clinical audit systems is compulsory, but is accepted without question as part of the clinical learning process.

(6) Safety rules are never compromised by economic considerations. If a serious issue emerges that indicates a tension between ethics and economic considerations, it is resolved at the highest levels in the organisation. In the hospital world, such issues might

include decisions to stop admissions when bed occupancy is too high or when staffing levels are under safety limits. While there is room for sensible flexibility in managing emergency situations, organisations ignore persistent alert signals at their peril. Wilful blindness is a constant danger. 'How this could this have happened and we did not notice' is a common comment made to committees of inquiry.

(7) The health and safety of staff has the same priority as it does for patients and visitors. The organisation has a robust and codified approach to occupational health and makes adequate investments.

(8) The organisation has robust and rehearsed plans in place to respond to civil emergencies and pandemics.

Leadership

The best organisations have wise, stable and experienced leadership teams that are a visible example of their organisation's culture and ethics. Leaders operate with a strong moral compass. They are trusted by staff and the clinical community and have earned the respect of patient groups. They inspire rather than bully and are strong enough to demand adherence to the organisation's values and codes of acceptable conduct. They always strike the right balance between providing quality services and dealing with economic pressures. They are prudent and financially aware. They are sensibly ambitious for their organisation but never compromise patient safety. They manage to bridge any perceived gaps between the political targets of the day and professional ethics. Quality and safety are at the core of their belief system.

Hubris, excessive pride or over-confidence, is a constant danger for managerial and clinical leaders with significant power. It is not easy to deal with such individuals as they occupy senior positions and have little personal insight. Boards have a special responsibility to first identify these problems and then either help or remove the individuals concerned. Many talented managers or clinicians can change their behaviour with the proper support.

Good healthcare service leaders never lose their respect for medicine and its ethical traditions. Unlimited clinical freedom is rarely possible in modern healthcare systems on either economic or quality assurance grounds. Nevertheless, physicians must be able to exercise their clinical experience and instincts with as much freedom as possible when they decide how to treat individual patients with the caveat that they must record their reasons for departing from an approved treatment pathway and wherever possible consult the patient or the patient's family. With proper consent and prudent care, innovation will still be possible.

Organisational Change

Reorganising whole healthcare systems carries with it substantial dangers and needs to be approached with great care. The true price of organisational change is rarely correctly assessed and the invisible costs of disrupted quality programmes and the loss of organisational memory are almost never included in the equation. One classic international error was closing mental health asylums before community care was properly established, tested and funded.

Arguments about the centralisation of specialist hospital services, such as children's heart surgery, in order to secure (allegedly) better clinical outcomes and stronger service viability are occurring in all jurisdictions. Local communities and healthcare professionals who may face losing a valued and accessible service need to be shown clear evidence of what the advantages of such reorganisations are if they are to support rather than resist such moves. Professional opinions, issued in lofty tones, are not as strong as hard evidence. Many local communities simply see such moves as more cost cutting.

Judgements about the pace at which organisational changes are undertaken are crucial to the ultimate success of any process. There are occasions when swift and decisive change is appropriate; stability does not mean that organisations should be static, but for the most part, too many reforms are rushed and ill-prepared, which can generate chaos and contribute to failure.

Radical changes to clinical processes and ward configurations in hospitals need to be planned and implemented with great care and patience. Too many of these initiatives have ended up creating conflict and confusion. A switch to remote consultation in general practice, which might be the next major change in primary and outpatient care, needs to be thought through properly.

In some cases, organisational change is, however, essential. In many jurisdictions, social care needs urgent and radical reform and linking much more closely with healthcare. The costs of not taking on what is undeniably a huge challenge are likely to be higher in the long run than the status quo.

Serial Killers and Angels of Death

Serial killers in the healthcare professions are luckily very rare indeed, but this means that when cases do occur, they are extremely difficult to identify, stop and prosecute. The perpetrators often move between institutions or care settings and become expert in hiding or falsifying their records and professional history. Unforgivably, in some cases where suspicions — but not firm proof — arise, employers quietly allow the offenders to move on. In other cases, they occupy positions of authority that makes it difficult for their conduct to be investigated. Some, like Dr. Harold Shipman, who murdered so many, were very popular with their patients until their crimes were uncovered. The principal barrier to preventing such behaviour is the fundamental belief held by most of the healthcare community that deliberately harming patients is simply unthinkable. Sadly, rare though it is, the unthinkable does happen.

Any unusual or unexpected series of events that causes harm to patients is a signal that something is wrong and should cause alarm bells to ring in any quality assurance system. Abnormally high mortality rates, either amongst a physician's patients or within a hospital or care home, should be closely investigated. The use of dangerous drugs like diamorphine, a popular weapon used by serial killers, needs constant monitoring. High-level reviews of unusual patient mortality rates have proved to be of value in some circumstances but are no substitute for routine and continuous local reviews of patient deaths. Improvements to the systems for how deaths are recorded are likely to improve detection rates.

In some cases, so-called 'angels of deaths' have decided to undertake the 'mercy killing' of patients in great suffering or close to death. This is often used as a justification for murder in healthcare systems but is still an illegal act in all but a few jurisdictions. Pain relief, using dangerous drugs, is permissible in terminal care provided that it is not hidden, is properly recorded, has no criminal motive and when practical is dispensed with the consent of the patient or their relatives. When patients die in such situations, murder is always the last option to be investigated when all other options have failed to produce an explanation.

The police are only involved when the suspicion of murder becomes the only probable explanation for an unexplained event. They are often called in by a hospital or other healthcare organisation with great reluctance. In most cases, specialist police teams are needed to investigate suspicious events in a healthcare setting.

There is no guaranteed failsafe method that can protect an organisation against the deliberate and considered plans of an individual determined — or addicted — to doing harm. Constant vigilance and an open and transparent organisation culture, where unusual events are always reported and investigated, is the best and most effective preventative measure.

Regulatory Bodies and Inspectors

Most countries have adopted the principle of self-regulation for the healthcare professions. However, critics do not think that the professions have covered themselves in glory in this role; failing to properly protect the public as well as they might have done by being too focussed on protecting the reputation of the profession they are regulating. In my view, these criticisms are too harsh and on balance self-regulation is likely to be more effective than external control by binding professions to standards that they have set. However, some reforms are warranted. Regulation bodies should not be made up of only healthcare professions but also incorporate independent voices. These should not be token appointments, but a substantive presence. Optics matter and more balanced bodies will result in greater trust. Most regulatory bodies do now publish the outcomes of their disciplinary hearings and decisions, which is a helpful step towards greater transparency.

In a globalised world, the migration of healthcare professionals to different jurisdictions has become increasingly common. There is therefore a need for the bodies that regulate national healthcare systems to seek far greater international cooperation in terms of sharing information and coming to common positions on essential issues.

Healthcare professions are, for the most part, regulated separately and as a consequence, different standards of practice and ethics are commonplace. This is increasingly inappropriate in the modern healthcare world where teamwork is becoming the cornerstone of excellent care. Some degree of integration or at least the sharing of basic principles is needed. This may also reduce the current substantial costs related to maintaining multiple different regulation bodies for the various healthcare professions.

When healthcare professionals are investigated for potential wrongdoing, the regulators should share with their employers a duty of care. The reasons for regulators to discipline professionals come under two basic categories: (1) incompetent clinical practice and (2) behaviour that brings the profession into disrepute. The latter is by far the most common and includes issues such as dishonesty, criminal convictions, inappropriate relationships with patients and abuse of either patients or colleagues. Incompetent practice can be corrected with additional training and close supervision but inappropriate behaviour demands that the individual shows both insight and remorse. The policy adopted by some regulators to accept a practitioner's admission of an honest mistake and to stipulate that further training or learning is undertaken is good practice.

Of course, in some cases, the negligent behaviour is of such seriousness that the professional must be struck off. Relicensing physicians who have been removed from the professional register for misconduct or incompetent practice is a complicated process and it must be ensured that adequate recompense and real improvements are evident. What is not at all acceptable is the unethical practice, common in some US states, of dumping practitioners that have been struck off into the prison system to treat patients in a second-class service.

Regular revalidation for practitioners, utilised by some but not all regulators, can be seriously burdensome. Many professional health-care leaders doubt its value in improving the quality of healthcare. On the other hand, a licence for life is also unsatisfactory. New means of ensuring that professionals remain up to date with the latest develop-ments in this rapidly evolving field, while retaining their skills, need to be explored.

The value of external inspectors, which now exist in many coun-tries, is increasingly being questioned on the grounds that they are firstly, not very effective and secondly, extremely expensive. I am not as sure that they should be removed. They have uncovered some instances of very poor practice such as those discovered at Mid Staffordshire and in Western Australia. Some, and particularly those from professional colleges, have been reluctant to publish their find-ings whilst other inspection processes have become hopelessly bureaucratic. They work better when their focus is on making the inspection an impetus for learning rather than blame. The creation of an ombudsman for patient safety, a position that now exists in Finland, is worth serious consideration. It also chimes with the recent Cumberlege report that recommends the appointment of a commis-sioner for patient safety.

System failure — rather than the actions of an individual — can on occasion be the primary cause of harm. An inexperienced doctor working in a high-pressure setting without adequate support is an example of a situation where the system is at fault.

Staffing Issues

The view held by many in rural communities that any healthcare pro-fessional is better than none at all does not stand up to proper scru-tiny. Poor healthcare professionals produce poor clinical results for patients wherever they practise. When there is a failure to recruit a suitably qualified and experienced professional to a vacant post, the future of a whole local service is at risk. Community leaders should be invited to join in a risk assessment if a less qualified individual is appointed to decide whether a service should be changed. Continuing to provide services with depleted staff numbers or in the absence of key staff is dangerous practice and rarely in the true interests of local patients. There are usually options available other than closure including additional support from other centres.

Many of the case studies in this book identify poor recruitment processes as a cause of later problems. These processes must be particularly thorough if the candidates are being recruited from other countries where qualifications and experience may be of a lower standard. Ideally, background checks should always be completed prior to a decision to employ but where this is not possible they should be completed as quickly as possible. Licensing checks should, of course, be mandatory and the checking process should be regularly audited. Quietly parting company with a seriously incompetent or dangerous healthcare professional (or manager) should not be acceptable employer behaviour. Some of the serial killers discussed in this book would have been picked up far earlier if their employers had been more transparent.

Healthcare providers that employ large numbers of temporary staff or locums have a duty to ensure that they are properly inducted and supervised until their competence and understanding of the respective organisation's code of ethics and conduct is well understood. High levels of locums in the clinical staff should trigger serious alarms.

In some jurisdictions, health and safety laws are being applied more vigorously in healthcare settings and extended to cover injuries to patients with very high fines or even criminal charges for breaches. Public safety is paramount, but prevention is better than regulation. Many safety precautions, such as removing ligature points on mental health wards or regularly monitoring radiation levels in radiology and radiotherapy units are straightforward and should be the norm.

Occupational healthcare services play an important role in protecting the safety of patients and staff. Healthcare organisations need to follow the example of the airline industry in being proactive in detecting high stress levels amongst staff. The appointment of a board-level Director of Safety/Occupational Health in hospitals is an idea worthy of further consideration.

Personal protection equipment must be readily available to staff who need it and supply chains must be secure and reliable. When wearing protective equipment, staff must remember the value of a human face and a sympathetic smile.

Those staff known to be at risk of danger due to their health profile or ethnicity should not be deployed to clinical areas where they may be endangered. This has been a proven failing during the COVID-19 pandemic. Occupational healthcare services should identify such individuals in advance of a crisis.

The growing problem of violence towards staff working in healthcare settings must be stamped out. Zero tolerance policies are the way forward and the use of security personnel at peak times in high-risk departments such as A&E is to be utilised to ensure staff safety.

Patients

Patient groups should always be listened to with respect. They should never be ignored or cast as the enemy no matter how challenging the issues are. If adverse or 'never' events have occurred, patient groups should be included in investigations to ensure that they can see for themselves what happened, what action has been taken and why it will never happen again. All jurisdictions would be wise to introduce a legal duty of candour. An acknowledgement that harm has been done to a patient, if it is provided fully and speedily, will often lead to a sensible mediated settlement where damages are deemed to be required.

Hospitals and care homes need to be infection secure. The current pandemic has illustrated that there is a pressing need to re-evaluate the current policies on visitors in order to reduce the risk of infection. Modern technology presents usable alternatives for communication and contact between patients and their relatives in all but the most exceptional circumstances, such as late terminal care.

Patient confidentiality is an important ethical principle that must be defended at all costs. Patient records and data should be protected by watertight legal action. There have been many cases where unscrupulous staff or corporations have breached the trust that patients place in their health organisations for profit.

Patient Consent

Patients have a right to be consulted and their permission sought before any clinical procedure is undertaken. For the most part, patients trust the healthcare professionals treating them to act in their best interests but this must not be taken for granted. Patients — or, if that is not possible, their families — need to be fully involved in consent decisions, particularly when significant risk is involved. Do-not-resuscitate orders must go through the proper processes and the guidance to staff on how to obtain consent must be clear and unambiguous. Patients can be part of the quality and safety checking process if they are informed of the expected clinical pathway, by questioning any omissions and variations. This is relatively straightforward for routine non-emergency surgery and should be widely adopted.

Places of Risk

Long-stay institutions, whether large or small, present a risk to patients if they become isolated and closed from the wider community. Being 'out of sight and out of mind' is dangerous. The wider use of CCTV within such homes or high-security units is essential in some circumstances. For example, children's homes are often a target for sexual predators and need exceptional levels of oversight and support. CCTV cameras should be routinely deployed at the entry and exit points of care homes where confused patients are resident. They should also be installed in acute psychiatric units. Some hospitals now commonly place CCTV cameras at the exit points from maternity wards.

Hospitals that have allowed high rates of bed occupancy (anything over 85%) to become the norm are dangerous for both patients and staff for a variety of reasons. High occupancy rates often signal a wider system failure that cannot be easily resolved by the organisation.

Risk for patients is often present at the boundaries of care. In a healthcare system that is functioning well, seamless transitions are typical and are central to excellent care. However, when organisations do not work together as they should because of conflicting objectives, perverse incentives or personality clashes, problems begin to become visible. Higher authorities need to have the will and capacity to intervene when a lack of collaboration presents dangers for patients.

Tensions between professional groups, such as those this book has highlighted in maternity care, create potential hazards for women and must be exposed and resolved. When working relationships break down between professionals, their leaders must confront the issues with the individuals involved. External mediation is often helpful.

However, it would be wrong to identify poor working relationships between obstetricians and midwives as the principal reason for the poor outcomes in this specialty. Poor staffing levels, skill deficiencies, poor antenatal care and bad judgements about where women can most safely deliver babies all play their part. Maternity care is clearly not as safe as it could be, even in developed countries, and should be the focus of vigorous quality improvement programmes.

Quality Programmes

Quality programmes have become a core strategy in all healthcare organisations. They have a tendency to reduce their effectiveness over time and need regular refreshment and updating. Changes of leadership also can put specific programmes at risk. Targeting zero is evidently a challenge, as are 'get it right first time' initiatives, but they are perfectly reasonable in the context of healthcare settings. If incentives and penalties are in operation in quality programmes, they need to be regularly checked for unintended consequences. Penalties levied by the NHS on local authorities for delays in finding placements for patients awaiting discharge from hospital were abandoned as ineffective because they damaged local collaboration. In some jurisdictions, performance-related payment systems run into the billions. Information about the radiation risks of imaging tests on patients proved to be more powerful in influencing the behaviour of clinicians to reduce their ordering of examinations than financial targets.

When alarms are sounded about the functioning of a medical device, the responsible authorities often struggle to know which patients to contact to warn that they might be at risk. Joint, and other medical device registers, with identified patients, are a sensible idea as they enable immediate and direct contact with the affected patients, which is far more effective than issuing general warnings to physicians. These registers can also contribute to clinical research programmes designed to check the effectiveness of clinical outcomes over time. The joint registers enabled orthopaedic surgeons to better understand which implants lasted the longest and at what point checks should be implemented to assess any deterioration in performance. Some hospital quality programmes now require medical examiners to review all deaths in hospital that adds materially to learning and provides some defence against undetected repeated mistakes or crimes. These appointments are in addition to the role played by coroners.

Staff morale is firmly linked to the quality of care provided to patients and should also be measured in quality assessments.

Problems in Clinical Practice

Practitioners, as we have seen, need to keep up to date with modern clinical practice, but employers need to create the opportunities for this to happen.

Diagnostic and treatment errors can be reduced with systematic checks and adherence to safety protocols, particularly in high-risk areas such as operating theatres. Most pathology errors occur outside laboratories either prior to testing or in the interpretation of the results. The fact that screening tests have a small, inbuilt error rate needs to be communicated to the public more widely. A second diagnostic test is a vital element in obtaining a good second opinion.

Medication errors are still far too common in all healthcare settings and better monitoring is needed to reduce them. For example, the prescribing of antibiotics should be audited much more closely in both primary and secondary care. Antibiotic resistance is becoming a growing and major international risk to life. The procedures for accessing and administering dangerous and controlled drugs also need to be tightened and should include double-checking as a standard. The prescribing of highly addictive opioids is now widespread in many countries, and given the societal damage that these drugs wreak, their use should be further scrutinised and preventative action taken.

Medical equipment can become lethal for both the users and those being treated if it is not properly maintained, calibrated and replaced at the end of its safe operating life. Particular attention needs to be paid to radiotherapy, ultrasound and robotic instruments. A safety register for such equipment should become mandatory and include the manufacturer's end of safe life data. With the increasing use of advanced and hi-tech equipment in hospitals, there is a growing need for specialised biomedical engineers to become part of safety teams.

Managers and clinicians need to be cautious of an over-reliance on clinical computer systems. They are not infallible and can occasionally produce hazardous outcomes for patients. Safety teams might also be boosted by the addition of an expert in clinical computing.

Speeding up clinical trials for new drugs and treatments is clearly desirable if it can be done safely. However, changes to well-established protocols — as are now being proposed for potential vaccines for COVID-19 — need to be done with the upmost care and with mandatory retrospective evaluation. Historically, a number of drugs granted accelerated approval by the US Food and Drug Administration were later shown to present serious problems for patients.

Mental Health Services

Mental health services are under-resourced in most healthcare systems. When many jurisdictions made the radical change from asylum care to care in the community, the new services were insufficiently prepared. Patient abuse and institutionalisation — two of the most cited reasons for this major change in approach — still occur in community settings. Many mental healthcare professionals consider that there is still both a place and need for safe long-term care either in community homes or modern asylums that are well connected to their local communities and healthcare professional networks.

The science that underpins psychiatry is still developing but great advances have been made and there is now much that can be done to restore mental health, relieve painful symptoms and realign disrupted lives. As is the case for patients with some physical diseases, learning to live with the symptoms is sometimes the only way forward.

Prisoners with poor mental health are badly served in most jurisdictions. Too often, prison has become a dumping ground for the mentally ill.

The Sexual Exploitation of Children

The sexual exploitation of children and vulnerable adults in health and social care settings is more common than anyone would wish. Identifying children at risk in order to prevent abuse will require exceptional levels of intra-organisation collaboration and intelligence sharing. Children who have been victims need multi-service support if they are to move on successfully to new lives as survivors.

The historical lessons that can be learnt from the UK Child Migration Programme, which relocated thousands of children to the British colonies, need to be borne in mind as countries now accept unaccompanied children from the Middle East and war and conflict zones. Governments need to fully understand and take responsibility for their role as the corporate parent and take exceptional care in placing children with new families or in social care settings. Governments cannot simply place children and then forget them. That would be a scandal waiting to happen.

Fraud and Corruption

Endemic fraud and corruption can only be reduced with politically led culture change. Long-standing corrupt and fraudulent practices (such as improper patient charging) require long-term solutions. National and regional anti-corruption teams seem to be achieving success in some countries. International cooperation is the most effective way of policing counterfeit drug scams that continue to proliferate online, often by organised crime syndicates. The extent to which fake drugs have been able to enter into the global supply chain is alarming. In some jurisdictions, organised crime has been allowed to infiltrate healthcare systems; a development that quickly reduces quality standards as the single-minded pursuit of profit takes hold.

The pharmaceutical and medical device industries need to walk the talk with regard to their own codes of conduct and claims of ethical standards. The self-regulation of big pharma has largely proved to be ineffective. Fines for the poor manufacture of drugs or for marketing medications way beyond the uses for which they have been licensed need to be increased exponentially so that they are not regarded, as is now the case with some companies, as a cost of doing business. The ban on the public advertising of prescription drugs that operates in Europe and many other countries, but not in the US, should remain in place and be extended wherever possible.

Another norm in the way that pharmaceutical and medical device companies go about their business is bestowing 'gifts' to their potential customers in the healthcare industry. It would be sensible to ban all such gifts, no matter how small. If research grants, gifts or free samples are judged appropriate, they should always be made transparently to healthcare organisations or companies rather than to individuals. Declarations of interest should be embedded in the corporate codes of conduct of all health organisations.

Infrastructure projects, such as the building of new hospitals, have been at the centre of a number of healthcare scandals over the years. Again, depending on the jurisdiction, elements of the organised crime community may be involved. All such projects need close supervision.

Fiddling the figures when reporting the state of an organisation's financial situation in order to maintain funding has been exposed in several high-profile cases. In addition, falsifying the performance of an organisation in terms of achieving quality targets, such as reductions in patient waiting lists, is really fraud by another name. It should not be regarded as a semi-legitimate exercise in gaming the rules.

Health and the Law

Given that healthcare organisations should acknowledge a duty of care to those that have been harmed whilst in their care, patients should not have to turn to the courts for compensation. A swift and honest admission of guilt and a demonstration that action has been taken to prevent a reoccurrence of a mistake will often satisfy patients and relatives or lead to a mediated settlement. However, on a systems level, some of the major failures that affected so many people, such as the thalidomide drug and contaminated blood scandals, demonstrate the need for governments to manage and contribute to compensation schemes.

Some of the countries that operate no-blame compensation schemes that do not require proof of negligence seem to be valued by patients but also have their critics who claim that they are not overly generous.

Wilful neglect, a new crime in England and Wales since 2015, applies in all health and social care settings. Individual practitioners, professional leaders and managers should all be aware of the consequences, as conviction under this law could well lead to a prison sentence.

Managing and Managers

Complex modern healthcare systems, hospitals and primary care providers all need skilled managers to run effectively. When managers fail, they not only damage their organisations but also put patients at risk. The best-in-class healthcare service managers all have a clear vision, are honest and focus on the safety and rights of patients.

Managers should foster open and transparent organisations, which tend to be the safest, the best to work in and provide space for innovation and learning. Patients are best served when staff feel a genuine pride in the organisation in which they serve and both understand and practise its core values.

Managers need to have encyclopaedic knowledge of what is happening in their organisations. There can be no areas that are off limits, or cliques that protect their own turf. They have to gain and retain the confidence and respect of clinical staff but still act decisively and, if necessary, ruthlessly, when problems arise. Sometimes this requires real courage.

Rationing, resource allocation and priority-setting is inevitable in all healthcare systems, given the gap between what medicine can realistically offer and what individuals and governments are prepared to pay. Bad choices harm vulnerable patients and do little to advance the overall health of communities. Rationing should therefore be both scientifically and values based. In some cases, unnecessary tests and procedures can be reduced in the interests of both patient safety and economics. Stopping investment into treatments or drugs that have no proven worth is evidently also legitimate.

The experiment of using private finance as a means of injecting capital into healthcare systems has largely failed. It can only work if there is a long-term adjustment to revenue flows and operating costs. A new building is of little value if the funds to operate it do not exist.

Governments and managers need to plan for emergencies like the COVID-19 pandemic in the same way they anticipate other civil emergencies.

In almost all countries the glamour and excitement of the acute sector has left mental health and social care lagging far behind in terms of investment and how these services are perceived. Politicians have felt safe in ignoring how these sectors are funded, simply dealing with scandals as and when they occur. However, as with many facets of health, the COVID-19 pandemic may have started to move the needle. The plight of care homes, presented with a huge influx of hospital patients, many of whom had not been tested for the virus, led to huge spikes of infections and thousands of deaths. That the situation was completely mismanaged seems clear, but it displayed clearly to most of the public that the sector is run by devoted staff, often on the minimum wage, and left to sink or swim in a national emergency.

The need for more integrated health and social care is self-evident for both economic and quality-of-life reasons. Perhaps now is the time that we may begin to see it happen.

The ethical and professional duties that are placed on everyone that works in the healthcare sector are onerous, and so they should be. As this book has made clear, the unthinkable happens more often than we would like and constant vigilance is vital for safety.

Endnotes

Chapter One

1. They hoped to save £325,000 through this reorganisation. Edwards, B. (2013). *The Stafford Inquiries: A Collapse in the Culture of Care.* Amazon Kindle.
2. Evidence to Francis Inquiry by Terrence Deighton, quoted in *ibid.*
3. This and other patient stories can be found in the report of the public inquiry into Mid Staffordshire Hospitals: Report of the Mid Staffordshire NHS Foundation Trust Public Inquiry (2013). *House of Commons Papers* [commonly referred to as The Francis Report] (London: UK, The Stationery Office).
4. The Health Commission (2009). *Investigation into Mid Staffordshire NHS Foundation Trust* (London: UK, The Health Commission).
5. '[A] result of 100 for any hospital or diagnostic group in a hospital, means that mortality is exactly as expected, when measured against comparators. A result higher than 100 indicates a higher than expected mortality rate; a result lower than 100 indicates a lower than expected mortality rate. The figures are revised on a monthly basis when Trusts review and revise their data. *Report of the Mid Staffordshire NHS Foundation Trust Public Inquiry* (House of Commons papers).
6. BMJ (2011). Royal College of Surgeons failed to follow up on its critical report on Mid Staffordshire trust, inquiry hears. *BMJ* **343**: d4189
7. *Ibid.*
8. A patient story from: Report of the Mid Staffordshire NHS Foundation Trust Public Inquiry (2013). *House of Commons Papers* [commonly referred to as The Francis Report] (London: UK, The Stationery Office).

9. Commission for Healthcare Audit and Inspection (2009). *Investigation into Mid Staffordshire NHS Foundation Trust* (London: Healthcare Commission).

10. Gainsbury, S. (2017). *The Bottom Line: Understanding the NHS Deficit and Why It Won't Go Away* (London: The Nuffield Trust).

11. Special measures apply when NHS Trusts have serious quality failures or financial problems and there are concerns that the existing leadership cannot make the necessary improvements without support. They consist of a series of interventions designed to remedy the problems within a reasonable time frame.

12. Davies, G. (2005). *Queensland Public Hospitals Commission of Inquiry Report* (Brisbane: Queensland Public Hospitals Commission of Inquiry).

13. In 2010, Dr. Patel appealed his convictions. In a plea deal, he pleaded guilty to fraud and the other charges were dropped. In 2015 he was barred from ever practising medicine in Australia again.

14. A review by the Australian Orthopaedic Association advised that a safe service required four specialist orthopaedic surgeons.

15. *C. Difficile* is bacteria that can affect the bowel and cause diarrhoea.

16. The Healthcare Commission (2007). *Investigation into Outbreaks of C. Difficile at Maidstone and Tunbridge Wells NHS Trust* (London: Healthcare Commission).

17. *Ibid.*

18. Australian Institute of Health and Welfare (2020). Bloodstream infections associated with hospital care 2018–19, AIHW, February 20. Retrieved from: https://www.aihw.gov.au/reports/health-care-quality-performance/bloodstream-infections-associated-with-hospital-care/contents/introduction

19. European Society of Clinical Microbiology and Infectious Diseases (2019). High prevalence of healthcare associated infections and low testing rates found in European hospitals and long-term care facilities, *MedicalXpress*, April 13. Retrieved from: https://medicalxpress.com/news/2019-04-high-prevalence-healthcare-associated-infections-eu.html

20. The Local.se (2018). Finance minister calls for inquiry into hospital scandal, February 7. Retrieved from: https://www.thelocal.se/20180207/finance-minister-calls-for-new-karolinska-hospital-inquiry

21. They found no evidence to proceed.

22. Ciralsky, A. (2016). The celebrity surgeon who used love, money and the Pope to scam an NBC News producer, *Vanity Fair*, February. Retrieved

from: https://www.vanityfair.com/news/2016/01/celebrity-surgeon-nbc-news-producer-scam

23. Karolinska Institute, The Macchiarini Case: Timeline. Retrieved from: https://news.ki.se/the-macchiarini-case-timeline

24. Rostlund, L., and Gustafsson, A. (2019). *Konsulterna: Kampen om Karolinska* (Stockholm: Adlibris).

25. Schreiber, M. (2019). Researchers are surprised by the magnitude of Venezuela's health crisis, NPR, April 5. Retrieved from: https://www.npr.org/sections/goatsandsoda/2019/04/05/709969632/researchers-are-surprised-by-the-magnitude-of-venezuelas-health-crisis

26. University of North Carolina (2019). 172 Rural hospital closures: January 2005-Present, The Cecil G. Sheps Centre for Health Services Research. Retrieved from: https://www.shepscenter.unc.edu/programs-projects/rural-health/rural-hospital-closures/

27. In 2017, the US invested 17.9% of its GDP on health.

28. Yasunga, H. (2008). The catastrophic collapse of morale amongst hospital physicians in Japan. *Risk Management and Health Policy* 1: 1–6.

29. Investment levels increased from a low of 8.2% of GDP in 2008 to 10.9% of GDP in 2017.

30. The Japan Times (1999). Fatal IV drip spurs malpractice probe in Hiroo, March 16. Retrieved from: https://www.japantimes.co.jp/news/1999/03/16/national/fatal-iv-drip-spurs-malpractice-probe-in-hiroo/#.XtvJQ6d7EWo

31. Jacob, S. (2014). Physician autonomy is under siege and morale is declining, *D Magazine*, June 30. Retrieved from: https://www.dmagazine.com/healthcare-business/2014/06/physician-autonomy-is-under-siege-and-morale-is-declining/

32. Hlavinka, E. (2019). Doc's depression, medical errors go hand in hand, *Medpage Today*, November 27. Retrieved from: https://www.medpagetoday.com/psychiatry/depression/83607

33. Killick, P., and Brougham. C. (2017). Independent Review into the circumstances surrounding the discharge, transfer and death of a patient and the HSE's responses to and investigations to the same. A report for Health Services Executive, Verita, London.

34. Laming, W. H. (2003). *The Victoria Climbie Inquiry. Report of an Inquiry by Lord Laming* (Cm. 5730) (London: The Stationery Office).

35. Smith, R. (2016). Turning round failing hospitals. *BMJ*. Retrieved from: https://blogs.bmj.com/bmj/2016/03/23/richard-smith-turning-round-failing-hospitals/

36. By 2018, comparisons of avoidable deaths by locality (clinical commissioning groups) became available in England. The highest rates were found in the northwest of England (Manchester and Blackpool) and the lowest in Surrey in the South of England. Office of National Statistics (2019). *Avoidable Mortality in the UK: 2017* (London: Office of National Statistics).

37. Makary, M., and Daniel, M. (2016). Medical error — the third leading cause of death in the US. *BMJ*, May 3 **353**: i2139.

38. Sipherd, R. (2018) The third leading cause of death in US most doctors don't want you to know about? *CNBC*, February 22. Retrieved from: https://www.cnbc.com/2018/02/22/medical-errors-third-leading-cause-of-death-in-america.html

39. Emily Jerry Foundation, *Emily's Story*. Retrieved from: https://emilyjerryfoundation.org/emilys-story/

40. Examples include giving the wrong blood type or operating on the wrong limb.

41. Wagner, C., Smits, M., Sorra, J., and Huang, C. C. (2013). Assessing patient safety culture in hospitals across countries. *International Journal for Quality in Health Care* **25**(3): 213–221.

42. Care Quality Commission (2013). Our strategy for 2013–2016, April 18. Retrieved from: https://www.cqc.org.uk/news/stories/our-strategy-2013-2016

43. Blackwell, T. (2017). Inside Canada's secret world of medical error: 'There is a lot of lying, there's a lot of cover-up'. *National Post*, July 7. Retrieved from: https://nationalpost.com/health/inside-canadas-secret-world-of-medical-errors-there-is-a-lot-of-lying-theres-a-lot-of-cover-up

Chapter Two

1. Including a Rolls Royce Silver Cloud automobile.

2. An opioid painkiller

3. There were a total of six Shipman Inquiry Reports starting in 2002.

4. The Government response was published in 2007, titled 'Learning from tragedy, keeping patient's safe: Overview of the Government's action programme in response to the recommendations of the Shipman Inquiry', CM 7014 (London: HMSO).

5. He later worked at Cincinnati's VA Hospital and Cincinnati's Drake Memorial Hospital.

6. He forged a fact sheet from the Illinois Department of Corrections stating that he had been convicted of a misdemeanour and was sentenced to six months rather than three years for felony poisoning.
7. During his trial, he claimed his confession had been beaten out of him.
8. Pavel Veprek, Head of the Czech Health Forum, which promotes healthcare reforms.
9. Later increased on appeal to 12 years.
10. A short-acting synthetic muscle relaxant.
11. She has been committed to a high secure hospital.
12. Department of Health (1994). *The Allitt Inquiry: Independent Inquiry Relating to Deaths and Injuries on the Children's Ward at Grantham and Kesteven General Hospital During the Period February to April 1991* (London: HMSO).
13. He had qualified as a nurse in the Philippines.
14. Operation Roxburg.
15. The nurse involved later sued the Police.

Chapter Three

1. Flott, K., Fontana, G., and Darzi, A. (2019). *The Global State of Patient Safety* (London: Imperial College London).
2. La Pietra, L., Calligaris, L., Molendini, L., Quattrin, R., and Brusaferro, S. (2005). Medical errors and clinical risk management: State of the art. *ACTA Otorhinolaryngologica Italica* 25(6): 339–346.
3. Schwendimann, R., Blatter, C., Dhaini, S., *et al.* (2018). The occurrence, types, consequences and preventability of in-hospital adverse events — a scoping review. *BMC Health Services Research* 18: 521.
4. Slawomirski, L., Auraaen, A., and Klazinga, N. (2017). *The Economics of Patient Safety: Strengthening a Value-based Approach to Reducing Patient Harm at National Level* (Bonn: OECD).
5. Graber, M. L. (2013). The incidence of diagnostic error in medicine. *BMJ Quality & Safety* 22(Suppl 2): ii21–ii27.
6. Chronic obstructive pulmonary disease.
7. Graber, M. L. (2013). The incidence of diagnostic error in medicine. *BMJ Quality & Safety,* 22 (Suppl 2): ii21–ii27.
8. Emslie, S., Knox, K., and Pickstone, M. (Eds.) (2002). *Improving Patient Safety: Insights from American, British and Australian Healthcare* (Welwyn Garden City, Hertfordshire, UK: ECRI).
9. *Ibid.*

10. The drug was not taken off the Canadian approved list until March 1962.
11. Thalidomide Trust UK. About Thalidomide. Retrieved from: https://www.thalidomidetrust.org/about-us/about-thalidomide/
12. The UK government contributed £20 million.
13. Hawkins, B. (2019). A bitter pill, *ABC News Australia*, July 17. Retrieved from: https://www.abc.net.au/news/2019-03-11/thalidomide-survivors-demand-recognition-over-disaster/10724268?nw=0
14. Reuters (2020). Sanfoni investigated over epilepsy drug linked to birth defects, *Reuters Business News*, February 4. Retrieved from: https://www.reuters.com/article/us-sanofi-depakine/sanofi-investigated-over-epilepsy-drug-linked-to-birth-defects-idUSKBN1ZY0NW
15. (EU) 2017/745; and (EU) 2017/746.
16. FDA (2019). FDA takes action to protect patients from risk of certain textured breast implants; requests Allergan voluntarily recall certain breast implants and tissue expanders from market, July 24. Retrieved from: https://www.fda.gov/news-events/press-announcements/fda-takes-action-protect-patients-risk-certain-textured-breast-implants-requests-allergan
17. Allergan (2019). A continued commitment to patients, BIOCELL replacement warranty. Retrieved from: https://allergan-web-cdn-prod.azureedge.net/actavis/actavis/media/allergan-pdf-documents/biocell-replacement-warranty.pdf
18. The Daily Telegraph (2013). Calls for a crackdown on cosmetic surgery, April 23. Retrieved from: https://www.telegraph.co.uk/news/health/news/10014195/Calls-for-crackdown-on-cosmetic-surgery.html
19. Carteret, A.-M. (1992). *L'affaire du Sang* (Paris: Editions La Decouverte).
20. The company denied it had campaigned for a delay until it was ready to market its product.
21. Department of Health (2002). *Report of the Tribunal of Inquiry into the Infection with HIV and Hepatitis C of Persons with Haemophilia and Related Matters (Lindsay Tribunal)* (Dublin: Government of Ireland).
22. The proceedings and evidence to the Infected Blood Inquiry are available online: https://www.infectedbloodinquiry.org.uk
23. Crumlin Hospital is the only healthcare centre in Ireland that runs its own donation centre.

24. Hunter, N. (2020). Blood scandal spectre still looms, Irishhealthpro. com, February 14. Retrieved from http://www.irishhealth.com/article. html?id=10415

25. WHO. Health care associated infections: FACT SHEET. Retrieved from: https://www.who.int/gpsc/country_work/gpsc_ccisc_fact_ sheet_en.pdf

26. Methicillin-resistant *Staphylococcus aureus.*

27. Calikoglu, S., Murray, R., and Feeney, D. (2012). Hospital pay-for-performance programs in Maryland produced strong results, including reduced hospital-acquired conditions. *Health Affairs* **31**(12): 2649–2658.

28. Wakesmith Solicitors (2017). Hospital acquired infection case study 2017. Retrieved from: https://www.wake-smith.co.uk/hospital-acquired-infection-case-study

29. Pollack, A. (2010). Rising threat of infections unfazed by antibiotics, *The New York Times,* February 26. Retrieved from: https://www. nytimes.com/2010/02/27/business/27germ.html

30. Gibson, E. (2019). Five die from flu caught in hospital, Newsroom. co.nz., December 18. Retrieved from: https://www.newsroom. co.nz/2019/12/18/953648/influenza-outbreaks-striking-the-elderly-in-hospital

31. Reilly, B. M., and Evans, A. T. (2009). Much ado about (doing) nothing. *Annals of Internal Medicine* **150**(4): 270–271.

32. Greenfield, P. (2018). NHS wields axe on 17 'unnecessary procedures, *The Guardian,* June 30. Retrieved from: https://www.theguardian. com/society/2018/jun/29/nhs-wields-the-axe-on-17-unnecessary-procedures

33. Choosing Wisely US (2020). Case study: Shedding light on excess imaging, January 22. Retrieved from: https://www.choosingwisely. org/resources/updates-from-the-field/case-study-shedding-light-on-excess-imaging/

34. Choosing Wisely US (2020). Recommendations for clinicians. Retrieved from: https://www.choosingwisely.co.uk/i-am-a-clinician/recommendations/

35. Dubé, D.-E. (2017). Canadians undergo more than 1 million potentially unnecessary medical tests, treatments a year, April 6. Retrieved from: https://globalnews.ca/news/3359201/canadians-undergo-more-than-1-million-potentially-unnecessary-medical-tests-treatments-a-year-report/

36. Haymond, S. (2016). What everyone should know about lab tests: They aren't always correct and they aren't always useful, *Scientific American*, May 9. Retrieved from: https://blogs.scientificamerican. com/guest-blog/what-everyone-should-know-about-lab-tests/

37. Graber, M. L. (2013). Incidence of diagnostic error in medicine. *BMJ Quality and Safety* 22: ii21–ii27.

38. Brooks, L. (1999). 11 deaths after late diagnoses at NHS breast cancer unit, *The Guardian*, April 14. Retrieved from: https://www.theguardian. com/uk/1999/apr/14/libbybrooks

39. Graber, M. L. (2013). The incidence of diagnostic error in medicine. *BMJ Quality & Safety* 22(Suppl 2): ii21–ii27.

40. Cooper, G. (1998). Eight women die in smear test blunders, *The Independent*, January 21. Retrieved from: https://www.independent. co.uk/news/eight-women-die-in-smear-test-blunders-1141800.html

41. BBC (2018). Irish cervical check scandal; Mother settles case for €7.5m, June 29. Retrieved from: https://www.bbc.com/news/ world-europe-44659869

42. Petticrew, M. P., Sowden, A. J., Lister-Sharp, D., and Wright, K. (2000). False-negative results in screening programmes: Systematic review of impact and implications. *Health Technology Assessment* 4(5): 1–120.

43. Committee of Inquiry into Allegations Concerning the Treatment of Cervical Cancer at National Women's Hospital and into Other Related Matters [The Cartwright Report] (1988) (Government Printing Office: New Zealand).

44. See also: Bryder, L. (2018). *The Rise and Fall of the National Women's Hospital* (Auckland: Auckland University Press).

45. New Zealand Herald (2018). Auckland District Health Board apologises for deadly medical experiment, August 26. Retrieved from: https://www.nzherald.co.nz/nz/news/article.cfm?c_id=1&objectid= 12113964

46. Bryder, L. (2018). *The Rise and Fall of the National Women's Hospital* (Auckland: Auckland University Press).

47. CMO (2013). *Chief Medical Officer Annual Report 2012: Children and Young People's Health* (London: UK Government).

48. The European Commission (2017). *EU One Health Action Plan against Antimicrobial Resistance (AMR)* (Brussels: European Commission).

49. Associated Press (2019). Michigan sues four firms including Walgreens over deadly opioid epidemic, *The Guardian*, December 17. Retrieved from: https://www.theguardian.com/us-news/2019/dec/17/michigan-sues-walgreens-companies-drugs-opioids-painkillers

50. Kalkman, G. A., *et al.* (2019). Trends in use and misuse of opioids in the Netherlands: A retrospective, multi-source database study. *The Lancet Public Health* **4**(10): e498–e505.

51. Krumholz, H. M. and Ross, J. S. (2017). Taking shortcuts in drug testing can put patients at risk, National Public Media (NPR), April 4. Retrieved from: https://www.npr.org/sections/health-shots/2017/04/04/522583228/taking-shortcuts-in-drug-testing-can-put-patients-at-risk

52. Eli Lilly was the parent company of Dista, who promoted the drug in the UK.

53. House of Commons debate (1988) Hansard, March 17, Vol. 129, cc1319–cc1326.

54. Blunt, C. J. (2018). The avoidable scandal. Benoxaprofen and theories of medical evidence, March 15. Retrieved from: http://cjblunt.com/the-avoidable-scandal-benoxaprofen-and-theories-of-medical-evidence/

55. *Ibid.*

56. Staines, R. (2019). France's Servier finally goes on trial over Mediator safety scandal, Pharmaphorum, September 23. Retrieved from: https://pharmaphorum.com/news/frances-servier-finally-goes-on-trial-over-mediator-safety-scandal/

57. Mullard, A. (2013). Mediator scandal engulfs French compensation body. *The Lancet* **381**(9880): P180. Retrieved from: https://www.thelancet.com/journals/lancet/article/PIIS0140-6736(13)61106-X/fulltext

58. Elliott, R. A., Camacho, E., Campbell, F., Jankovic, D., Martyn-St James, M., Kaltenthaler, E., Neves., and De Faria, R. I. (2018). *Prevalence and Economic Burden of Medication Errors in The NHS in England: Rapid Evidence Synthesis and Economic Analysis of the Prevalence and Burden of Medication Error in the UK* (Policy Research Unit in Economic Evaluation of Health and Care Interventions (EEPRU)).

59. Davis, N. M., and Cohen M. R. (1981). *Medication Errors: Causes and Prevention* (Philadelphia, PA: Strickly Co).

60. Tariq, R. A., and Scherbak, Y. (2020). *Medication Errors* (Treasure Island, FL, USA: StatPearls Publishing).

61. Kohn, L. T., Corrigan, J. M., and Donaldson, M. S. (2000). *To Err is Human: Building a Safer Health System* (Washington, D.C.: National Academy Press).

62. World Health Organization (2016). *Medication Errors: Technical Series On Safer Primary Care* (Geneva: World Health Organization).

63. Roughead, E. E., Semple, S. J., and Rosenfeld, E. (2016). The extent of medication errors and adverse drug reactions throughout the patient journey in acute care in Australia. *International Journal of Evidence-based Healthcare* **14**(3): 113–122.

64. NHS Improvement (2019). The NHS patient safety strategy, July 2. Retrieved from: https://improvement.nhs.uk/resources/patient-safety-strategy/

65. NICE UK. (2009). Medicine's Adherence: Involving patients in decisions about prescribed medicines and supporting adherence. Clinical Guidance [CG 76], January 28. Retrieved from: https://www.nice.org.uk/guidance/cg76

66. The fee in 2019 was £28 per MUR with a limit of £400 per year.

67. Cheragi, M. A., Manoocheri, H., Mohammadnejad, E., and Ehsani, S. R. (2013). Types and causes of medication errors from nurse's viewpoint. *Iranian Journal of Nursing and Midwifery Research* **18**(3): 228–231.

68. Weeks, G., George, J., Maclure, K., and Stewart, D. (2016). Non-medical prescribing versus medical prescribing for acute and chronic disease management in primary and secondary care. *The Cochrane Database of Systematic Reviews* **11**(11): doi: 10.1002/14651858. CD011227.pub2.

69. Bedford, H (2011). *Childhood Immunisation: Achievements and Challenges* (London: UCL Institute of Child Health).

70. Rao, T. S., and Andrade, C. (2011). The MMR vaccine and autism: Sensation, refutation, retraction, and fraud. *Indian Journal of Psychiatry* **53**(2): 95–96.

71. Kmietowicz, Z. (2010). Wakefield is struck off for the "serious and wide-ranging findings against him." *BMJ* **340**: c2803.

72. BBC News (2018). Chinese firm fined $1.3bn for illegal production of rabies vaccine, October 17. Retrieved from: https://www.bbc.com/news/world-asia-china-45886388

73. Smith, R. (2014). Hundreds die each year in NHS due to faulty machines, *Daily Telegraph*, July 25. Retrieved from: https://www. telegraph.co.uk/news/health/news/10988112/Hundreds-die-each-year-in-NHS-due-to-faulty-machines-report.html

74. New Zealand Herald (2019). Over 55 Hawke's Bay patients face HIV, hepatitis tests after sterilised surgical equipment fail, February 13. Retrieved from: https://www.nzherald.co.nz/spotlight/news/article. cfm?c_id=1504095&objectid=12203422

75. Donaldson, L. (2002). An organisation with a memory. *Clinical Medicine* 2(5): 452–457.

76. Newmarker, C. (2014). 7 recent medical device failures catching FDA's eye, *Medical Device and Diagnostic Industry*, March 14. Retrieved from: https://www.mddionline.com/7-recent-medical-device-failures-catching-fdas-eye

77. Kirsh, D. (2019). The grim story behind seven of medtechs worst failures, *Medical Design and Outsourcing*, April 19. Retrieved from: https://www.medicaldesignandoutsourcing.com/the-grim-stories-behind-seven-of-medtechs-worst-failures/

78. Smith, R. (2014). Hundreds die each year in NHS due to faulty machines, *Daily Telegraph*, July 25. Retrieved from: https://www. telegraph.co.uk/news/health/news/10988112/Hundreds-die-each-year-in-NHS-due-to-faulty-machines-report.html

79. Cohen, D. (2012). How safe are metal on metal implants? *BMJ* **344**: e1410.

80. *Ibid.*

81. National Joint Registry for England, Wales, Northern Ireland and the Isle of Man. 15th Annual Report 2018. Retrieved from: https://www. hqip.org.uk/resource/national-joint-registry-15th-annual-report-2018/#.Xt5qsqd7E5s

82. Llamas, M. (2019). Transvaginal mesh verdicts and settlements, *Drugwatch*. Retrieved from: https://www.drugwatch.com/transvaginal-mesh/verdict-settlement/

83. The Lancet [Editorial] (2018). Patient safety in vaginal mesh surgery. *The Lancet*. Retrieved from: https://www.thelancet.com/journals/lancet/article/PIIS0140-6736(18)32480-2/fulltext

84. Llamas, M. (2019). Transvaginal mesh verdicts and settlements, *Drugwatch*. Retrieved from: https://www.drugwatch.com/transvaginal-mesh/verdict-settlement/

85. Gornall, J. (2018). How mesh became a four letter word. *BMJ* **363**: k4137.

86. Osborne, H., Devlin, H., and Barr, C. (2018). The implant files, *The Guardian*, Society, November 25.

87. Bogdanich, W. (2010). Radiation offers new cures and a way to do harm, *The New York Times*, January 23. Retrieved from: https://www. nytimes.com/2010/01/24/health/24radiation.html

88. Papows, J. (2010). *Glitch: The Hidden Impact of Faulty Software* (Upper Saddle River, NJ: Prentice-Hall).

89. Gornall, J. (2018). How mesh became a four letter word. *BMJ* **363**: k4137.

90. Rose, B. W. (1994). Fatal dose: Radiation deaths linked to AECL computer errors, *CCNR*. Retrieved from: http://www.ccnr.org/ fatal_dose.html

91. The Herald, Scotland (1993). Blunder led to cancer deaths, September 30. Retrieved from: https://www.heraldscotland.com/ news/12717319.blunder-led-to-cancer-deaths/

92. Johnston, R. (2019). Database of radiological incidents and related events, Johnston's Archive, August 24. Retrieved from: http://www. johnstonsarchive.net/nuclear/radevents/index.html

93. World Health Organization (2008). *Radiotherapy Risk Profile: Technical Manual* (Geneva: World Health Organization).

94. Ballas, L. K., Elkin, E. B., Schrag, D., Minsky, B. D., and Bach, P. B. (2006). Radiation therapy facilities in the United States. *International Journal of Radiation Oncology, Biology, Physics* **66**(4): 1204–1211.

95. A new machine cost around £2 million in 2020.

96. Bogdanich, W. (2010). Radiation offers new cures and a way to do harm, *The New York Times*, January 23. Retrieved from: https://www. nytimes.com/2010/01/24/health/24radiation.html

97. Roser, M., and Ritchie, H. (2020). Maternal mortality, OurWorldInData. org. Retrieved from: https://ourworldindata.org/maternal-mortality

98. MBRRACE-UK (2019). Mothers and babies: Reducing risk through audit and confidential inquiries across the UK. Retrived from: https:// www.npeu.ox.ac.uk/mbrrace-uk

99. Morris, J. (2018). Understanding the health of babies and expectant mothers, Nuffield Trust, November 6. Retrieved from: https://www. nuffieldtrust.org.uk/resource/understanding-the-health-of-babies-and-expectant-mothers

100. Department of Health (2016). Safer maternity care: Next steps towards the national maternity ambition. Retrieved from: https://assets.publishing.service.gov.uk/government/uploads/system/uploads/attachment_data/file/560491/Safer_Maternity_Care_action_plan.pdf

101. Healthcare Quality Improvement Partnership (HQIP). A-Z of clinical outcome programmes 2020. Retrieved from: https://www.hqip.org.uk/clinical-outcome-review-programmes/#.Xt-W0Kd7E5s

102. Hoyert, D. L., and Miniño, A. M. (2020). Maternal mortality in the United States: Changes in coding, publication and data release 2018 *National Vital Statistics Reports* **69**(2): 1–18.

103. Gaskin, I. M. (2008). Maternal death in the United States: A problem solved or a problem ignored? *The Journal of Perinatal Education* **17**(2): 9–13.

104. Now called the Centre for Maternal and Child Enquiries (CMACE).

105. Kirkup, B. (2015). *The Report of the Morecambe Bay Investigation* (London: The Stationery Office).

106. Campbell, D. (2007). National Patient Safety Report [quoted in] The tragic cost of NHS baby blunders, *The Observer*, September 23. Retrieved from: https://www.theguardian.com/society/2007/sep/23/health.medicineandhealth

107. Australian Health Practitioner Regulation Agency (2017). Update on the status of investigations — health practitioners associated with Djerrwarrh Health Services, AHPRA, March 10. Retrieved from: https://www.ahpra.gov.au/News/2017-03-10-media-statement.aspx

108. King, C. (2016). Bacchus Marsh Hospital: Coroner finds significant failings in care in baby death cases, *ABC News Australia*, May 4. Retrieved from: https://www.abc.net.au/news/2016-05-05/bacchus-marsh-baby-deaths-case-coroner-releases-findings/7385182

109. Victoria State Government (2020). Targeting zero: The review of hospital safety and quality assurance in Victoria. Retrieved from: https://www.dhhs.vic.gov.au/publications/targeting-zero-review-hospital-safety-and-quality-assurance-victoria

110. In 2019, there were 160 midwife led units in England with the majority located alongside hospital maternity units.

111. FIGO (2018). C-Sections: How to stop the epidemic, November 7. Retrieved from: https://www.figo.org/news/c-sections-how-stop-epidemic

112. Boerma, T., Ronsmans, C., Melesse, D. Y., Barros, A., Barros, F. C., Juan, L., Moller, A. B., Say, L., Hosseinpoor, A. R., Yi, M., de Lyra Rabello Neto, D., and Temmerman, M. (2018). Global epidemiology of use of and disparities in caesarean sections. *Lancet (London, England)* **392**(10155): 1341–1348.

113. Sowden, A., Aletras, V., Place, M., Rice, N., Eastwood, A., Grilli, R., Ferguson, B., Posnett, J., and Sheldon, T. (1997). Volume of clinical activity in hospitals and healthcare outcomes, costs, and patient access. *Quality in Health Care* **6**(2): 109–114.

114. Meadows, C. I. S., Rattenbury, W., and Waldmann, C. (2011). Centralisation of specialist critical care services. *Journal of the Intensive Care Society* **12**(2): 87–89.

115. Stewart, G. D., Long, G., and Tulloh, B. R. (2006). Surgical service centralisation in Australia versus choice and quality of life for rural patients. *The Medical Journal of Australia* **185**(3): 162–163

116. Bhattarai, N., *et al.* (2019). Preferences for emergency medical services: Discrete choice experiment. *BMJ Open* **9**: e030966.

117. OECD (2009). *OECD Economic Surveys: New Zealand 2009* (Paris: OECD).

118. Morris, S., *et al.* (2014). Impact of centralising acute stroke services in English metropolitan areas on mortality and length of hospital stay: Difference-in-differences analysis. *BMJ* **349**: g4757.

119. Christiansen, T., and Vrangbæk, K. (2018). Hospital centralization and performance in Denmark — Ten years on. *Health Policy (Amsterdam, Netherlands)* **122**(4): 321–328.

120. Elrod, J. K., and Fortenberry, J. L. (2017). The hub-and-spoke organization design: An avenue for serving patients well. *BMC Health Services Research* **17**: 457.

121. Meadows, C. I. S., Rattenbury, W., and Waldmann, C. (2011). Centralisation of specialist critical care services. *Journal of The Intensive Care Society* **12**(2): 87–89.

122. Devarakonda, S. (2016). Hub and spoke model: Making rural healthcare in India affordable, available and accessible. *Rural Remote Health* **16**(1): 1–8.

123. Kennedy, I. (2001). *Learning from Bristol: The Report of the Public Inquiry into Children's Heart Surgery at the Bristol Royal Infirmary, 1984–1995* (London: The Stationery Office).

124. Adams, S., and Smith, R. (2010). Nobody disciplined after baby deaths, *Daily Telegraph*, July 28. Retrieved from: https://www.

telegraph.co.uk/news/health/news/7917445/Nobody-disciplined-after-baby-deaths.html

125. The NHS in England performs fewer than 4000 operations a year.
126. Hamilton, L. (2017). Reconfiguration of clinical services in the NHS in the "too difficult" box, Royal College of Surgeons of England, February 7. Retrieved from: https://www.rcseng.ac.uk/news-and-events/blog/heart-surgery-reconfiguration/
127. Kennedy, I. (2001). *Learning from Bristol: The Report of the Public Inquiry into Children's Heart Surgery at the Bristol Royal Infirmary, 1984–1995* (London: The Stationery Office).
128. Vonlanthen, R., *et al.* (2018). Toward a consensus on centralization in surgery. *Annals of Surgery* **268**(5): 712–724.
129. National Congenital Heart Disease Audit (2019). Understanding children's heart surgery outcomes. Retrieved from: https://www.hqip.org.uk/wp-content/uploads/2019/09/Ref-129-Cardiac-NCHDA-Summary-Report-2019-FINAL.pdf
130. Lundström, N. R., Berggren, H., Björkhem, G., Jögi, P., and Sunnegårdh, J. (2000). Centralization of pediatric heart surgery in Sweden. *Pediatric Cardiology* **21**(4): 353–357.
131. Alexander, H. (2019). 'Inward looking': Governance review slams feuding children's hospitals, *Sydney Morning Herald*, July 4. Retrieved from: https://www.smh.com.au/national/nsw/inward-looking-governance-review-slams-feuding-children-s-hospitals-20190703-p523rt.html
132. ABC News (2019). D marchese, May 30; Mayers, L. (2019). Cartel behaviour, May 29.
133. Symonds, P., Naftalin, N., and Shaw, P. (2003). A smear on Audit: Implications of the Leicester cervical smear audit. *BJOG* **110**(7): 646–648.
134. Bewick, M., and Haynes, S. (2018). Independent review of Cardiac Surgery Service: St Georges Hospital NHS Trust, IQ4U. Retrieved from: https://www.stgeorges.nhs.uk/wp-content/uploads/2018/08/Independent-review-of-cardiac-surgery — St-George's-University-Hospitals....pdf
135. Woo, Y. L., Kyrgiou, M., Bryant, A., Everett, T., and Dickinson, H. O. (2012). Centralisation of services for gynaecological cancer. *Cochrane Database of Systematic Reviews* **2012**(3): doi: 10.1002/14651858. CD007945.pub2.
136. Linton, S. (2020). Leading cancer hospital faces being stripped of child services amid safety fears, *Independent*, January 31. Retrieved

from: https://www.independent.co.uk/news/health/royal-marsden-child-cancer-safety-nhs-england-a9311176.html

137. NHS England Board meeting 30/1/2020. Retrieved from: https://www.england.nhs.uk/wp-content/uploads/2020/01/nhs-england-improvement-public-board-agenda-300120.pdf

138. Royal College of Surgeons (2015). The state of surgery in Wales. Retrieved from: https://www.rcseng.ac.uk/library-and-publications/rcs-publications/docs/state-of-surgery-wales/

139. NHS Improvement (2018). Surgical never events. Retrieved from: https://improvement.nhs.uk/documents/3213/Learning_from_surgical_Never_Events_FINAL.pdf. Similar reports are available for earlier years.

140. Optical coherence tomography — a non-invasive procedure.

141. Mackenzie Bean, M. (2019). 5 most common sentinel events so far in 2019, Becker's Healthcare, August 14. Retrieved from: https://www.beckershospitalreview.com/quality/5-most-common-sentinel-events-so-far-in-2019.html

142. Adams, K., Drees, J., and Dyrda, L. (2020). Patient experience 'never events' from 16 execs at Cleveland Clinic, Providence & more, Beckers Healthcare, May 20. Retrieved from: https://www.beckershospitalreview.com/digital-transformation/patient-experience-never-events-from-16-execs-at-cleveland-clinic-hca-providence-more.html

143. Cumberlege, J. (2020). First do no harm: The report of the Independent Medicines and Medical Devices Safety Review. Retrieved from: https://www.immdsreview.org.uk/Report.html

144. Foetal Valproate Spectrum Disorder (FVSD).

145. See footnote 36.

146. Christiansen, T., and Vrangbæk, K. (2018). Hospital centralization and performance in Denmark — Ten years on. *Health Policy* 122(4): 321–328.

Chapter Four

1. In 2019, the Board had 26 members.

2. NYSED, Office of the Professions (2014). New law changes entry level education requirement for licensure as a physical therapist. Retrieved from: http://www.op.nysed.gov/prof/pt/ptnews.htm

3. Published by the American College of Physicians.

4. Organización Medica Colegial de España (2016). *Good Medical Practice: Guidelines for a Professional Performance of Excellence* (Madrid: CGCOM).

5. As of 2017.

6. Canadian Nursing Association (2017). Available at: https://www.cna-aiic.ca/~/media/cna/page-content/pdf-en/code-of-ethics-2017-edition-secure-interactive

7. 98% of graduates from US medical schools pass first time. The first time pass rate for overseas graduates is 78%.

8. Fauber, J., and Wynn, M. (2019). Malpractice, mistakes and misconduct: Doctors who surrender a medical license in one state can practice in others, *USA Today*, December 16. Retrieved from: https://eu.usa-today.com/story/news/2018/11/30/medical-board-license-failures-doctor-malpractice-move-states/2159948002/

9. Pharmacists, physiotherapists and general nurses.

10. EU (2005). *Directive 2005/36/EC of the European Parliament and of the Council of 7 September 2005 on the Recognition of Professional Qualifications* (Text with EEA relevance).

11. Mivacron is a neuromuscular blocking drug used in anaesthesia.

12. Gic, J. A. (2007). "The physician and the nurse," in *The Medical Malpractice Survival Handbook* (ACLM) (Maryland Heights, MI: Mosby/Elsevier), pp. 111–116.

13. Nursing and Midwifery Council (NMC) (2019). NMC announces new online system for overseas applicants, October 7. Retrieved from: https://www.nmc.org.uk/news/press-releases/nmc-announces-new-online-system-for-overseas-applicants/.

14. Dyer, C. (2014). UK doctor who worked in the US after being struck off by GMC has license withdrawn. *BMJ* **348**: g1613.

15. In 2019 there were 290,000 doctors licensed to practise in the UK.

16. BMA Medical Ethics Department (2013). *Everyday Medical Ethics and Law* (Chichester: Wiley Blackwell).

17. NMC (2019). Fitness to Practise Committee, October 7–10. Retrieved from: https://www.nmc.org.uk/globalassets/sitedocuments/ftpoutcomes/2019/october-2019/reasons-evans-ftpcsh-66094-20191010.pdf

18. Medical Practitioner Tribunal Service (2019). Public Record Determination: GMC Reg: 5160300, September 26. Retrieved from:

https://www.mpts-uk.org/hearings-and-decisions/medical-practitio-ners-tribunals/dr-lidia-hristeva-sept-19

19. Medical Practitioner Tribunal Service (2019). Public Record Determination: GMC Reg: 4366977, October 2. Retrieved from: https://www.mpts-uk.org/hearings-and-decisions/medical-practitioners-tribunals/dr-leopold-reinecke-sep-19

20. Health and Care Professions Tribunal Service (2019). Reg: RA75022, December 19.

21. Health and Care Professions Tribunal Service (2019). *Conduct and Competence Committee.* Reg: BS42055.

22. Nursing Council of Hong Kong (2016). Disciplinary Inquiry No NC/279/7/B, May.

23. Ahpra (2011). Retrieved from: https://www.ahpra.gov.au/Publications/Panel-Decisions/Panel-hearing-summary-2011-0025.aspx

24. Ahpra (2012). Decision of the Chiropractic Board of Australia. 2012.0082, May 3. Retrieved from: https://www.ahpra.gov.au/Publications/Panel-Decisions/Panel-hearing-summary-2012-0082.aspx

25. Samanta, A., and Samanta, J. (2019). Gross negligence manslaughter and doctors: Ethical concerns following the case of Dr Bawa-Garba. *Journal of Medical Ethics* **45**(1): 10–14.

26. Samanta, A., and Samanta, J. (2006). Charges of corporate manslaughter in the NHS. *BMJ (Clinical Research Education)* **332**(7555): 1404–1405.

27. Taylor, D., and Mackenzie, G. (2013). Staying focused on the big picture: Should Australia legislate for corporate manslaughter based on the United Kingdom model? *Criminal Law Journal* **37**(2): 99–113.

28. Medical Practitioners Tribunal Service (2019). Public Record of Determinations, Reg: 7341253, September 20.

29. Medical Practitioners Tribunal (2019). GMC Ref: 4684583, September 23.

30. Medical Practitioners Tribunal Service (2017). Reg: 6085223, July 25.

31. Medical Practitioners Tribunal (2019). Reg: 6142895, August 16.

32. Nursing and Midwifery Council (UK) (2019). Suspension Order Index, October. Retrieved from: https://www.nmc.org.uk/concerns-nurses-midwives/hearings/hearings-sanctions/suspension-orders-index/suspension-orders-2019/

33. Bosely, S., and Meikie, J. (2010). Locum GP struck off medical register for fatal overdose, *The Guardian*, June 18. Retrieved from:

https://www.theguardian.com/society/2010/jun/18/gp-daniel-ubani-struck-off

34. Medical Practitioners Tribunal (2019). Public Record of Determination. GMC Reference: 4327121, August 2.
35. Medical Practitioner Tribunal Service (2019). Public Record of Determination. GMC Reg: 6076892, October 31.
36. Medical Practitioner Tribunal Service (2019). Public Record of Determination. GMC Reg: 6110999, June 6.
37. Ahpra (2019). Medical practitioner disqualified for a serious breach of professional conduct, December 30. Retrieved from: https://www.medicalboard.gov.au/News/2019-12-27-Medical-practitioner-disqualified-for-a-serious-breach-of-professional-conduct.aspx
38. The Daily Telegraph (2020). GP who molested women at his surgery handed three life sentences, February 7. Retrieved from: https://www.telegraph.co.uk/news/2020/02/07/gp-molested-women-surgery-handed-three-life-sentences/
39. Ahpra (2012). Panel hearing summary 2012.0066. Retrieved from: https://www.ahpra.gov.au/Publications/Panel-Decisions/Panel-hearing-summary-2012-0066.aspx
40. Greysen, S. R., Chretien, K. C., Kind, T., Young, A., and Gross, C. P. (2012). Physician violations of online professionalism and disciplinary actions: A national survey of state medical boards. *JAMA* **307**(11): 1141–1142.
41. Medical Practitioners Tribunal (2019). Public Record of Determination. GMC Reg: 4371034, October 18.
42. See: www.practitionerhealth.nhs.net
43. McClure, M., McIntosh, E., and Oved, M. C. (2018). This Alberta doctor's drinking cost him his US medical license twice, *Star Metro Calgary*, May 1. Retrieved from: https://www.thestar.com/news/canada/2018/05/01/this-alberta-doctors-drinking-cost-him-his-us-medical-licence-twice.html
44. New Zealand Health Practitioners Disciplinary Tribunal 2019. Case Med 19/442P.
45. See: https://www.end-opioid-epidemic.org/resources/california-acep-safe-prescribing-guidelines/
46. Department of Justice. US Attorney's Office. District of New Jersey (2020). Doctor described as 'Candy Man' and 'El Chapo of Opioids' admits distributing opioids to patients, February 24. Retrieved from: https://www.justice.gov/usao-nj/pr/doctor-described-candy-man-and-el-chapo-opioids-admits-distributing-opioids-patients

47. BBC News. (2019). Majid Mustafa: 'Deplorable' dentist struck off for wife drug plot, December 5. Retrieved from: https://www.bbc.com/news/uk-england-humber-50674022

48. British Columbia College of Nursing Professionals (2018). Disciplinary Notices, March 27. Retrieved from: https://www.bccnp.ca/bccnp/Announcements/Pages/Announcement.aspx?AnnouncementID=11

49. Medical Practitioners Tribunal Service (2017). GMC 7037071, September 6. Retrieved from: https://www.mpts-uk.org/hearings-and-decisions/medical-practitioners-tribunals/dr-justine-mcintyre-sept-19

50. NMC (2019). Fitness to Practice Committee, October 7. Retrieved from: https://www.nmc.org.uk/globalassets/sitedocuments/ftpoutcomes/2019/october-2019/reasons-watson-ftpcsm-67314-20191007.pdf

51. Ahpra (2013). Nursing and Midwifery Board of Australia. Panel Hearing Summary 2013.0173. Retrieved from: https://www.ahpra.gov.au/Publications/Panel-Decisions/Panel-hearing-summary-2013-0173.aspx

52. Ahpra Nursing and Midwifery Board of Australia (2017). Nurse disqualified for 12 months for professional misconduct, May 19. Retrieved from: https://www.nursingmidwiferyboard.gov.au/News/2017-05-19-nurse-disqualified.aspx

53. NMC (2019). Fitness to Practise Committee, December 15. Retrieved from: https://www.nmc.org.uk/globalassets/sitedocuments/ftpoutcomes/2019/october-2019/reasons-cabia-ftpcsor-60757-20191029.pdf

54. General Pharmaceutical Council (2019). Fitness to Practise Committee. Reg: 2047435, October 10. Retrieved from: https://www.pharmacyregulation.org/content/vincent-kwadzo-torku

55. General Pharmaceutical Council (2019). Fitness to Practise Committee. Reg: 5028384, September 26. Retrieved from: https://www.pharmacyregulation.org/content/nicholas-bawden

56. James, G. (2020). *Report of the Independent Inquiry into the Issues Raised by Paterson* (London: House of Commons HC 31).

57. Hartley-Brewer, J. (2000). Downfall of surgeon who ruined lives, *The Guardian*, June 2. Retrieved from: https://www.theguardian.com/uk/2000/jun/02/juliahartleybrewer

58. Health organisations contribute an annual fee to fund NHS Resolution.

59. Malouf, G. (2016). How does Australia measure up with medical negligence? Gerard Malouf & Partners, November 16. Retrieved from: https://www.gerardmaloufpartners.com.au/publications/how-does-australia-measure-up-with-medical-negligence/

60. Ahpra (2017). Medical practitioner disqualified for ten years for professional misconduct, July 17. Retrieved from: https://www.medicalboard.gov.au/News/2017-07-17-disqualified.aspx

61. The Local DK (2017). Danish doctor negligence case to be retried by Supreme Court, November 9. Retrieved from: https://www.thelocal.dk/20171109/danish-doctor-negligence-case-to-be-retried-by-supreme-court

62. Of the 126 cases that went through this process in 2018, 66 were closed as there were no grounds for concern about public safety.

63. Professional Standards Authority for Health and Social Care (2018). NMC Lessons Learnt Review May 2018. Retrieved from: https://www.professionalstandards.org.uk/publications/detail/nmc—lessons-learned-review-may-2018

64. Grindlay, D. (2018). Doctors deemed incompetent and stripped of registration after years of work, *ABC Wimmera*, August 3. Retrieved from: https://www.abc.net.au/news/2018-08-03/foreign-trained-rural-doctors-facing-crackdown-despite-shortage/10066748

65. *Ibid.*

66. Skolnick, A. A. (1998). Critics denounce staffing jails and prisons with physicians convicted of misconduct. *JAMA* **280**(16): 1391–1392.

67. Svorney, S. (2004). Licensing doctors: Do economists agree? *Econ Journal Watch* **1**(2): 279–305.

68. These reflective subjects may change over time.

69. Tazzyman, A. *et al.* (2019). Reforming regulatory relationships. The impact of medical revalidation on doctors, employers and the General Medical Council in the UK. *Regulation and Governance* **13**(4): 593–608.

70. Between December 2012 and July 2016, 33,148 doctors left the UK register.

71. Collins, A. (2016). Is revalidation pushing doctors out of the profession? *BMJ* **355**: i5630.

72. Only 11% of concerns raised with the GMC are referred to an Independent Tribunal.

73. See Chapter Seven for more on corruption in Pakistan.

Chapter Five

1. Budzowska, J. (2020). Extrajudicial compensation proceedings for injured patients in Sweden and Poland, BFP Law Firm, January 19.

Retrieved from: https://personalinjurylawyers.pl/extrajudicial-compensation-proceedings-for-injured-patients-in-sweden-and-in-poland/

2. Physicians working privately contribute directly to the insurance fund.
3. See footnote 1.
4. Chisholm, D. (2019). *North and South*, July, n. 400, 44–50.
5. Wallis, K. A. (2017). No-fault, no difference: No-fault compensation for medical injury and healthcare ethics and practice. *The British Journal of General Practice: The Journal of the Royal College of General Practitioners* **67**(654): 38–39.
6. Latner, A. W. (2016). Could Denmark be the blueprint for an American medical malpractice overhaul? Clinical Advisor, January 5. Retrieved from: https://www.clinicaladvisor.com/home/my-practice/legal-advisor/could-denmark-be-the-blueprint-for-an-american-medical-malpractice-overhaul/
7. NHS Resolution (2019). Annual report and accounts 2018 to 2019, August 9. Retrieved from: https://www.gov.uk/government/publications/nhs-resolution-annual-report-and-accounts-2018-to-2019
8. Mello, M. M., Chandra, A., Gawande, A. A., and Studdert, D. M. (2010). National costs of the medical liability system. *Health Affairs (Project Hope)* **29**(9): 1569–1577.
9. Standing Committee of the Hospitals of the European Union (HOPE) (2004). Insurance and Malpractice. HOPE. Retrieved from: http://www.hope.be/wp-content/uploads/2015/11/71_2004_OTHER_Insurance-and-malpractice-report.pdf
10. US$250,000 in 2019.
11. NHS Resolution (2019). Lesley Elder v George Eliot Hospital, England, April 2018, NHS Resolution Annual Report and Accounts 2018–2019. Retrieved from: https://assets.publishing.service.gov.uk/government/uploads/system/uploads/attachment_data/file/824345/NHS_Resolution_Annual_Report_and_accounts_print.pdf
12. NHS Resolution (2019). Darnley v Croydon, Supreme Court, London. NHS Resolution Annual Report and Accounts 2018–2019. Retrieved from: https://assets.publishing.service.gov.uk/government/uploads/system/uploads/attachment_data/file/824345/NHS_Resolution_Annual_Report_and_accounts_print.pdf
13. Wright Hassall LLP., Whyman, J. (2019). Our most notable medical negligence cases since 2019, Lexolology.com, August 27. Retrieved

from: https://www.lexology.com/library/detail.aspx?g=7426ab64-6002-41e9-abde-2b4b48a56ecc

14. Leighton Law (2019). 12 most famous medical malpractice cases — Dirty dozen of medical mistakes, Leighton Law. Retrieved from: https://leightonlaw.com/12-famous-medical-malpractice-cases/

15. Campion, E. W. (2003). A death at Duke. *The New England Journal of Medicine* **348**(12): 1083–1084.

16. Wright Hassall LLP., Whyman, J. (2019). Our most notable medical negligence cases since 2019, Lexolology.com, August 27. Retrieved from: https://www.lexology.com/library/detail.aspx?g=7426ab64-6002-41e9-abde-2b4b48a56ecc

17. Leighton Law (2019). 12 most famous medical malpractice cases — Dirty dozen of medical mistakes, Leighton Law. Retrieved from: https://leightonlaw.com/12-famous-medical-malpractice-cases/

18. NHS Improvement (2018). Surgical never events, December 9. Retrieved from: https://improvement.nhs.uk/documents/2266/Never_Events_list_2018_FINAL_v5.pdf

19. Associated Press (1995). Hospital settles case of amputation error, *The New York Times*, May 12. Retrieved from: https://www.nytimes.com/1995/05/12/us/hospital-settles-case-of-amputation-error.html

20. EuroScore II predicts the probability of in-hospital mortality after cardiac surgery and is widely used.

21. NHS (2020). Independent mortality review of cardiac surgery at St Georges Hospital, NHS England. Retrieved from: https://www.england.nhs.uk/london/wp-content/uploads/sites/8/2020/03/SGUH-Independent-Mortality-Review-March-2020.pdf

22. Field, P. R., Gangemi, G., and Kinsley, T. (2007). Under the knife and completely aware: A case of intraoperative awareness. The National Centre for Case Study Teaching in Science. Retrieved from: https://sciencecases.lib.buffalo.edu/collection/detail.html/?case_id=688&id=688

23. Celizic, M. (2017). 'I don't want this to happen to anyone else', *Today*, October 4. Retrieved from: https://www.today.com/health/i-dont-want-happen-anyone-else-1C9418865

24. Leighton Law (2020). $1,000,000 settlement — Neglect resulting in subdural hematoma (Key West). Retrieved from: https://leightonlaw.com/1000000-settlement-neglect-resulting-in-subdural-hematoma-key-west/

25. High Court of Australia (2003). Cattanach v Melchior. HCA38 (2003) 215CLR 1. Retrieved from: https://www.globalhealthrights.org/wp-content/uploads/2013/02/HC-2003-Cattanach-v.-Melchior.pdf

26. Vaginal birth after caesarean section.

27. NHS Litigation Authority (2012). *Ten Years of Maternity Claims: An Analysis of NHS Litigation Authority Data*, Case Study 5, p. 68 (London: NHS Litigation Authority).

28. Congressional Committee on Commerce; Sub-Committee on Oversight and Investigations (2000). Assessing the operation of the National Practitioner Data Bank. House Hearing, 106 Congress, March 16. Retrieved from: https://www.govinfo.gov/content/pkg/CHRG-106hhrg62975/html/CHRG-106hhrg62975.htm

29. Canadian Patient Safety Institute (2014). One woman's misfortunes show importance of patient voice, October 28. Retrieved from: https://www.patientsafetyinstitute.ca/en/toolsResources/Member-Videos-and-Stories/Pages/Kapka-Petrov.aspx

30. Augustus Cullen Law LLP. ACL settle medical negligence action for failure to diagnose dislocated elbow. Retrieved from: https://www.aclsolicitors.ie/news-events/current-news/recently-completed-medical-negligence-cases

31. NHS Resolution (2019). Case of Note: ZZZ v Yeovil District Hospital NHS Foundation Trust (High Court, 26 June 2019, Garnham, J.), October 21. Retrieved from: https://resolution.nhs.uk/2019/10/21/case-of-note-zzz-v-yeovil-district-hospital-nhs-foundation-trust-high-court-26-june-2019-garnham-j/

32. Butcher, R. (2018). Simon Bramhall: Surgeon who branded initials on patients' livers spared jail, *The Independent*, January 12. Retrieved from: https://www.independent.co.uk/news/uk/crime/simon-bramhall-latest-surgeon-liver-branding-patients-prison-sentence-spared-jail-a8155096.html

33. David Rohde, D. (2000). Doctor who carved initials gets probation, *The New York Times*, April 26. Retrieved from: https://www.nytimes.com/2000/04/26/nyregion/doctor-who-carved-initials-gets-probation.html

34. Ferner, R. E., and McDowell, S. E. (2006). Doctors charged with manslaughter in the course of medical practice, 1795–2005: A literature review. *Journal of the Royal Society of Medicine* **99**(6): 309–314.

35. These numbers do not include doctors charged with criminal abortion.

36. Curnow, A. (1996). Death under anaesthetic: The case of Dr Adomako. *Medicine, Science and the Law* **36**: 188–193.

37. The Royal College of Surgeons of England Bulletin (2014). Letter to the Editor: Making Sense of the Sellu case. *Annals of the Royal College of Surgeons England [Supplement]* **96**: 118–119.

38. Loff, B., and Cordner, S. (2000). Melbourne doctor found guilty of manslaughter over death of young girl. *The Lancet* **356**(9245): 1909–2000.

39. Health Care Complaints Commission, NSW Medical Tribunal (2008). Dr Arthur Garry Gow — Conditions imposed on registration. Retrieved from: https://www.hccc.nsw.gov.au/decisions-orders/media-releases/2008/Dr-Arthur-Garry-Gow---conditions-imposed-on-registration

40. Scholefield, A. (2007). Why are medical manslaughter cases so rare in Australia? Australian Doctor, September 15. Retrieved from: https://www.ausdoc.com.au/views/why-are-medical-manslaughter-cases-so-rare-australia

41. Leung, G. K. K. (2018). Medical manslaughter in Hong Kong — How, why and why not? *Hong Kong Medical Journal* **24**(4): 384–390.

42. Dyer, C. (2003). Doctor sentenced for manslaughter of leukaemia patient. *BMJ* **327**: 697.

43. Telegraph Media Group (2013). Jet set doctor who could have saved a dying man with a one-minute test is jailed, *The Telegraph*, February 12. Retrieved from: https://www.telegraph.co.uk/news/uknews/crime/9865199/Jet-set-doctor-who-could-have-saved-a-dying-man-with-a-one-minute-test-is-jailed.html

44. Manchester Evening News (2007). Surgeon who killed patient is freed by judge, February 15. Retrieved from: https://www.manchestereveningnews.co.uk/news/greater-manchester-news/surgeon-who-killed-patient-is-freed-1113083.

45. NHS Resolution (2019). *Annual Report and Accounts 2018/2019*, pp. 54 (London: The Stationery Office).

46. Meeres-Young, I. (2020). Tragic and avoidable baby death at Watford General Hospital, Field Fisher. Retrieved from: https://www.fieldfisher.com/en/injury-claims/case-studies/tragic-and-avoidable-baby-death-at-watford-general-hospital

47. Wright Hassall LLP., Whyman, J. (2019). Our most notable medical negligence cases since 2019, Lexolology.com, August 27. Retrieved from: https://www.lexology.com/library/detail.aspx?g=7426ab64-6002-41e9-abde-2b4b48a56ecc

48. Schmeilzl, B. (2019). Medical malpractice lawsuits in Germany, Cross Channel Lawyers, February 20. Retrieved from: https://www.cross-channellawyers.co.uk/medical-malpractice-lawsuits-in-germany/

Chapter Six

1. Cognitive behaviour therapy.
2. Formerly referred to as mental handicap.
3. Schizophrenia is a mental illness that affects the way that people think and has severe impact on daily life. The symptoms include hallucinations, delusions and disorganised thinking.
4. BMA (2015). What mental health means to me. Edited version of an account by a junior doctor, submitted to the BMA Writing Competition.
5. Lurie, S. (2014) Why can't Canada spend more on mental health? *Health* 6: 684–690.
6. WHO (2007). Breaking the vicious cycle between ill-health and poverty. Retrieved from: https://www.who.int/mental_health/policy/development/1_Breakingviciouscycle_Infosheet.pdf?ua=1
7. Szasz, T. S. (1961). *The Myth of Mental Illness: Foundations of a Theory of Personal Conduct* (Idaho Falls, ID: Hoeber-Harper).
8. Sweere, J. J. (2004). *Golden Rules for Vibrant Health in Body and Spirit: A Holistic Approach to Health and Wellness* (Laguna Beach, CA: Basic Health Publications).
9. Department of Health and Social Security (1971). *Better Services 1971: Better Services for the Mentally Handicapped.* Cmnd 4683 (DHSS) (London: HMSO); Department of Health and Social Security (1975). *Better Services 1975: Better Services for the Mentally Ill.* Cmnd 6233 (DHSS) (London: HMSO).
10. Eide, S. (2018). Systems under strain: Deinstitutionalization in New York State and City, November 28. Manhattan Institute. Retrieved from: https://www.manhattan-institute.org/deinstitutionalization-mental-illness-new-york-state-city
11. He later became Chancellor of the Exchequer in the UK.
12. DHSS (1969). *Report of the Committee of Inquiry into Allegations of Ill-treatment of Patients and Other Irregularities at the Ely Hospital, Cardiff,* Cmnd 3975 (London: HMSO).
13. Dr. Lawlor moved to Australia, where he continued to practise.
14. BMA (1976). BMA demands full inquiry into consultant's suspension. *British Medical Journal* 2(6041): 958.

15. McAllen, J. (2019). History repeating: New Zealand's mental health Inquiries, *RNZ*. Retrieved from: https://www.rnz.co.nz/programmes/news-extras/story/2018668626/history-repeating-new-zealand-s-mental-health-inquiries

16. Barbui, C., Papola, D., and Saraceno, B. (2018). Forty years without mental hospitals in Italy. *International Journal of Mental Health Systems* **12**: 43.

17. Hill, A. (2012). Winterbourne View care home staff jailed for abusing residents, *The Guardian*, October 26. Retrieved from: https://www.theguardian.com/society/2012/oct/26/winterbourne-view-care-staff-jailed

18. Usually referred to as the Chelmsford Royal Commission.

19. Roth, D. (2017). Chemical restraint at Callan Park hospital for the insane before 1900, Australian Policy and History Network, November 14. Retrieved from: https://aph.org.au/2017/11/chemical-restraint-at-callan-park-hospital-for-the-insane-before-1900/

20. McAllen, J. (2018). History repeating: New Zealand's mental health Inquiries, October 27. Retrieved from: https://www.rnz.co.nz/programmes/news-extras/story/2018668626/history-repeating-new-zealand-s-mental-health-inquiries

21. Mason, K., *et al.* (1988). *Report of the Committee of Inquiry into Procedures in Certain Psychiatric Hospitals in Relation to Admission, Discharge or Release on Leave of Certain Classes of Patients* (Wellington: Government Printer).

22. Gallen Inquiry (1983). *Report of the Committee of Inquiry into Procedures at Oakley Hospital and Related Matters* (Wellington: Government Printer).

23. A region-wide network of medium secure units was also developed in the UK.

24. Palmer, R. (2009). The devil's in the detail, *Dominion Post*, July 29. Retrieved from: http://www.stuff.co.nz/dominion-post/2500232/The-devils-in-the-detail

25. Knoll, J. L. (2012). Inpatient suicide: Identifying vulnerability in the hospital setting, *The Psychiatric Times*, May 22. Retrieved from: https://www.psychiatrictimes.com/view/inpatient-suicide-identifying-vulnerability-hospital-setting

26. Large, M., Myles, N., Myles, H., Corderoy, A., Weiser, M., Davidson, M., and Ryan, C. J. (2018). Suicide risk assessment among psychiatric inpatients: A systematic review and meta-analysis of high-risk categories. *Psychological Medicine* **48**(7): 1119–1127.

27. The Science Museum (2019). 'Heroic Therapies' in Psychiatry, London. Retrieved from: https://www.sciencemuseum.org.uk/objects-and-stories/medicine/heroic-therapies-psychiatry

28. Spencer, J. L. (2015). The West Virginia Lobotomy Project (1952–1955): How the Mountain State became the proving ground for one of psychiatry's most notorious procedures. James Spencer, Cross Lanes. Ms 2019-049. West Virginia Archives and History.

29. See: https://www.cuh.nhs.uk/neurosciences/your-treatment/deep-brain-stimulation

30. Fallon, P., Bluglass, R., Edwards, B., and Daniels, G. (1999). *Report of the Committee of Inquiry into the Personality Disorder Unit at Ashworth Hospital. January 1999.* Cm 4194 (London: Stationery Office).

31. The Stepping Up Initiative. Steve Leifman — A judge on the mental health frontlines in Miami. Retrieved from: https://stepuptogether.org/people/steve-leifman

32. Athwal, H. (2004). Rocky Bennett — Killed by institutional racism? Institute of Race Relations, February 18. Retrieved from: http://www.irr.org.uk/news/rocky-bennett-killed-by-institutional-racism/

33. Norfolk, Suffolk and Cambridgeshire Strategic Health Authority (2003). *Independent Inquiry into the Death of David Bennett* (Cambridge: SHA).

34. Schraer, R. (2019). Theresa May: Did she solve her seven burning injustices? *BBC News*, May 24. Retrieved from: https://www.bbc.com/news/uk-politics-48380610

35. BBC Northern Ireland (2020). Muckamore Abbey Hospital: Timeline of abuse allegations, *BBC*, January 23. Retrieved from: https://www.bbc.com/news/uk-northern-ireland-49498971

36. Lessenberry, J. (2018). Michigan's mental health scandal, *Detroit Metro Times*, March 7. Retrieved from: https://www.metrotimes.com/detroit/michigans-mental-health-scandal/Content?oid=9900977

37. Bill of Rights Institute and Justice US Supreme Court. Olmstead v. United States (1928). 277 US. 438

38. Down from a high point of 50,000 beds in 1978.

39. Corbett, R. (2016). After the Institutions: Why Ontario's decision to shut long-term care facilities haunt some to this day, *Ottowa Citizen*, 25 November. Retrieved from: http://everycanadiancounts.com/after-the-institutions-why-ontarios-decision-to-shut-long-term-care-facilities-haunts-some-to-this-day/

40. Ontario Ombudsman (2016). *Nowhere to Turn: Investigation into the Ministry of Community and Social Services' Response to Situations of Crisis Involving Adults with Developmental Disabilities* (Ottowa: Ontario Ombudsman).

41. Maurice Duplessis was the Premier of Quebec between 1936–1939 and 1944–1959.

42. See: https://www.dementiastatistics.org/statistics-about-dementia/

43. See: https://www.dementia.org.au

44. Barnes, S. (2020). More than 25,000 dementia patients sectioned in past five years amid warnings that they are being locked up to 'control' their behaviour, *The Telegraph*, February 7. Retrieved from: https://www.telegraph.co.uk/news/2020/02/07/25000-dementia-patients-sectioned-past-five-years-amid-warnings/

45. Mayo Clinic (2019). Dementia — diagnosis and treatment. Retrieved from: https://www.mayoclinic.org/diseases-conditions/dementia/diagnosis-treatment/drc-20352019

46. OHO (2017). The report into the circumstances surrounding the deaths of mentally ill patients: Gauteng Province, Office of the Health Ombudsman. Retrieved from: http://healthombud.org.za/publications/reports/report-into-the-circumstances-surrounding-the-deaths-of-mentally-ill-patients-gauteng-province/

47. Hodal, K., and Hammond, R. (2018). Emaciated, mutilated, dead: The mental health scandal that rocked South Africa, *The Guardian*, October 14. Retrieved from: https://www.theguardian.com/global-development/2018/oct/14/emaciated-mutilated-dead-the-mental-health-scandal-that-rocked-south-africa

48. Chrisafis, A. (2018). France is 50 years behind: The 'state scandal' of French autism treatment, *The Guardian*, February 8. Retrieved from: https://www.theguardian.com/world/2018/feb/08/france-is-50-years-behind-the-state-scandal-of-french-autism-treatment

49. *Ibid.*

50. Rehan, M. A., Kuppa, A., Ahuja, A., Khalid, S., Patel, N., Budi Cardi, F. S., Joshi, V. V., Khalid, A., and Tohid, H. (2018). A strange case of dissociative identity disorder: Are there any triggers? *Cureus* 10(7): e2957.

51. Maden, T., and Tyrer, P. (2003). Dangerous and severe personality disorders: A new personality concept from the United Kingdom. *Journal of Personality Disorders* 17(6): 489–496.

52.   NHS England. Thomas and David's story. Retrieved from: https://www.england.nhs.uk/personal-health-budgets/phbs-in-action/patient-stories/thomas-and-davids-story/

53.   Triggle, N. (2019). Whorlton Hall: Hospital 'abused' vulnerable adults, *BBC News*, May 22. Retrieved from: https://www.bbc.com/news/health-48367071

54.   Mares, S., Newman, L., Dudley, M., and Gale, F. (2002). Seeking refuge, losing hope: Parents and children in immigration detention. *Australasian Psychiatry* 10(2): 91.

55.   Greenstein, L. (2017). PTSD and trauma: Not just for veterans, National Alliance on Mental Illness, November 8. Retrieved from: https://www.nami.org/Blogs/NAMI-Blog/November-2017/PTSD-and-Trauma-Not-Just-for-Veterans

56.   The number involved in the UK is thought to be about 2 million.

57.   American Psychiatric Association, Patient Story: PTSD. Retrieved from: https://www.psychiatry.org/patients-families/ptsd/patient-story-ptsd

58.   Sisti D. A., Segal, A. G., and Emanuel, E. J. (2015). Improving long-term psychiatric care: Bring back the asylum. *JAMA* 313(3): 243–244.

59.   Ferracuti, S., Pucci, D., Trobia, F., Alessi, M. C., Rapinesi, C., Kotzalidis, G. D., and Del Casale, A. (2019). Evolution of forensic psychiatry in Italy over the past 40 years (1978–2018). *International Journal of Law and Psychiatry* 62: 45–49.

60.   Care Quality Commission Report (2018). Mental Health Rehabilitation Inpatient Services: Ward types, bed numbers and use by clinical commissioning groups and NHS Trusts, CQC, March. Retrieved from: https://www.cqc.org.uk/sites/default/files/20180301_mh_rehabilitation_briefing.pdf

61.   Transform Drug Policy Foundation, Drug decriminalisation in Portugal: Setting the record straight. Retrieved from: https://transformdrugs.org/drug-decriminalisation-in-portugal-setting-the-record-straight/

Chapter Seven

1.   Transparency International (2016). Corruption in the Pharmaceutical Sector: Diagnosing the Challenges. Retrieved from: https://www.transparency.org.uk/publications/corruption-in-the-pharmaceutical-sector/

2.   OECD (2017). *Tackling Wasteful Spending in Health* (Paris: OECD).

3. Sparrow, M. K. (2000). *License to Steal: How Fraud Bleeds America's Health Care System* (Denver: Westview Press).

4. Pennsylvania Insurance Fraud Prevention Authority. Health insurance fraud. Retrieved from: https://www.helpstopfraud.org/Types-of-Insurance-Fraud/Health

5. Wikipedia. HCA Healthcare. Retrieved from: https://en.wikipedia.org/wiki/HCA_Healthcare

6. US Attorney's Office, District of South Carolina (2015). HCA settles allegations of billing for unnecessary tests, November 17. Retrieved from: https://www.justice.gov/usao-sc/pr/hca-settles-allegations-billing-unnecessary-lab-tests-and-double-billing-fetal-testing

7. US Department of Justice (2020). Chicago woman found guilty for role in $7 million scheme to defraud Medicare, February 14. Retrieved from: https://www.justice.gov/opa/pr/chicago-woman-found-guilty-role-7-million-scheme-defraud-medicare

8. United States Attorney's Office, District of New Jersey (2020). Former pharmacy employee admits role in multi-million dollar illegal kickback scheme, February 10. Retrieved from: https://www.justice.gov/usao-nj/pr/former-pharmacy-employee-admits-role-multi-million-dollar-illegal-kickback-scheme

9. Department of Justice, Office of Public Affairs (2019). South Florida health care facility owner convicted for role in largest health care fraud scheme ever charged by Department of Justice, May 4. Retrieved from: https://www.justice.gov/opa/pr/south-florida-health-care-facility-owner-convicted-role-largest-health-care-fraud-scheme-ever

10. BMJ (2014). Corruption ruins the doctor-patient relationship in India. *BMJ* **348**: g3169.

11. Beech, H. (2013). How corruption blights China's health care system, *Time*, August 2. Retrieved from: https://world.time.com/2013/08/02/corruption-blights-chinas-healthcare-system/

12. Wan, A. (2013). Managers sacked at Shaanxi hospital after child trafficking allegation, *South China Morning Post*, August 4. Retrieved from: https://www.scmp.com/news/china/article/1294354/managers-sacked-shaanxi-hospital-after-child-trafficking-allegation

13. Directorate-General for Migration and Home Affairs (European Commission) and ECORYS (2017). Updated study on corruption in the healthcare sector. Retrieved from: https://op.europa.eu/en/publication-detail/-/publication/9537ddb7-a41e-11e7-9ca9-01aa75ed71a1

14. *Ibid.*

15. Abba, T. (2019). Wait list mismanagement reveals corruption in Italy's public health care system, *La Stampa*, June 16. Retrieved from: https://www.lastampa.it/esteri/la-stampa-in-english/2018/01/19/news/wait-list-mismanagement-reveals-corruption-in-italy-s-public-health-care-system-1.33969346

16. The Canadian Press (2018). Ex-Manager sentenced to 39 months in prison in MUHC fraud scandal, *Global News*, December 17. Retrieved from: https://globalnews.ca/news/4769802/ex-manager-sentenced-to-39-months-prison-in-muhc-fraud-scandal/

17. Poulson, J. (1981). *The Price* (London: Michael Joseph).

18. Hargreaves, B. (2019). EU Industry loses €16.5 billion in sales to counterfeit drugs, Outsourcing-Pharma.com, June 18. Retrieved from: https://www.outsourcing-pharma.com/Article/2019/06/18/Economic-cost-of-counterfeit-drugs

19. Haq, I., and Esuka, O. M. (2018). Blockchain technology in the pharmaceutical industry to prevent counterfeit drugs. *International Journal of Computer Applications* **180**(25): 8–12.

20. Day, M. (2011). Mafia corruption linked to 126 hospital deaths, *The Independent*, October 4. Retrieved from: https://www.independent.co.uk/news/world/europe/mafia-corruption-linked-to-126-hospital-deaths-2365585.html

21. ANSA (2015). 9 probed over San Raffaele fraud, June 16. Retrieved from: https://www.ansa.it/english/news/general_news/2015/06/16/9-probed-over-san-raffaele-fraud_1be92690-d57c-4e04-b40f-115f32edc057.html

22. Goyal, M., Mehta, R. L., Schneiderman, L. J., and Sehgal, A. R. (2002). Economic and health consequences of selling a kidney in India. *JAMA* **288**(13): 1589–1593.

23. Evans, R. (2017). Pakistani police rescue 24 from organ trafficking gang, *BBC*, January 24. Retrieved from: https://www.bbc.com/news/health-38722052

24. Dyer O. (2002). GP struck off after offering to "fix" kidney sale. *BMJ (Clinical Research Edition)* **325**(7363): 510.

25. Erin C. A., and Harris J. (2003). An ethical market in organs. *Journal of Medical Ethics* **29**: 137–138.

26. NHS Blood and Transplant Authority (2015). NHS Blood and Transplant reveals nearly 49,000 people in the UK have had to wait for a transplant in the last decade, November 20. Retrieved from: https://www.organdonation.nhs.uk/get-involved/news/nearly-

49-000-people-in-uk-have-had-to-wait-for-a-transplant-in-the-last-decade/

27. See: https://endtransplantabuse.org
28. WHO (2013). Deadly medicines contamination in Pakistan, WHO Global Alert. Retrieved from: https://www.who.int/features/2013/pakistan_medicine_safety/en/
29. Farmer, B. (2019). Pakistan's government dissolves medical registration body in crackdown on fraud and corruption, *Daily Telegraph*, October 25. Retrieved from: https://www.telegraph.co.uk/global-health/science-and-disease/pakistans-government-dissolves-medical-registration-body-crackdown/
30. Minion, L. (2018). New Health Engine scandal raises scrutiny of digital health consent practices as Health Minister orders urgent review, *Healthcare IT*, June 25. Retrieved from: https://www.health-careit.com.au/article/new-healthengine-scandal-raises-scrutiny-digital-health-consent-practices-health-minister
31. Chang, D. (2017). Feds bust dozens for ID theft, including former Jackson Health secretary, *Miami Herald*, January 31. Retrieved from: https://www.miamiherald.com/news/health-care/article129792849.html
32. Bandell, B. (2013). Former South Miami Hospital worker pleads guilty to identity theft, *South Florida Business Journal*, July 16. Retrieved from: https://www.bizjournals.com/southflorida/news/2013/07/16/former-south-miami-hospital-worker.html
33. Committee on Standards in Public Life (1995). The seven principles of public life: An overview of the 'Nolan Principles', which are the basis of the ethical standards expected of public office holders. Retrieved from: https://www.gov.uk/government/publications/the-7-principles-of-public-life
34. See: https://www.justice.gov/opa/pr/generic-drug-manufacturer-ranbaxy-pleads-guilty-and-agrees-pay-500-million-resolve-false
35. United States Attorney's Office, Eastern District of Pennsylvania (2013). Janssen Pharmaceuticals pleads guilty and is sentenced for misbranding, January 3. Retrieved from: https://www.justice.gov/usao-edpa/pr/janssen-pharmaceuticals-pleads-guilty-and-sentenced-misbranding
36. United States Department of Justice (2012). GlaxoSmithKline to plead guilty and pay $3 billion to resolve fraud allegations and failure to report safety data, July 2. Retrieved from: https://www.justice.

gov/opa/pr/glaxosmithkline-plead-guilty-and-pay-3-billion-resolve-fraud-allegations-and-failure-report

37. United States Department of Justice (2010). Pharmaceutical giant Astra Zeneca to pay $520m for off-label drug marketing, April 27. Retrieved from: https://www.justice.gov/opa/pr/pharmaceutical-giant-astrazeneca-pay-520-million-label-drug-marketing

38. McGreal, C. (2019). Billionaire founder of opioid firm guilty of bribing doctors to prescribe drug, *The Guardian*, May 2. Retrieved from: https://www.theguardian.com/us-news/2019/may/02/john-kapoor-opioids-billionaire-founder-guilty-of-bribing-doctors-to-prescribe

39. General for Migration and Home Affairs (European Commission) and ECORYS (2017). Updated study on corruption in the healthcare sector. Available at: https://op.europa.eu/en/publication-detail/-/publication/9537ddb7-a41e-11e7-9ca9-01aa75ed71a1

40. Press Association (2015). Ex-UN consultants jailed for bribes over drugs supplied to 'starving Africans', *The Guardian*, September 23. Retrieved from: https://www.theguardian.com/uk-news/2015/sep/23/un-guido-bakker-sijbrandus-scheffer-jailed-contracts-drugs-congo

41. Grogan, K. (2012). Abbott pays $1.6 billion to settle Depakote investigation, *Pharma Times*, May 8. Retrieved from: http://www.pharmatimes.com/news/abbott_pays_$1.6_billion_to_settle_depakote_investigation_977357

42. Kmietowicz, Z. (2009). Eli Lilly pays record $1.4bn for promoting off-label use of olanzapine. *BMJ (Clinical Research Edition)* **338**: b127.

43. Kennedy, B. (2015). Sector responds to shocking £83m pharmacist fraud claims, *Community Pharmacist News*, September 25.

44. Vivian, J. C. (2012). Pharmacy fraud, waste and abuse, *US Pharmacist* 37(6): 68–70.

45. Prescription Medicines Code of Practice Authority (2018). PMCPA Annual Report 2017, December 4. Retrieved from: https://www.pmcpa.org.uk/about-us/media/news/pmcpa-annual-report-2017/

46. Competition and Markets Authority (2019). Nortriptyline investigation: Anti-competitive agreement and conduct. Case Reference 50507.2, June 18. Retrieved from: https://www.gov.uk/cma-cases/pharmaceutical-sector-suspected-anti-competitive-agreements-and-conduct-50507-2

47. Pearl, R. (2018). Shame, scandal plague healthcare providers in 2018, *Forbes*, December 10. Retrieved from: https://www.forbes.com/sites/robertpearl/2018/12/10/shame-scandal/#79723e546807

48. Black, Asian and Minority Ethnic.

49. Nationwide Employment Lawyers (2014). Hospital whistleblower awarded £230,000 in damages. Retrieved from: https://natemplaw.co.uk/portfolio/hospital-whistleblower-awarded-230000-in-compensation/

50. The system will be phased out in 2020.

51. Select Committee on Public Accounts (1998). Sixty-Second Report. Retrieved from: https://publications.parliament.uk/pa/cm199798/cmselect/cmpubacc/657/65705.htm

52. Lawton, A., Rayner, J., and Lasthuizen, K. (2013). *Ethics and Management in the Public Sector* (New York, NY: Routledge).

53. Edwards, B. (2019). *Ministers of the NHS: The Toughest Job in Government* (Amazon Kindle).

54. See: https://www.ccc.wa.gov.au/news-media/news/report-reveals-senior-health-employee-claimed-more-half-million-dollars-overtime

55. Ozkan, J. (2019). Piero Anversa and cardiomyocyte regeneration: Harvard University probe into scientific misconduct raises questions that won't go away. *European Heart Journal* 40(13): 1036–1037.

Chapter Eight

1. Paolucci, E. O., Genuis, M. L., and Violato, C. (2001). A meta-analysis of the published research on the effects of child sexual abuse. *The Journal of Psychology*, 135(1): 17–36.

2. Kershaw, R. P. (2020). Countering child sex exploitation and abuse, Australian Federal Police, February 19. Retrieved from: https://www.afp.gov.au/news-media/national-speeches/countering-child-sexual-exploitation-and-abuse-national-press-club

3. Dodd, V. (2016). Recorded child sex abuse cases increase by more than 30%, *The Guardian*, March 9. Retrieved from: https://www.theguardian.com/society/2016/mar/09/recorded-child-sex-abuse-cases-increase-by-more-than-30

4. Curtis, R., Terry, K., Dank, M., Dombrowski, K., and Khan, B. (2008). *The Commercial Sexual Exploitation of Children in New York City* (New York: Center for Court Innovation).

5. Tim Swarens, T. (2018). Who buys a trafficked child for sex? Otherwise ordinary men, *USA Today*, January 30. Retrieved from: https://eu.

usatoday.com/story/opinion/nation-now/2018/01/30/sex-trafficking-column/1073459001/

6. EU Migration and Home Affairs. Child sexual abuse. Retrieved from: https://ec.europa.eu/home-affairs/what-we-do/policies/organized-crime-and-human-trafficking/child-sexual-abuse_en

7. Valman B. (1988). Implications of the Cleveland inquiry. *BMJ (Clinical Research Education)* **297**(6642): 151–152.

8. US State Department (2019). Trafficking in Persons Report June 2019. Retrieved from: https://www.state.gov/wp-content/uploads/2019/06/2019-Trafficking-in-Persons-Report.pdf

9. Artz, L., Ward, C. L., Leoschut, L., Kassanjee, R., and Burton, P. (2018). The prevalence of child sexual abuse in South Africa: The Optimus Study South Africa. *South African Medical Journal (Suid-Afrikaanse tydskrif vir geneeskunde)* **108**(10): 791–792.

10. Knaus, C. (2017). More than 2,200 Australians reported abuse in orphanages or children's homes, *The Guardian*, March 7. Retrieved from: https://www.theguardian.com/australia-news/2017/mar/07/more-than-2200-child-abuse-survivors

11. Jay, A. (2014). Independent inquiry into child sexual exploitation in Rotherham (1997–2013). Retrieved from: https://www.rotherham.gov.uk/downloads/download/31/independent-inquiry-into-child-sexual-exploitation-in-rotherham-1997---2013

12. Smith, J. (2016). *The Dame Janet Smith Review Report: An Independent Review into the BBC's Culture and Practices during the Jimmy Savile and Stuart Hall Years* (London: BBC).

13. Many of the hospitals where Savile had worked had their own local inquiries.

14. Alexis Jay (who had led the inquiry in Rotherham) was the fourth Chair of the body. The first three had all resigned because of alleged conflicts of interest or dissatisfaction with the process.

15. Daigle, K., and Dodds, P. (2017). UN Peacekeepers: How a Haiti child sex ring was whitewashed, *The Associated Press*, May 26. Retrieved from: https://apnews.com/96f9ff66b7b34d9f971edf0e92e2082c/UN-Peacekeepers:-How-a-Haiti-child-sex-ring-was-whitewashed

16. BBC News (2018). Oxfam Haiti sex claims: Charity 'failed in moral leadership', February 11. Retrieved from: https://www.bbc.com/news/uk-43020875

17. Froese, I. (2018). Nearly 1,300 students victims of sexual offenses by school staff over the last 2 decades, Canadian study says, *CBC News*, June 14. Retrieved from: https://www.cbc.ca/news/canada/

manitoba/child-sexual-abuse-study-comprehensive-1300-victims-
1.4705643

18. NHS England (2018). Strategic direction for sexual assault and abuse
services, April 12. Retrieved from: https://www.england.nhs.uk/pub-
lication/strategic-direction-for-sexual-assault-and-abuse-services/

19. Irzin, C. (2000). *The Truth About Child Sex Abuse* (London:
Routledge).

20. Associated Press (2019). Clergy accused of child sexual abuse still
working with kids unsupervised, *The New York Post*, October 4.
Retrieved from: https://nypost.com/2019/10/04/clergy-accused-
of-child-sexual-abuse-still-working-with-kids-unsupervised/

21. ProPublica (2012). Sins of omission: How the Catholic Church
shielded credibly accused priests, March 6. Retrieved from: https://
www.propublica.org/series/sins-of-omission

22. Wikipedia. Commission to Inquire into Child Abuse. Retrieved from:
https://en.wikipedia.org/wiki/Commission_to_Inquire_into_Child_
Abuse

23. Niechcial, J. (2010). *Lucy Faithfull: Mother to Hundreds* (Cambridge:
Compositions by Carn).

24. See: https://www.childabuseinquiry.scot/

25. Operation Augusta (2004–2005) and Operation Span (2010–2012).

26. Scheerhout, J. (2019). Who is Maggie Oliver? The detective who
resigned over the treatment of 'Amber', *Greater Manchester News*, July
29. Retrieved from: https://www.manchestereveningnews.co.uk/
news/greater-manchester-news/margaret-oliver-rochdale-police-
grooming-13027067

27. Shropshire Star (2017). West Mercia chaplain reinstated after inquiry over
comments on child sex exploitation, January 10. Retrieved from: https://
www.shropshirestar.com/news/emergency-services/2017/01/10/
west-mercia-police-chaplain-reinstated-after-inquiry-over-comments-on-
child-sex-exploitation/

Chapter Nine

1. Peter Ubel, P. (2016). The bureaucratic hassles physicians face are
extraordinary, kevinMD.com, August 25. Retrieved from: https://
www.kevinmd.com/blog/2016/08/bureaucratic-hassles-physicians-
face-extraordinary.html

2. Creswell, J., and Abelson, R. (2014). Hospital chain said to scheme to
inflate bills, *The New York Times*, January 23. Retrieved from: https://

www.nytimes.com/2014/01/24/business/hospital-chain-said-to-scheme-to-inflate-bills.html

3. The King's Fund (2011). Myth four: The NHS has too many managers. Available at: https://www.kingsfund.org.uk/projects/health-and-social-care-bill/mythbusters/nhs-managers

4. Michael, E. (2020). A third of US health care spending stems from administrative costs, *Healio*, January 6. Retrieved from: https://www.healio.com/news/primary-care/20200106/a-third-of-us-health-care-spending-stems-from-administrative-costs

5. Edwards, N., Marshall, M., McLellan, A., and Abbasi, K. (2003). Doctors and managers: A problem without a solution? *BMJ (Clinical Research Education)* **326**(7390): 609–610.

6. Navarro, V., Muntaner, C., Borrell, C., Benach, J., Quiroga, A., Rodríguez-Sanz, M., Vergés, N., and Pasarín, M. I. (2006). Politics and health outcomes. *Lancet (London, England)* **368**(9540): 1033–1037.

7. Edwards, B. (2018). *Ministers of Health: The Toughest Job in Government* (Amazon Kindle).

8. Edwards, B., and Fall, M. (2005). *The Executive Years of the NHS* (Oxford: Radcliffe Publishing).

9. Edwards, B. (2019). *Ministers of the NHS: The Toughest Job in Government* (Amazon Kindle).

10. See Chapter Three for more detail.

11. Bryder, L. (2014). *The Rise and Fall of the National Women's Hospital* (Auckland: Auckland University Press).

12. See Chapter Three for more detail.

13. See: https://www.ccdhb.org.nz/about-us/board-meetings-and-papers/ccdhb-and-hvdhb-public-board-papers-12-february-2020.pdf

14. NHS RightCare is a national programme that delivers operational and contracting guidance to reduce unwarranted variations in care.

15. Porter, M., and Tiesberg, E. O. (2006). *Redefining Health Care: Creating Value-based Competition on Results* (Cambridge, MA: Harvard Business Press).

16. See: https://valuebasedcareaustralia.com.au

17. BBC News. (2016). Sherwood Forest NHS Trust reveals £1bn PFI overspend, November 2. Retrieved from: https://www.bbc.com/news/uk-england-nottinghamshire-20173727

18. Humphries, J., and Thorp, L. (2018). Liverpool's 'new' Royal hospital stands empty — How did it come to this and when will it be finally be finished? *Liverpool Echo*, August 8. Retrieved from: https://www.

liverpoolecho.co.uk/news/liverpool-news/liverpools-new-royal-hospital-stands-15000342

19. Davies, A. (2018). CEO of troubled Sydney hospital resigns two days after opening, *The Guardian*, November 21. Retrieved from: https://www.theguardian.com/australia-news/2018/nov/21/ceo-of-troubled-sydney-hospital-resigns-two-days-after-opening

20. Corderoy, A. (2016). Our hospitals are being privatised: Is anyone paying attention? *The Guardian*, September 19. Retrieved from: https://www.theguardian.com/commentisfree/2016/sep/20/our-hospitals-are-being-privatised-is-anybody-paying-attention

21. Kirkup, W. (2018). Report of the Liverpool Community Health Independent Review (The Kirkup Review). Retrieved from: https://improvement.nhs.uk/documents/2403/LiverpoolCommunity Health_IndependentReviewReport_V2.pdf

22. Vize, R. (2018). Liverpool NHS scandal shows how culture of denial harms patients, *The Guardian*, February 10. Retrieved from: https://www.theguardian.com/healthcare-network/2018/feb/10/liverpool-nhs-scandal-shows-how-culture-of-denial-harms-patients

23. This was the NHS Trust Development Authority.

24. See: www.airedale-trust-nhs.uk

25. Royal Papworth Hospital, Cambridge, UK.

26. See the case studies in Chapter Three.

27. Lacina, L. (2020). What's needed now to protect health workers: WHO COVID-19 briefing, World Economic Forum, April 10. Retrieved from: https://www.weforum.org/agenda/2020/04/10-april-who-briefing-health-workers-covid-19-ppe-training/

28. These are NHS and nursing home total numbers, not including private sector hospitals.

29. Public Health England (2020). COVID-19: Review of disparities in risks and outcomes, June 2. Retrieved from: https://www.gov.uk/government/publications/covid-19-review-of-disparities-in-risks-and-outcomes

30. Cook, T., Kusumovic, E., and Lennane, S. (2020). Deaths of NHS staff from COVID-19 analysed. *Health Service Journal* April 22. Retrieved from: https://www.hsj.co.uk/exclusive-deaths-of-nhs-staff-from-covid-19-analysed/7027471.article

31. France 24. (2020). Italy says number of doctors killed by coronavirus passes 100, April 9. Retrieved from: https://www.france24.com/en/20200409-italy-says-number-of-doctors-killed-by-coronavirus-passes-100

32. The Guardian (2020). Lost on the frontline. Retrieved from: https://www.theguardian.com/us-news/2020/jun/17/covid-19-coronavirus-healthcare-workers-deaths

33. Hogan, G. (2020). Brooklyn hospital workers protest, demanding equipment to prevent more staff deaths, NPR, April 16. Retrieved from: https://www.npr.org/2020/04/16/836424351/brooklyn-hospital-workers-protest-demanding-equipment-to-prevent-more-staff-deat

34. Henley, J. (2020). 'He sacrificed himself': Tributes to first doctor to die from coronavirus in France, *The Guardian*, March 22. Retrieved from: https://www.theguardian.com/world/2020/mar/22/he-sacrificed-himself-tributes-to-first-french-doctor-to-die-from-coronavirus

35. Recent reports for 2016 show that needle stick injuries in the US have reduced, with less than 0.7% of cases requiring more than one day off work.

36. Institute of Medicine (US) Committee on the Adequacy of Nursing Staff in Hospitals and Nursing Homes; Wunderlich, G. S., Sloan, F., and Davis, C. K. (eds.) (1996). "Staffing and Work-Related Injuries and Stress," Chapter 7 in *Nursing Staff in Hospitals and Nursing Homes: Is It Adequate?* (Washington, DC: National Academies Press). Retrieved from: https://www.ncbi.nlm.nih.gov/books/NBK232675/

37. See: https://www.osha.gov/dsg/hospitals/

38. Dowler, C. (2011). Nurses suffer more than 8,800 serious industrial injuries in three years, *The Nursing Times*, August 30. Retrieved from: https://www.nursingtimes.net/roles/nurse-managers/exclusive-nhs-nurses-suffer-more-than-8800-serious-industrial-injuries-in-three-years-30-08-2011/

39. Health and Safety Authority (2015). Summary of workplace injury, illness and fatality statistics: 2014–2015. Retrieved from: https://www.hsa.ie/eng/Publications_and_Forms/Publications/Corporate/HSA_Statistics_Report_2014-2015.pdf

40. Silva, K. (2017). Woman falls up Charters Towers hospital stairs gets $1.6m pay out, *ABC*, February 28. Retrieved from: https://www.abc.net.au/news/2017-03-01/hospital-fall-compensation-pay-out-charters-towers/8312092

41. Johnson, S. (2019). Violence in the NHS: Staff face routine assault and intimidation, *The Guardian*, September 9. Retrieved from: https://www.theguardian.com/society/2019/sep/04/violence-nhs-staff-face-routine-assault-intimidation

42. ITV (2018). Health Secretary reveals new measures to better protect NHS staff, October 31. Retrieved from: https://www.itv.com/news/2018-10-31/health-secretary-reveals-new-measures-to-better-protect-nhs-staff/

43. See: http://www.legislation.gov.uk/ukpga/2018/23/contents/enacted

44. See footnote 41.

45. Department of Health and Social Care (2018). Paramedics to be given body cameras to protect them from abuse. Retrieved from: https://www.gov.uk/government/news/paramedics-to-be-given-body-cameras-to-protect-them-from-abuse

46. IOSH Magazine (2018). Government announce measures to tackle attacks on NHS staff, November 5. Retrieved from: https://www.ioshmagazine.com/government-announces-measures-tackle-attacks-nhs-staff

47. Kurter, H. L. (2019). Health care remains America's most dangerous profession due to workplace violence. *Forbes*, November 24. Retrieved from: https://www.forbes.com/sites/heidilynnekurter/2019/11/24/healthcare-remains-americas-most-dangerous-profession--due-to-workplace-violence-yet-hr-1309-bill-doesnt-stand-a-chance/#449b45d43bc6

48. The Joint Commission (2018). Sentinel Event Alert 59: Physical and verbal violence against health care workers. Retrieved from: https://www.jointcommission.org/en/resources/patient-safety-topics/sentinel-event/sentinel-event-alert-newsletters/sentinel-event-alert-59-physical-and-verbal-violence-against-health-care-workers/

49. United States Government Accountability Office (2016). Workplace Safety and Health: Additional efforts needed to help protect healthcare workers from workplace violence. Retrieved from: https://www.gao.gov/assets/680/675858.pdf

50. Groenewold, M. R., Sarmiento, R., Vanoli, K., Raudabaugh, W., Nowlin, S., and Gomaa, A. (2018). Workplace violence injury in 106 US hospitals participating in the Occupational Health Safety Network (OHSN), 2012–2015. *American Journal of Industrial Medicine* 61(2): 157–166.

51. Australian Bureau of Statistics (2018). Work-related injuries, Australia. Jul 2017–Jun 2018, October 30. Retrieved from: https://www.abs.gov.au/ausstats/abs@.nsf/mf/6324.0

52. NSW Bureau of Crime Statistics and Research. Retrieved from: https://www.bocsar.nsw.gov.au/Pages/bocsar_pages/Assaults-on-hospital-premises.aspx

53.   Thompson, G. (2019). Rates of violence against nurses in hospitals increasing rapidly, *ABC*, June 11. Retrieved from: https://www.abc.net.au/news/2019-06-11/rates-of-violence-against-nurses-rising-rapildy/11196716

54.   Thompson, G. (2019). Rates of violence against nurses in hospitals increasing rapidly, *ABC*, June 11. Retrieved from: https://www.abc.net.au/news/2019-06-11/rates-of-violence-against-nurses-rising-rapildy/11196716

55.   Black, C. (2008). Working for a healthier tomorrow: Work and health in Britain. Department for Work and Pensions. Retrieved from: https://www.gov.uk/government/publications/working-for-a-healthier-tomorrow-work-and-health-in-britain

56.   These fines increased to £5 million in 2020.

57.   Lewis, J. (2008). Occupational health's duty of care to employees, *Personnel Today*, March 7. Retrieved from: https://www.personnelto-day.com/hr/occupational-healths-duty-of-care-to-employees/

58.   Brodies LLP (2019). Guilty plea for healthcare provider's breach of health and safety law, *Lexology*, February 22. Retrieved from: https://www.lexology.com/library/detail.aspx?g=f1cd1b5d-318e-462e-b5f8-3c002d51ec5a

59.   Public Law Today (2018). NHS trusts and health and safety fines, March 29. Retrieved from: https://www.publiclawtoday.co.uk/healthcare-law/174-healthcare-features/37504-nhs-trusts-and-health-and-safety-fines

60.   NHS Employers (2020). New death in service benefits announced for NHS staff, April 27. Retrieved from: https://www.nhsemployers.org/news/2020/04/death-in-service

61.   Hansard: House of Commons Debates (1993). Vol 221, cc 143–150, March 15. Available at: https://publications.parliament.uk/pa/cm/cmvo221.htm

62.   Klein R. (1994). Lessons from the financial scandals in Wessex and the West Midlands. *BMJ (Clinical Research Edition)* **308**(6923): 215–216.

63.   See: http://www.healthpayrollinquiry.qld.gov.au

64.   NBR (2018). Something is rotten in the state of New Zealand's healthcare, April 5. Retrieved from: https://www.nbr.co.nz/opinion/something-rotten-state-new-zealand's-healthcare

65.   The Health Foundation (2018). How much has the backlog in maintenance of NHS estates increased? October 30. Retrieved from: https://www.health.org.uk/chart/how-much-has-the-backlog-in-maintenance-of-nhs-estates-increased

66. Hall, C. (2002). Hospital Chief quits in waiting list 'fiddles', *The Telegraph*, May 4. Retrieved from: https://www.telegraph.co.uk/news/uknews/1393119/Hospital-chief-quits-in-waiting-list-fiddles.html

67. D. J. Bowles and Associates (2012). Investigation into Management Culture in NHS Lothian. Retrieved from: http://www.nhslothian.scot.nhs.uk/MediaCentre/PressReleases/2012/Documents/Lothian_report_for_Cab_Sec_10th_May.pdf

68. Hansard, House of Commons (1997). North Yorkshire Ambulance Trust debate. Vol 296 cc817-26, June 25. Retrieved from: https://api.parliament.uk/historic-hansard/commons/1997/jun/25/nirth-yorkshire-ambulance-trust

69. Clover, B. (2019). 'Defensive' Trust removed patient criticism from Royal College report, *HSJ*, July 18. Retrieved from: https://www.hsj.co.uk/quality-and-performance/defensive-trust-removed-patient-criticism-from-royal-college-report/7025579.article

70. See: https://www.leapfroggroup.org/data-users/leapfrog-hospital-safety-grade

71. New South Wales Health Care Complaints Commission (2003). Special Commission of Inquiry into the Campbelltown and Camden Hospitals. Retrieved from: https://researchdata.edu.au/special-commission-inquiry-camden-hospitals/166830

72. Andres, G. I. (2015). NHS apology given to West London mental health whistleblower, Damian McCarthy Employment Law, November 24. Retrieved from: https://damianmccarthy.com/nhs-apology-given-to-west-london-mental-health-whistleblower/

73. Faunce, T. A., and Bolsin, S. N. (2004). Three Australian whistleblowing sagas: Lessons for internal and external regulation. *The Medical Journal of Australia* 181(1): 44–47.

74. Moser, J. (2009). Texas nurses under fire for whistleblowing. *American Journal of Nursing* 109(10): 19.

75. Lakhani, N. (2012). NHS watchdog claimed that whistleblower Kay Sheldon was 'mentally ill', *The Independent*, August 15. Retrieved from: https://www.independent.co.uk/life-style/health-and-families/health-news/exclusive-nhs-watchdog-claimed-that-whistleblower-kay-sheldon-was-mentally-ill-8046640.html

76. Marrs, C. (2014). Kay Sheldon on tackling problems in the CQC, *Civil Service World*, November 25. Retrieved from: https://www.civilserviceworld.com/news/article/kay-sheldon-on-tackling-problems-in-the-cqc

77. Campbell, D., and Weaver, M. (2019). Hospital hired fingerprint experts to unmask whistleblower, report finds, *The Guardian*, January 30. Retrieved from: https://www.theguardian.com/society/2020/jan/30/hospital-hired-fingerprint-experts-to-unmask-whistleblower-report-finds

78. Faunce, T. A., and Bolsin, S. N. (2004). Three Australian whistleblowing sagas: Lessons for internal and external regulation. *The Medical Journal of Australia* 181(1): 44–47.

79. Gagging clauses cannot be used to prevent protected disclosure, e.g. on issues such as patient safety.

80. Edwards, B., and Fall, M. (2005). *The Executive Years of the NHS. The England Account 1985–2003* (Cambridge: The Nuffield Trust).

81. See: http://www.hope.be/wp-content/uploads/2015/11/58_2000_HOPE-REPORT_Hospital-and-health-care-rationing.pdf

82. Rivett, G. New Influences and New Pathways 1988–1997, in Rivett, G. (ed.) *The History of the NHS* (London: Nuffield Trust). Retrieved from: https://www.nuffieldtrust.org.uk/health-and-social-care-explained/the-history-of-the-nhs/

83. Gainsbury, S. (2017). The bottom line: Understanding the NHS deficit and why it won't go away, The Nuffield Trust, August 31. Retrieved from: https://www.nuffieldtrust.org.uk/research/the-bottom-line-understanding-the-nhs-deficit-and-why-it-won-t-go-away

84. The Royal Society of Medicine (2017). New analysis links 30,000 excess deaths in 2015 to cuts in health and social welfare, February 17. Retrieved from: https://www.rsm.ac.uk/media-releases/2017/new-analysis-links-30-000-excess-deaths-in-2015-to-cuts-in-health-and-social-care/

85. Personal account by the Author.

86. Adapted from: Durr, K. (2005). *Ethics in Health Services Management.* Fourth Edition (Baltimore, MD: Health Professions Press).

87. Shapiro, E. (1996). *Fad Surfing in the Boardroom. Reclaiming the Courage to Manage in the Age of Instant Answers* (Oxford: Capstone).

88. Personal experiences of the Author in his time with Trent and West Midlands NHS Regions.

89. Personal interview with the Author.

90. Rego, A. and Araújo, B. (2019). Ethics guiding the actions of the hospital manager. *Journal of Hospital Administration* 8(2): doi: 10.5430/jha.v8n2p14.

91. Owen D. (2008). Hubris syndrome. *Clinical Medicine (London, England)* **8**(4): 428–432.

92. Jones, S. (2020). Spain: Doctors struggle to cope as 514 die from coronavirus in one day, *The Guardian*, March 24. Retrieved from: https://www.theguardian.com/world/2020/mar/24/spain-doctors-lack-protection-coronavirus-covid-19

93. WHO (2018). *Managing Epidemics. Key Facts About Major Deadly Diseases* (Geneva: WHO).

94. See above.

95. Track and trace is a standard public health response to find people that have been in contact with an infected person so that they can self-isolate. It needs to be rapidly increased in scale to be effective in a pandemic.

Chapter Ten

1. Combined costs for health and social care.

2. These country studies summarise work found in: Robertson, R., Gregory, S., and Jabbal, J. (2014). *The Social Care and Health Systems of Nine Countries* (London: The King's Fund).

3. *Ibid.*

4. *Ibid.*

5. *Ibid.*

6. *Ibid.*

7. *Ibid.*

8. Nuffield Trust (2020). Delayed transfers of care, May 1. Retrieved from: https://www.nuffieldtrust.org.uk/resource/delayed-transfers-of-care

9. Wall, M., and Horgan-Jones, J. (2019). The old country: Get ready for an ageing Ireland, *The Irish Times*, August 24. Retrieved from: https://www.irishtimes.com/life-and-style/health-family/the-old-country-get-ready-for-an-ageing-ireland-1.3993009

10. Kauranan, A. (2019). Care home scandal nudges Finland's voters back towards Social Democrats, *Reuters*, April 8. Retrieved from: https://www.reuters.com/article/us-finland-election-welfare/care-home-scandal-nudges-finlands-voters-back-toward-social-democrats-idUSKCN1RK1BL

11. Social Work England (2020). Fitness to Practice Committee. Reg number SW74722, January 29. Retrieved from: https://www.social-

workengland.org.uk/media/2941/ftpsor-meeting-john-ftp57265-20200129-1-002.pdf

12. Australian Association of Social Workers (2014). Evidence of harm caused by social workers: Australia and overseas examples, September 1. Retrieved from: https://www.aasw.asn.au/document/item/6565

13. Health and Care Professions Council Tribunal Service. Registration 72651, Hearing, March 8, 2018.

14. See: https://www.unhcr.org/asylum-in-the-uk.html

15. Connolly, A., and Stewart, J. (2019). Bupa's aged care homes failing standards across Australia, *ABC*, September 13. Retrieved from: https://www.abc.net.au/news/2019-09-12/bupas-aged-care-homes-failing-standards-across-australia/11501050?nw=0

16. Jones, S. (2019). Spanish police rescue elderly people from 'house of horrors', *The Guardian*, March 8. Retrieved from: https://www.theguardian.com/world/2019/mar/08/spanish-police-rescue-elderly-people-from-alleged-house-of-horrors

17. Parsons, A. (2016). Care Home Briefing 154 — Home guilty of corporate manslaughter but hospital prosecution fails, RadcliffesLeBrasseur LLC, February. Retrieved from: https://www.rlb-law.com/briefings/care-homes/care-home-guilty-of-corporate-manslaughter-but-hospital-prosecution-collapses/

18. Calder, R. (2018). State family services head 'deeply troubled' by ACS scandal, *New York Post*, August 21. Retrieved from: https://nypost.com/2018/08/21/state-family-services-head-deeply-troubled-by-acs-scandal/

19. In the UK, the state became involved in the year 1834 under the Poor Laws.

20. Morris, S. (2017). How 'house of horror' investigation brought Jersey abuse to light, *The Guardian*, July 7. Retrieved from: https://www.theguardian.com/uk-news/2017/jul/03/haut-de-la-garenne-house-of-horror-investigation-brought-jersey-abuse-to-light

21. Independent Jersey Care Inquiry (2017). Frances Oldham QC's summary statement, August 17. Retrieved from: http://www.jerseycareinquiry.org/SiteAssets/Pages/default/Report%20Launch%20Speech.pdf

22. Royal Commission into Institutional Responses to Child Sexual Abuse (2013). Retrieved from: https://www.childabuseroyalcommission.gov.au

23. Narey, M. (2016). Residential Care in England: Report of Sir Martin Narey's independent review of children's residential care, July. Retrieved from: https://assets.publishing.service.gov.uk/government/uploads/system/uploads/attachment_data/file/534560/Residential-Care-in-England-Sir-Martin-Narey-July-2016.pdf

24. Greenfield, P. and Marsh, S. (2018). Vulnerable children treated 'like cattle' in care home system, *The Guardian*, November 10. Retrieved from: https://www.theguardian.com/society/2018/nov/10/vulnerable-children-treated-like-cattle-in-care-home-system

25. The cost of children's homes in England in 2015 was £750 million.

26. Children have migrated to the colonies for much of the 20th century.

27. Jay, A., Evans, M., Frank, I., and Sharpling, D. (2018). Child Migration Programmes Investigation Report, March. Retrieved from: https://www.iicsa.org.uk/publications/investigation/child-migration

28. Chenery, S. (2011). 'I can still hear the kid's screams', *Sydney Morning Herald*, June 12. Retrieved from: https://www.smh.com.au/national/i-can-still-hear-the-kids-screams-20110611-1fyap.html

29. See footnote 27.

30. The policy was officially adopted across the entire US–Mexico border from April 2018 until June 2018, but continued unofficially until at least October 2019.

31. BBC (2016). North Wales child abuse scandal, March 17. Retrieved from: https://www.bbc.com/news/uk-wales-north-east-wales-35502574

32. Waterhouse, R. (2000). Lost in care: Report of the tribunal of inquiry into the abuse of children in care in Gwynedd and Clywd since 1974. (HC 201 1999–2000).

Index

Academic fraud, 204
Adams, John Bodkin, 28
Airedale Hospital, 234
Antibiotics, 59
Aremu, Peters O., 108, 204
Ashley, Jack, 62
Ashworth High Security Hospital, 167
Assault on a patient, 118
Asylums, 160
   Ely Hospital, Wales, 161
   Kingseat Hospital, 162
   Normansfield Hospital, 161
Autism in France, 174
   Chavy, Catherine, 175

Babes, Maria, 277
Baidoo, Isaac, 110
Bailey, Simon, 208
Bainbridge, Jonathan, 112
Bawa-Garba, H., 109
Bawden, Nicholas, 120
Bennett, David 'Rocky', 169
Benoxaprofen (Opren), 61
Birmingham, 258
Blood contamination, 50

Bramhall, Simon, 149
Breast implants, 49
   Mas, Jean-Claude, 49
Butler Sloss Inquiry, 209

Caesarean sections, 80
Cancer services, 89
   Royal Marsden, 90
Centralisation of specialist services, 81
Chief Biomedical Engineer, 68
Child abuse involving clergy, 214
Child B, 256
Child Migrants Trust, 281
Children's homes, 278
China, 102
Choosing Wisely, 54
   San Francisco Health Network, 54
   Top five actions, 55
Cleveland Clinic, 235
Clinical freedom, 220
Clinical trials, 58
Corporate parent, 282
Counterfeit drugs, 189
Covey, Amelia Anne, 238

COVID-19 pandemic, 23
Cullen, Charles, 37
Cunningham, Richard, 116

Danish compensation system, 136
Davies, Sally, 59
Delagente, Robert, 117
Dementia, 172
Depakine, 49
Dhillon, Dilip, 113
Diagnostic errors, 56
Duplessis children, 172

Eason, Darrie, 142
Elder, Leslie, 138
El-Keria, Amy, 244
Esformes, Philip, 185
Ethical problems, 258

Feller, Mitchell Dean, 116
Fit and proper person test, 262
Forgery, 118
Francis, Robert, 6
Fraser, Linda Elaine, 276
Furness Hospital, 76

Gedz, Liana, 149
Gibson, Vicky, 135
Good professional practice, 100
Great Ormond Street Hospital,
    249
Guimarães, Edson Izidoro, 30
Gupta, Manish, 112
Gururaj, Pandeshwar, 110

Hahnemann University Hospital, 17
Hancox, Debora, 194
Harassment, 114
    Gheorghiu, Serban, 114

Harvard Medical Practice Study, 45
Harvey, Donald, 31
Haut de la Garenne, 278
Health and misconduct, 115
Health Engine, 193
Hennessy, John, 281
High reliability organisations, 47
Hong Kong Nursing Council, 102
Hospital-acquired infections, 52
Hristeva, Lidia, 106

Infected Blood Inquiry, 51
Insurance fraud, 184
Isaacs, Larry Mitchell, 103
Istanbul Declaration, 192
Italian psychiatric reform, 162

Jangwa, Ernest, 110
Jay report into child sexual
    exploitation, 210
John, Roanna Althia, 275
Johnson, Thomas, 176
Joint replacements, 69

Kale, Sharmila, 111
Kapoor, John, 196
Karl, Richard, 105
Karolinska University Hospital, 13
    Budget deficit, 15
    Rostlund and Gustafsson, 15
    Value-based Healthcare, 14
Keogh, Bruce, 85
Kickbacks, 184
King, Willie, 141
Kovvali, Bala, 151

Lainz Angels of Death, 35
Lansley, Andrew, 228
Leapfrog Group, 250

Ledward, Rodney, 122
Letter, Stephan, 37
Levy, Graham, 240
Life Esidimeni, 173
Lobotomy, 166
Lucy Faithfull Foundation, 216

Macchiarini, Paola, 14
Maidstone and Tunbridge Wells
   NHS Trust, 11
     Health Commission Inquiry, 11
     No isolation facilities, 11
Malevre, Christine, 36
Managerial fads, 260
Managerial leaders, 222
Maternity, 75
McGill University Health Centre,
   188
McIntyre, Justine, 118
Mediator, 63
Medical devices, 68
Medical equipment, 67
Medication errors, 64
Melchior, K. A., 143
Miami-Dade County Jail, 168
Muckamore Abbey Hospital, 170
Mulhem, Feda, 151
Mustafa, Majid, 117

Narey, Martin, 280
National Practitioner Database,
   104
National Women's Hospital, 229
Nesset, Arnfinn, 34
'Never' or Sentinel Events, 90
Newton, Angelita, 185
NHS Lothian, 248
NHS Resolution, 137
Nobel, Joel, 47

North Yorkshire Ambulance
   Service, 248

Ohebshalom, Zachary, 185
Oliver, Margaret, 216
Opioids, 60
Organisational blindness, 6
Organisational change, 227
Organisational culture, 233
Organ trafficking, 190
Oxfam, 213

Paediatric cardiac surgery, 84
   Professional hubris, 84
Papalii, John, 164
Parodi, Stephen, 12
Patel, Jayant, 8
Paterson, Ian, 120
Payroll fraud, 204
Perkins, Zymere, 278
Petrov, Kapka, 146
Petrov, Maxim, 30
Pharmaceutical industry, 195
   Depakote, 197
   Paxil, 196
   Ranbaxy USA, 195
   Risperdal, 196
   Seroquel, 196
   Zyprexa, 198
Post-traumatic stress disorder, 178
Poulson, John, 188
Professional self-regulation, 99
Public sector ethos, 194
Puente, Angela Hernandez, 263
Punjab Institute of Cardiology, 192

Queensland Public Hospitals, 7
   Bundaberg Base Hospital, 8
   Charles Hospital, 10

Charters Towers Hospital, 9
Hervey Bay Hospital, 9
Prince Charles Hospital, 10
Rockhampton Hospital, 10
Townsville Hospital, 9

Radiotherapy, 72
    Therac-25, 73
Razafindranazy, Jean-Jacques, 237
Regulation of managers, 126
Reid, Evelina Sophia, 194
Reinecke, Leopold, 107
Revalidation, 128
Romney plan, 17
Royal Liverpool Hospital, 231
Russian Federation, 16

Safety culture, 235
Safety of women, 93
Santilian, Jesica, 139
Savile, Jimmy, 211
Schizophrenia, 157
Screening errors, 56
    East Devon Breast Cancer, 57
    Irish Health Executive, 58
    Kent and Canterbury Screening
        Programme, 57
Shah, Manish, 113
Shali, Mohammed, 111
Shipman, Harold, 28
Shrewsbury Hospital, 77
Siddiq, Muhammad, 107
Sizemore, Sherman, 142
Smart, Lisa, 145
Smoking and lung cancer, 203
Social care, 269
    Australia, 270
    England, 272

Finland, 274
France, 270
Ireland, 274
Netherlands, 271
Sweden, 272
US, 271
Social workers, 275
Sparrowhawk, Connor, 244
Stafford Hospital, 1
    CURE the NHS, 3, 6, 7
    Julie Bailey, 2
    Organisational culture, 6
Staff safety, 236
Swango, Michael, 31
System failures, 109
Szasz, Thomas, 160

Tenney, Lisa, 240
Toppan, Jane, 34
Torku, Vincent Kwadzo, 120

Ubani, Daniel, 112
Unnecessary treatments and tests,
    53
Uzoh, Chizoba Christopher, 112

Vaccines, 66
Vaginal mesh, 71
    Linda Gross, 72
Vale of Leven Hospital, 12
Value-based healthcare, 230
Vasco-Knight, Paula, 200
Venezuela, 16

Waterhouse report, 283
Wellington Hospital, 229
Wessex Regional Health Authority,
    245

Whistleblowers, 250
  Campbelltown and Camden
    Hospitals, 251
  Canberra Hospital, 252
  Care Quality Commission, 253
  King Edward Memorial
    Hospital, 254
  Texas Medical Board, 252

United Lincolnshire NHS
  Trust, 254
West London Mental Health
  Trust, 251
Wilful blindness, 249
Winterbourne View Care Home, 163

Zelenka, Petr, 34

Printed in the United States
by Baker & Taylor Publisher Services